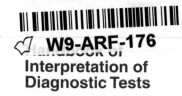

# Handbook of
# Interpretation of
# Diagnostic Tests

# Handbook of Interpretation of Diagnostic Tests

Jacques Wallach, M.D.
Clinical Professor of Pathology,
State University of New York
Health Science Center at Brooklyn;
Attending Pathologist,
Kings County Hospital Center,
Brooklyn, New York

**Lippincott - Raven**

P U B L I S H E R S

Philadelphia • New York

Acquisitions Editor: Richard Winters
Developmental Editor: Michelle LaPlante
Manufacturing Manager: Dennis Teston
Supervising Editor: Kimberly Swan
Production Editor: Jane Bangley McQueen, Silverchair Science + Communications
Cover Designer: Kevin Kall
Indexer: Betty Hallinger
Compositor: Lisa Cunningham, Silverchair Science + Communications
Printer: RR Donnelley, Crawfordsville

Printed in the United States of America

9 8 7 6 5 4 3 2 1

Library of Congress Cataloging-in-Publication Data

Wallach, Jacques B. (Jacques Burton), 1926–
　　Handbook of interpretation of diagnostic tests / Jacques Wallach.
　　　　p.　cm.
　　Includes index.
　　An abridgment of Interpretation of diagnostic tests. 6th ed. 1996.
　　ISBN 0-7817-1221-1
　　1. Diagnosis, Laboratory--Handbooks, manuals, etc.　I. Wallach,
Jacques B. (Jacques Burton), 1926–　Interpretation of diagnostic
tests. II. Title.
　　[DNLM: 1. Laboratory Techniques and Procedures--handbooks.　QY 39
W195h 1998]
　　RB38.2.W349　　1998
　　616.07'56--dc21
　　DNLM/DLC
　　for Library of Congress　　　　　　　　　　　　　　　　　97-51668
　　　　　　　　　　　　　　　　　　　　　　　　　　　　　　CIP

To Doris
and
To Kim, Lisa, and Tracy
and
To Gabriel, Jonah, Zachary, and Ariel

# Contents

# Preface

With the continued growth in the number and use of laboratory tests, the sixth edition of *Interpretation of Diagnostic Tests* has outgrown the pocket-sized format of prior editions. This more compact book is an attempt to restore the immediate use of a small, light book that conveniently fits into a coat pocket and is readily available for immediate reference. It cannot replace the wealth of information and data in the more detailed sixth edition.

This abridgment has been achieved by only including disorders frequently encountered in clinical practice. Illnesses with no diagnostically useful laboratory findings have been deleted or combined in one heading when important in differential diagnosis. Also omitted are less frequently used laboratory tests, findings that are not specific or helpful for the diagnosis of a particular condition, and most neonatal disorders and various hereditary and genetic conditions that require genetic studies for specific diagnosis.

Lists that are primarily clinical are not included in this edition. Details of tests that are chiefly of interest to the laboratorian rather than the clinician (e.g., blood cell morphology) are not included. Various disorders are summarized in tables that allow for simpler comparison of diseases (e.g., CSF findings in CNS diseases, thyroid function test changes in thyroid disorders, porphyrinurias) and faster differential diagnosis. In the style of dictionaries, disorders in this book are arranged alphabetically within organ system chapters (e.g., cardiovascular, respiratory) and further by subdivisions (e.g., under endocrine by adrenal, parathyroid, pituitary, thyroid); the test lists in Chapters 1–4 have also been arranged alphabetically. References and other data sources are omitted but can be found in the sixth edition. For more detailed information, the reader is referred to the sixth edition of *Interpretation of Diagnostic Tests*.

# Acknowledgments

I appreciate the thoughtful suggestions and criticisms from readers in many parts of the world and hope that this abridgment will continue to meet their needs for easily accessible, expeditive, useful, and effective information in their daily work as well as the larger *Interpretation of Diagnostic Tests* from which it is derived.

I thank the staff of Lippincott–Raven Publishers, especially Richard Winters, Senior Editor, for his sound advice; and Michelle LaPlante, Developmental Editor, and Jane Bangley McQueen, Nancy Winemiller, and staff at Silverchair Science + Communications, who diligently performed meticulous, difficult, day-to-day work on the manuscript; Betty Hollinger, who again prepared an outstanding index; and to other administrative persons who provided help and support behind the scenes.

I can never sufficiently express my gratitude to my wife, Doris, for all she has given me.

# Normal Values

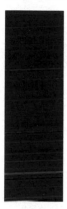

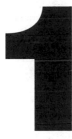

# Normal Blood Values

## Introduction to Normal Values (Reference Ranges)

The reader must always keep in mind that all values given in this book are to be used as general guidelines rather than rigid separations of normal from abnormal or diseased from healthy. Considerable variation in test results is due not only to instrumentation, methodology, and other laboratory techniques, but also to more subtle preanalytic factors such as position or condition of patient (e.g., supine or upright, fasting or postprandial), time of day, age, gender, climate, effect of diet or drugs, and characteristics of test population. It is therefore essential that the clinician use the reference ranges from the laboratory that is performing those particular tests, which have been determined for the laboratory's own procedures, patient population, and so forth. Too many misunderstandings occur from attempts to apply reference ranges of one laboratory to test results from another laboratory. Misinterpretation of laboratory data due to this error, as well as from overemphasizing the significance of borderline values, has caused immeasurable emotional pain and economic waste for innumerable patients.

Special notations should be made on the laboratory test request form when it is particularly germane to a test (e.g., time when blood is drawn is important when the tested component is subject to marked diurnal variation [cortisol, iron], relation to meals [glucose] or IV infusions [electrolytes], source of specimen [arterial or capillary rather than venous blood]). Many tests can be properly interpreted only when such information is known.

Some tests are performed too infrequently to be included in this list: Other tests have such wide reference ranges that interlaboratory use is limited.

A review of the texts, reference books, and current literature in clinical pathology often reveals surprising and considerable discrepancy between well-known sources. The following pages of normal laboratory values were summarized from my own experience as well as what seemed to be the best and most current sources of data available.

Some specialized analyte values appear with the disorder in question rather than in the section on normal values.

## General Principles

The purpose of all testing (e.g., laboratory, radiologic, electrocardiographic) is to reduce clinical uncertainty. The degree of reduction varies with the test characteristics and clinical situation. Modern medicine has superseded Voltaire's dictum that "the art of medicine consists of amusing the patient while nature cures the disease."

Many clinicians are still largely unaware of the reasoning they follow in seeking a diagnosis. They tend to use an empirical path that was previously successful or was learned in early training periods by observing their mentors during clinical rounds without appreciating the rationale for selecting, ordering, and interpreting laboratory tests; this is often absorbed in a subliminal, informal, or rote fashion. The need to control health care costs and many studies on the use of laboratory tests have emphasized the need for a selective approach.

Some important principles in using laboratory (and all other) tests are as follows:

1. Even under the best circumstances, no test is perfect (e.g., 100% sensitivity, specificity, predictive value). In any specific case, the results may be misleading. The most sensitive tests are best used to rule out a suspected disease so that the number of false-negative tests is minimal; thus a negative test tends to exclude the disease. The most specific tests are used to confirm or exclude a suspected disease and minimize the number of false-positive results. Sensitivity and specificity may be markedly altered by the coexistence of other disorders, or complications or sequelae of the primary disease.

2. Choosing tests should be based on the prior probability of the diagnosis being sought, which affects the predictive value of the test. This prior probability is determined by the history, physical examination, and prevalence of the suspected disorder (in that community at that time), which is why history and physical examination should precede the ordering of tests. The clinician need not know the exact prior probability of the disease: It is usually sufficient to estimate this as high, intermediate, or low. Moderate errors in estimating prior probability have only relatively limited effects on interpreting the tests. If the prior prevalence is high, a positive result tends to confirm the presence of the disease, but an unexpected negative result is not very useful in ruling out the disease. Conversely, when the prior prevalence is low, a normal result tends to rule out the disease, but an unexpected positive result is not very useful in confirming the disease.

3. In the majority of laboratory measurements, the combination of short-term physiologic variation and analytic error is sufficient to render the interpretation of single determinations difficult when the concentrations are in the borderline range. Any particular laboratory result may be incorrect for a large variety of reasons regardless of the high quality of the laboratory; all such results should be rechecked. If indicated, a new specimen should be submitted with careful confirmation of patient identification, prompt delivery to the laboratory, and immediate processing. In some circumstances, confirmation of test results at another laboratory may be appropriate.

4. Based on the statistical definition of *normal* as within the 95% range of values, 5% of independent tests will be outside this normal range in the absence of disease. If 12 tests are performed, at least one abnormal result will occur in 46% of normal persons; for 20 tests, 64% of normal persons will have at least one abnormal result. The greater the degree of abnormality of the test result, the more likely that a confirmed abnormality is significant or represents a real disorder. Most slightly abnormal results are due to preanalytic factors.

5. Tables of reference values represent statistical data for 95% of the population; values outside these ranges do not necessarily represent disease. Results may still be within the reference range but be elevated above the patient's baseline, which is why serial testing is important in a number of conditions. For example, in acute myocardial infarction, the increase in serum creatine kinase may be abnormal for that patient even though the value may be within the normal range.

6. An individual's test values tend to remain fairly constant over a period of years when performed in a good laboratory with comparable technology; comparison of results with previous values obtained when the patient was not ill (if available) are often a better reference value than normal ranges.

7. Multiple test abnormalities are more likely to be significant than single test abnormalities. When two or more tests for the same disorder are positive, the results reinforce the diagnosis, but when only one test is positive and the other is negative, the strength of the interpretation is diluted.

8. The degree of abnormality ("signal strength") is useful. Thus, a value increased 10 times the upper reference range is much more likely to be clinically significant than one that is only slightly increased.

9. Characteristic laboratory test profiles that are described in the literature and in this book represent the full-blown picture of the well-developed or far-advanced case, but all abnormal tests may be present simultaneously in only a small fraction (e.g., one-third) of patients with that condition. Even when a test profile (combination of tests) is characteristic of a particular disorder, other conditions or combination of disorders may produce exactly the same combination of laboratory test changes.

10. Excessive repetition of tests is wasteful, and the excess burden increases the possibility of laboratory errors. Appropriate intervals between tests should be dictated by the patient's clinical condition.

11. Tests should only be performed if they will alter the patient's diagnosis, prognosis, treatment, or management. Incorrect test values or isolated individual variations in results may cause "Ulysses syndrome" and result in loss of time, money, and peace of mind.

12. Clerical errors are far more likely than technical errors to cause incorrect results. Greatest care should be taken to completely and properly label and identify all specimens, which should *always* be accompanied by a test requisition form. Busy hospital laboratories receive inordinate numbers of unlabeled, unidentified specimens each day that are useless, burdensome, and sometimes dangerous because incorrect results may be reported.

13. Reference ranges vary from one laboratory to another; users should know what these ranges are for each laboratory they use and should also be aware of variations due to age, gender, race, size, and physiologic status (e.g., pregnancy, lactation) that apply to the particular patient. These normal ranges represent collected statistical data rather than classification of patients as having disease or being healthy. This collection of data is best illustrated in the use of *multitest* chemical profiles for screening individuals known to be disease-free. The probability of any given test being abnormal is about 2% to 5%, and the probability of disease if a screening test is abnormal is generally low (0% to 15%). The frequency of abnormal single tests is 1.5% (albumin) to 5.9% (glucose) and up to 16.6% (sodium).

14. The effect of drugs on laboratory test values must never be overlooked. The clinician should always be aware of what drugs the patient has been taking, including over-the-counter medications, vitamins, and iron, among others. These effects may produce false-negative as well as false-positive results. For example, vitamin C may produce a false-negative test for occult blood in the stool.

## Hematology—Reference Values

| | |
|---|---|
| Blood count, complete (CBC) | See Tables 1-1 and 1-2. |
| Carboxyhemoglobin | <5% of total |
| Ceruloplasmin | 23–43 mg/dL |
| Copper | 75–145 $\mu$g/dL |
| Delta-aminolevulinic acid | 1.5–7.5 mg/24-hr urine |
| ESR | |
| Wintrobe | |
| Males | 0–10 mm in 1 hr |
| Females | 0–15 mm in 1 hr |
| Neonate/child | 3–13 mm in 1 hr |
| Newborn | 0–2 mm in 1 hr |
| Westergren | |
| Males | 0–13 mm in 1 hr |
| Females | 0–20 mm in 1 hr |
| Erythropoietin | |
| Males | 17.2 mU/mL (mean) |
| Females | 18.8 mU/mL (mean) |

**Table 1-1.** Reference Ranges for Complete Blood Count at Various Ages*

| Age | RBC ($\times 10^6$/cu mm) | Hb (g/dL) | Hct (%) | MCV (fL) | MCH (pg) | RDW (%) |
|---|---|---|---|---|---|---|
| Newborn | 4.1–6.7 | 15.0–24.0 | 44–70 | 102–115 | 33–39 | 13.0–18.0 |
| 1–23 mos | 3.8–5.4 | 10.5–14.0 | 32–42 | 72–88 | 24–30 | 11.5–16.0 |
| 2–9 yrs | 4.0–5.3 | 11.5–14.5 | 33–43 | 76–90 | 25–31 | 11.5–15.0 |
| 10–17 yrs | | | | | | |
| Male | 4.2–5.6 | 12.5–16.1 | 36–47 | 78–95 | 26–32 | 11.5–14.0 |
| Female | 4.1–5.3 | 12.0–15.0 | 35–45 | 78–95 | 26–32 | 11.5–14.0 |
| >18 yrs | | | | | | |
| Male | 4.7–6.0 | 13.5–18.0 | 42–52 | 78–100 | 27–31 | 11.5–14.0 |
| Female | 4.2–5.4 | 12.5–16.0 | 37–47 | 78–100 | 27–31 | 11.5–14.0 |

*Mean platelet volume = 6.0–9.5 fL for all age groups. Platelets = 150,000–450,000/cu mm for all age groups. Mean corpuscular hemoglobin concentration = 32–36 gm/dL for all age groups.

Ferritin
    Newborns                                          25–200 ng/mL
    1 month                                            200–600 ng/mL
    2–5 months                                       50–200 ng/mL
    6 months to 15 yrs                           7–142 ng/mL
    Adult males                                       20–300 ng/mL
    Adult females                                    15–120 ng/mL
    Borderline (males or females)          10–20 ng/mL
    Iron excess                                        >400 ng/mL
Folate, erythrocyte
    <1 yr                                                  74–995 ng/mL
    1–11 yrs                                            96–362 ng/mL
    ≥ 12 yrs                                            180–600 ng/mL
Folate, serum                                       ≥ 3.5 $\mu$g/L
G6PD, erythrocyte
    2–17 yrs                                            6.4–15.6 U/gm Hb
    ≥ 18 yrs                                            8.6–18.6 U/gm Hb
Haptoglobins                                        Genetic absence in 1% of population
    Newborns                                          Absent in 90%; 10 mg/dL in 10%
    1–6 months                                       Gradual increase to 30 mg/dL
    6 months to 17 yrs                           40–180 mg/dL
    Adults                                                40–270 mg/dL
Hb electrophoresis
    Hb A
        0–30 days                                      10–40%
        6 months to adult                         >95%
    Hb $A_2$
        0–30 days                                      <1%
        1 yr to adult                                  1.5–3.0%
                                                              3.0–3.5% (borderline)
    Hb F                                                  <2%
    No abnormal Hb variants
Iron, liver tissue                                     530–900 $\mu$g/gm dry weight
Iron, serum
    Newborn                                            100–250 $\mu$g/dL
    Infant                                                  40–100 $\mu$g/dL
    Child                                                   50–120 $\mu$g/dL

**Table 1-2.** Reference Ranges for White Blood Cell Count at Various Ages (Differential Count in Absolute Numbers)

| Age | WBC (× 1000/cu mm) | Total Neutrophils* | Segs | Bands | Lymphs | Monos | Eos | Baso |
|---|---|---|---|---|---|---|---|---|
| Newborn | 9.1–34.0 | 6.0–23.5 | 6.0–20.0 | <3.5 | 2.5–10.5 | <3.5 | <2.0 | <0.4 |
| 1–23 mos | 6.0–14.0 | 1.1–6.6 | 1.0–6.0 | <1.0 | 1.8–9.0 | <1.0 | <0.7 | <0.1 |
| 2–9 yrs | 4.0–12.0 | 1.4–6.6 | 1.2–6.0 | <1.0 | 1.0–5.5 | <1.0 | <0.7 | <0.1 |
| 10–17 yrs | 4.0–10.5 | 1.5–6.6 | 1.3–6.0 | <1.0 | 1.0–3.5 | <1.0 | <0.7 | <0.1 |
| >18 yrs | 4.0–10.5 | 1.5–6.6 | 1.3–6.0 | <1.0 | 1.5–3.5 | <1.0 | <0.7 | <0.1 |

Segs = segmented neutrophils; Bands = band neutrophils; Lymphs = lymphocytes; Monos = monocytes; Eos = eosinophils; Baso = basophils.
*Total Neutrophils = Segs + Bands.

|  |  |
|---|---|
| Adults | |
| Male | 65–175 $\mu$g/dL |
| Female | 50–170 $\mu$g/dL |
| Iron, urine | 100–300 ng/24 hrs |
| Iron-binding capacity | 250–450 $\mu$g/dL |
| Percent saturation | 20–50% |
| LAP score | 40–100 |
| Lysozyme (muramidase), plasma | 0.2–15.8 $\mu$g/mL |
| Lysozyme (muramidase), urine | <3 mg/24 hrs |
| Methemoglobin | <3% of total |
| Myoglobin, serum | $\leq$ 90 ng/mL |
| Myoglobin, urine | 0–2 mg/mL |
| Osmotic fragility of RBC | Increased if hemolysis occurs in >0.5% NaCl |
| | Decreased if incomplete in 0.30% NaCl |
| Phosphofructokinase, erythrocyte | 3.0–6.0 U/gm Hb |
| Protoporphyrin, free erythrocyte (FEP) | <100 $\mu$g/dL packed RBCs |
| Pyruvate kinase, erythrocyte | 2.0–8.8 U/gm Hb |
| Reticulocyte count, percent | 0.5–1.85% of erythrocytes |
| Absolute | $29–87 \times 10^9$/L |
| Sideroblasts, marrow | $\geq$ 30% of normoblasts |
| Sideroblasts, ringed | None |
| Transferrin | 240–480 mg/dL |
| Unsaturated vitamin $B_{12}$–binding capacity | 870–1800 pg/mL |
| Urobilinogen, urine | <4 mg/24 hrs |
| Urobilinogen, stool | 50–300 mg/24 hrs |
| Vitamin $B_{12}$, serum | 190–900 ng/L |

## Blood Coagulation Tests—Reference Values

| Antithrombin III, plasma | | |
|---|---|---|
| Immunologic | 17–30 mg/dL | |
| Functional | 80–120% | |
| BT | 3.0–9.5 mins | |
| Clot retraction, qualitative | Begins in 30–60 mins; complete within 24 hrs, usually within 6 hrs | |

| Coagulation factor assay (Infants may not reach adult level until age 6 months) | **Activity** | **Plasma levels** |
|---|---|---|
| I (fibrinogen) | | |
| Males | | 180–340 mg/dL |
| Females | | 190–420 mg/dL |
| II (prothrombin) | 70–140% | 100 $\mu$g/mL |
| V (accelerator globulin) | 70–160% | 10 $\mu$g/mL |
| VII (proconvertin-Stuart) | 65–170% | 0.5 $\mu$g/mL |
| VIII (antihemophilic globulin) | 55–145% | 0.1 $\mu$g/mL |
| IX | 70–140% | 5 $\mu$g/mL |
| X (Stuart factor) | 70–140% | 10 $\mu$g/mL |
| XI | 65–145% | 5 $\mu$g/mL |
| XII (Hageman factor) | 60–160% | 30 $\mu$g/mL |
| XIII | 50–200% | 10 $\mu$g/mL |
| Factor VIII related antigen | 45–185% | |
| Coagulation factor VIII inhibitor | Negative | |
| Coagulation time (Lee-White) | 6–17 mins (glass tubes) | |
| | 19–60 mins (siliconized tubes) | |
| Euglobulin lysis | No lysis in 2 hrs | |

| | |
|---|---|
| Fibrinogen split products | Negative at >1:4 dilution |
| | Positive at >1:8 dilution |
| Fibrinolysins | No clot lysis in 24 hrs |
| Lupus anticoagulant (dilute Russell's viper venom time [dRVVT]) (P) | Negative |
| aPTT | 25–38 secs |
| Platelet aggregation | Full response to adenosine diphosphate, epinephrine, and collagen |
| Platelet antibody, serum | Negative |
| Platelet count | 140,000–340,000/cu mm (Rees–Ecker) |
| | 150,000–350,000/cu mm (Coulter counter) |
| Protein C activity (P) | 70–130% |
| Protein C antigen (P) | 60–125% |
| Protein S activity, total or free (P) | |
|    Males | 60–130% |
|    Females | 50–120% |
| PT, one stage | ±2 secs of control (control should be 11–16 secs) |
| Ristocetin cofactor (P) | 45–140% |
| Ristocetin-Willebrand factor | 45–140% |
| Thrombin time (TT) | ±5 secs of control |
| von Willebrand factor antigen, plasma | 45–165% |
| Whole blood clot lysis | No clot lysis in 24 hrs |

## Blood Chemistries—Reference Values

These values will vary depending on the individual laboratory as well as the methods and instruments used. Clinicians should compare the applicability of these data to their own situations.

| | |
|---|---|
| Acetone | 0.3–2.0 mg/dL |
| Ammonia | 9–33 U/L |
|    Newborn at term or premature | <50 U/L |
| Amylase (total) (Ektachem [Kodak, Rochester, NY]) | |
|    Age <18 yrs | 0–260 U/L |
|    Adults (age ≥ 18 yrs) | 35–115 U/L |
| Base, excess | |
|    Newborns | –10 to –2 mEq/L |
|    Infant | 7 to  1 mEq/L |
|    Child | –4 to +2 mEq/L |
|    Adult | –3 to +3 mEq/L |
| Bicarbonate | |

#### Age (yrs)

| Males | Females | |
|---|---|---|
| 1–2 | 1–3 | 17–25 mEq/L |
| 3–4 | 4–5 | 18–26 mEq/L |
| 4–5 | 6–7 | 19–27 mEq/L |
| 6–7 | 8–9 | 20–28 mEq/L |
| ≥ 8[a] | ≥ 10[a] | 21–29 mEq/L |

| | |
|---|---|
| Bilirubin (Ektachem) | |
|    Total | |
|       <1 day | <5.8 mg/dL |
|       1–2 days | <8.2 mg/dL |
|       3–5 days | <11.7 mg/dL |
|       >1 month | <1.0 mg/dL |

| | |
|---|---|
| Direct | |
|     1 month to adult | <0.6 mg/dL |
| Calcium | |
|   Total (Ektachem) | |
|     1–3 yrs | 8.7–9.8 mg/dL |
|     4–11 yrs | 8.8–10.1 mg/dL |
|     12–13 yrs | 8.8–10.6 mg/dL |
|     14–15 yrs | 9.2–10.7 mg/dL |
|     >16 yrs | 8.9–10.7 mg/dL |
|   Ionized | |
|     Males | |
|       1–19 yrs | 4.9–5.5 mg/dL |
|       ≥ 20 yrs[a] | 4.75–5.30 mg/dL |
|     Females | |
|       1–17 yrs | 4.9–5.5 mg/dL |
|       ≥ 18 yrs[a] | 4.75–5.30 mg/dL |
| Carbon dioxide | |
|   $CO_2$ | 17–31 mEq/L |
|   $pCO_2$ (whole blood) | |
|     Adults | 32–48 mm Hg |
|     Infants | 27–41 mm Hg |
| Ceruloplasmin | |
|   1–3 yrs | 24–46 mg/dL |
|   4–6 yrs | 24–42 mg/dL |
|   7–9 yrs | 24–40 mg/dL |
|   10–13 yrs | 22–36 mg/dL |
|   14–19 yrs | 14–34 mg/dL |
| Chloride | 96–109 mEq/L |
| Cholesterol | See Chapter 12. |
| Cholinesterase | |
|   Plasma | 7–25 U/mL |
|   RBC | 0.65–1.3 pH units |
| Copper | 75–145 µg/dL |
| CK (Ektachem) | |
|   1–3 yrs | 60–305 U/L |
|   4–6 yrs | 75–230 U/L |
|   7–9 yrs | 60–365 U/L |

| | Males (U/L) | Females (U/L) |
|---|---|---|
| 10–11 yrs | 55–215 | 80–230 |
| 12–13 yrs | 60–330 | 50–295 |
| 14–15 yrs | 60–335 | 50–240 |
| 16–19 yrs | 55–370 | 45–230 |

| | |
|---|---|
| CK isoenzymes | MB <5% |
| Creatinine | |
|   <1 wk | 0.6–1.1 mg/dL |
|   1–4 wks | 0.3–0.7 mg/dL |
|   1–12 months | 0.2–0.4 mg/dL |
|   >1 yr | 0.2–0.7 mg/dL |

**Age (yrs)**

| Males | Females | |
|---|---|---|
| 1–2 | 1–3 | 0.2–0.6 mg/dL |
| 3–4 | 4–5 | 0.3–0.7 mg/dL |
| 5–9 | 6–8 | 0.5–0.8 mg/dL |
| 10–11 | ≥ 9 | 0.6–0.9 mg/dL |
| 12–13 | 12–13 | 0.6–1.0 mg/dL |
| 14–15 | 14–15 | 0.7–1.1 mg/dL |
| ≥ 16 | ≥ 16 | 0.8–1.2 mg/dL |
| Cryoglobulins | | 0 |

Gamma-glutamyl transferase (GGT)
   (Ektachem)

| | Males (U/L) | Females (U/L) |
|---|---|---|
| 1–3 yrs | 6–19 U/L | |
| 4–6 yrs | 10–22 U/L | |
| 7–9 yrs | 13–25 U/L | |
| 10–11 yrs | 17–30 | 17–28 |
| 12–13 yrs | 17–44 | 14–25 |
| 14–15 yrs | 12–33 | 14–26 |
| 16–19 yrs | 11–34 | 11–28 |

Glucose (fasting)   60–100 mg/dL (depends on method)
Lactate (Ektachem)   6.3–18.9 mg/dL
Lactate dehydrogenase (LD) (Ektachem)

| | Males (U/L) | Females (U/L) |
|---|---|---|
| 1–3 yrs | 500–920 U/L | |
| 4–6 yrs | 470–900 U/L | |
| 7–9 yrs | 420–750 U/L | |
| 10–11 yrs | 432–700 | 380–700 |
| 12–13 yrs | 470–750 | 380–640 |
| 14–15 yrs | 360–730 | 390–580 |
| 16–19 yrs | 340–670 | 340–670 |

LD isoenzymes
   LD-1   17–28%
   LD-2   30–36%
   LD-3   19–25%
   LD-4   10–16%
   LD-5   6–13%
Lead
   Adults   <20 $\mu$g/dL
   ≤ 15 yrs   <10 $\mu$g/dL
Lipase   56–239 U/L
Lipid fractionation
   Cholesterol esters   60–75% of total
   Phospholipids   180 320 mg/dL
Magnesium (Ektachem)   1.7–2.3 mg/dL
Myoglobin   ≤ 90 ng/mL
Osmolality   275 295 mOsm/kg
Oxygen
   Saturation, arterial   96 100% of capacity
   Tension, $pO_2$ arterial; while breathing
      room air

| Age (yrs) | |
|---|---|
| Newborns | 60–75 mm Hg |
| <60 | >85 mm Hg |
| 60 | >80 mm Hg |
| 70 | >70 mm Hg |
| 80 | >60 mm Hg |
| 90 | >50 mm Hg |
| While breathing 100% oxygen | >500 mm Hg |

Oxygen dissociation, P50 (RBCs)   26–30 mm Hg
pH, arterial   7.36–7.44
pH, venous   7.32–7.38
Phenylalanine
   ≤ 1 wk   42–124 $\mu$mol/L
   <16 yrs   26–86 $\mu$mol/L
   ≥ 16 yrs   41–68 $\mu$mol/L
Phosphatase, alkaline (Ektachem)
   1–3 yrs   145–320 U/L
   4–6 yrs   150–380 U/L
   7–9 yrs   175–420 U/L

| | Males (U/L) | Females (U/L) |
|---|---|---|
| 10–11 yrs | 135–530 | 130–560 |
| 12–13 yrs | 200–495 | 105–420 |
| 14–15 yrs | 130–525 | 70–230 |
| 16–19 yrs | 65–260 | 50–130 |

Phosphate (Ektachem)

| | |
|---|---|
| <5 days | 4.6–8.0 mg/dL |
| 1–3 yrs | 3.9–6.5 mg/dL |
| 4–6 yrs | 3.7–5.4 mg/dL |
| 7–11 yrs | 3.7–5.6 mg/dL |
| 12–13 yrs | 3.3–5.4 mg/dL |
| 14–15 yrs | 2.9–5.4 mg/dL |
| 16–19 yrs | 2.8–4.6 mg/dL |

Potassium

| | |
|---|---|
| 1–15 yrs | 3.7–5.0 mEq/L |
| 16–59 yrs | 3.6–4.8 mEq/L |
| ≥ 60 yrs | 3.9–5.3 mEq/L |
| Prostatic acid phosphatase (PAP) | <3.7 ng/mL |

Prostate-specific antigen (PSA)
Males[b]

| | |
|---|---|
| Normal | <4.0 ng/mL |
| Borderline | 4–10 ng/mL |
| 40–49 yrs | 1.5 ng/mL |
| 50–59 yrs | 2.5 ng/mL |
| 60–69 yrs | 4.5 ng/mL |
| 70–79 yrs | 7.5 ng/mL |

| | Total (gm/dL) | Albumin (gm/dL) |
|---|---|---|
| Proteins, serum (Ektachem) | | |
| <5 days | 5.4–7.0 | 2.6–3.6 |
| 1–3 yrs | 5.9–7.0 | 3.4–4.2 |
| 4–6 yrs | 5.9–7.8 | 3.5–5.2 |
| 7–9 yrs | 6.2–8.1 | 3.7–5.6 |
| 10–19 yrs | 6.3–8.6 | 3.7–5.6 |

Globulin

| | |
|---|---|
| <1 yr | 0.4–3.7 gm/dL |
| 1–3 yrs | 1.6–3.5 gm/dL |
| 4–9 yrs | 1.9–3.4 gm/dL |
| 10–49 yrs | 1.9–3.5 gm/dL |

Prealbumin (transthyretin)

| | |
|---|---|
| <5 days | 6.0–21.0 mg/dL |
| 1–5 yrs | 14.0–30.0 mg/dL |
| 6–9 yrs | 15.0–33.0 mg/dL |
| 10–13 yrs | 20.0–36.0 mg/dL |
| 14–19 yrs | 22.0–45.0 mg/dL |

Electrophoresis

| | |
|---|---|
| Albumin | 3.1–4.3 gm/dL |

Globulin

| | |
|---|---|
| Alpha$_1$ | 0.1–0.3 gm/dL |
| Alpha$_2$ | 0.6–1.0 gm/dL |
| Beta | 0.7–1.4 gm/dL |
| Gamma | 0.0–1.6 gm/dL |
| Alpha$_1$-antitrypsin | >180 mg/dL |
| Z heterozygotes | 79–171 mg/dL |
| Z homozygotes | 19–31 mg/dL |
| Total complement | 25–110 units |
| C1 esterase inhibitor | 8–24 mg/dL |
| C1q complement component | 7–15 mg/dL |
| C2 (second component of complement) | 50–250% of normal |
| C3 (third component of complement) | 70–150 mg/dL |
| C4 (fourth component of complement) | 10–30 mg/dL |
| C5 (fifth component of complement) | 9–18 mg/dL |

| Immunoglobulins | IgG (mg/dL) | IgA (mg/dL) | IgM (mg/dL) |
|---|---|---|---|
| 0–4 months | 141–930 | 5–64 | 14–142 |
| 5–8 months | 250–1190 | 10–87 | 24–167 |
| 9–11 months | 320–1250 | 17–94 | |
| 1–3 yrs | 400–1250 | | |
| 1–2 yrs | | | 35–242 (females) |
| | | | 35–200 (males) |
| 2–3 yrs | | 24–192 | 41–242 (females) |
| | | | 41–200 (males) |
| 4–6 yrs | 560–1307 | 26–232 | |
| 7–9 yrs | 598–1379 | 33–258 | |
| 10–12 yrs | 638–1453 | 45–285 | |
| 13–15 yrs | 680–1531 | 47–317 | |
| 16–17 yrs | 724–1611 | 55–377 | |
| 4–17 yrs | | | 56–242 (females) |
| | | | 47–200 (males) |
| ≥ 18 yrs | 700–1500 | 60–400 | 60–300 |

| IgE | |
|---|---|
| <1 yr | 0.0–6.6 IU/mL |
| 1–2 yrs | 0.0–20.0 IU/mL |
| 2–3 yrs | 0.1–15.8 IU/mL |
| 3–4 yrs | 0.0–29.2 IU/mL |
| 4–5 yrs | 0.3–25.0 IU/mL |
| 5–6 yrs | 0.2–17.6 IU/mL |
| 6–7 yrs | 0.2–13.1 IU/mL |
| 7–8 yrs | 0.3–46.1 IU/mL |
| 8–9 yrs | 1.8–60.1 IU/mL |
| 9–10 yrs | 3.6–81.0 IU/mL |
| 10–11 yrs | 8.0–95.0 IU/mL |
| 11–12 yrs | 1.5–99.7 IU/mL |
| 12–13 yrs | 3.9–83.5 IU/mL |
| 13–16 yrs | 3.3–188.0 IU/mL |
| IgD | 0–14 mg/dL |
| Sodium | 135–145 mEq/L |

| Transaminase (Ektachem) | | |
|---|---|---|
| AST (SGOT) | | |
| 1–3 yrs | 20–60 U/L | |
| 4–6 yrs | 15–50 U/L | |
| 7–9 yrs | 15–40 U/L | |
| 10–11 yrs | 10–60 U/L | |
| | **Males (U/L)** | **Females (U/L)** |
| 12–15 yrs | 15–40 | 10–30 |
| 16–19 yrs | 15–45 | 5–30 |
| ALT (SGPT) | | |
| 1–3 yrs | 5–45 | |
| 4–6 yrs | 10–25 U/L | |
| 7–9 yrs | 10–35 U/L | |
| | **Males (U/L)** | **Females (U/L)** |
| 10–11 yrs | 10–35 | 10–30 |
| 12–13 yrs | 10–55 | 10–30 |
| 14–15 yrs | 10–45 | 5–30 |
| 16–19 yrs | 10–40 | 5–35 |

| BUN (Ektachem) | |
|---|---|
| 1–3 yrs | 5–17 mg/dL |
| 4–13 yrs | 7–17 mg/dL |
| 14–19 yrs | 8–21 mg/dL |
| Uric acid (Ektachem) | |
| 1–3 yrs | 1.8–5.0 mg/dL |
| 4–6 yrs | 2.2–4.7 mg/dL |
| 7–9 yrs | 2.0–5.0 mg/dL |

|  | Males (mg/dL) | Females (mg/dL) |
|---|---|---|
| 10–11 yrs | 2.3–5.4 | 3.0–4.7 |
| 12–13 yrs | 2.7–6.7 | 3.0–5.8 |
| 14–15 yrs | 2.4–7.8 | 3.0–5.8 |
| 16–19 yrs | 4.0–8.6 | 3.0–5.9 |

Viscosity (correlates with fibrinogen, HDL cholesterol) (viscosimeter)
Plasma                    $1.38 \pm 0.08$ relative units
Serum                     $1.26 \pm 0.08$ relative units

[a]Adult value.

[b]Values higher in black men than in white men. Increase with age.

## Normal Blood and Urine Hormone Levels

ACTH, plasma                                  $\leq 60$ pg/mL
Aldosterone, serum
   0–3 weeks                              16.5–154 ng/dL
   1–11 months                            6.5–86 ng/dL
   1–10 yrs
      Supine                         3.0–39.5 ng/dL
      Upright                        3.5–124 ng/dL
   $\geq 11$ yrs (morning specimen,
     peripheral vein)                   1–21 ng/dL
Aldosterone, urine
   0–30 days                              0.7–11 $\mu$g/24 hrs
   1–11 months                            0.7–22 $\mu$g/24 hrs
   $\geq 1$ yr                            2–16 $\mu$g/24 hrs

| Androstenedione, serum | Males (ng/mL) | Females (ng/mL) |
|---|---|---|
| 0–7 yrs | 0.1–0.2 | 0.1–0.3 |
| 8–9 yrs | 0.1–0.3 | 0.2–0.5 |
| 10–11 yrs | 0.3–0.7 | 0.4–1.0 |
| 12–13 yrs | 0.4–1.0 | 0.8–1.9 |
| 14–17 yrs | 0.5–1.4 | 0.7–2.2 |
| $\geq 18$ yrs | 0.3–3.1 | 0.2–3.1 |

Angiotensin-converting enzyme, serum (SACE)
   $\leq 1$ yr                            10.9–42.1 U/L
   1–2 yrs                                9.4–36 U/L
   3–4 yrs                                7.9–29.8 U/L
   5–9 yrs                                9.6–35.4 U/L
   10–12 yrs                              10.0–37.0 U/L
   13–16 yrs                              9.0–33.4 U/L
   17–19 yrs                              7.2–26.6 U/L
   $\geq 20$ yrs                          6.1–21.1 U/L

| Calcitonin, plasma | Males (pg/mL) | Females (pg/mL) |
|---|---|---|
| Basal | $\leq 19$ | $<14$ |
| Calcium infusion (2.4 mg calcium/kg) | $\leq 190$ | $\leq 130$ |
| Pentagastrin infusion (0.5 $\mu$g/kg) | $\leq 110$ | $\leq 30$ |

Catecholamine fractionation (free), plasma

|  | Supine (pg/mL) | Standing (pg/mL) |
|---|---|---|
| Norepinephrine | 70–750 | 200–1700 |
| Epinephrine | $\leq 110$ | $\leq 140$ |
| Dopamine | $<30$ (any posture) | |

Catecholamine fractionation, urine
   Epinephrine
      $<1$ yr                       $<2.5$ $\mu$g/24 hrs
      1–2 yrs                       $<3.5$ $\mu$g/24 hrs
      2–3 yrs                       $<6.0$ $\mu$g/24 hrs
      4–9 yrs                       0.2–10.0 $\mu$g/24 hrs
      10–15 yrs                     0.5–20.0 $\mu$g/24 hrs
      $\geq 16$ yrs                 0–20 $\mu$g/24 hrs

Norepinephrine

| | |
|---|---|
| <1 yr | 0–10 $\mu$g/24 hrs |
| 1 yr | 1–17 $\mu$g/24 hrs |
| 2–3 yrs | 4–29 $\mu$g/24 hrs |
| 4–6 yrs | 8–45 $\mu$g/24 hrs |
| 7–9 yrs | 13–65 $\mu$g/24 hrs |
| ≥ 10 yrs | 15–80 $\mu$g/24 hrs |

Dopamine

| | |
|---|---|
| <1 yr | <85 $\mu$g/24 hrs |
| 1 yr | 10–140 $\mu$g/24 hrs |
| 2–3 yrs | 40–260 $\mu$g/24 hrs |
| ≥ 4 yrs | 65–400 $\mu$g/24 hrs |

Chorionic gonadotropins, beta-subunit

Serum

| | |
|---|---|
| Females | <5 IU/L |
| Postmenopausal females | <9 IU/L |
| Males | <2.5 IU/L |
| CSF | ≤ 1.5 IU/L |

Cortisol, free, urine    24–108 $\mu$g/24 hrs

Cortisol (includes cortisol, corticosterone, 11-deoxycortisol for general
screening), plasma

| | |
|---|---|
| AM | 7–25 $\mu$g/dL |
| PM | 2–14 $\mu$g/dL |

Deoxycorticosteroids (for metyrapone
test), plasma

| | |
|---|---|
| AM | 0–5 $\mu$g/dL |
| PM | 0–3 $\mu$g/dL |

Dehydroepiandrosterone sulfate
(DHEA-S), serum

| | Males ($\mu$g/mL) | Females ($\mu$g/mL) |
|---|---|---|
| 0–30 days | | |
| Premature | 0.25–10.0 | 0.25–10.0 |
| Full-term | 0.25–2.0 | 0.25–2.0 |
| 1–16 yrs | <0.5 | <0.5 |
| ≥ 17 yrs | <0.0 | <3.0 |

Estradiol, serum

| | |
|---|---|
| Children | <10 pg/mL |
| Adult males | 10–50 pg/mL |
| Premenopausal adult females | 30–400 pg/mL |
| Postmenopausal females | <30 pg/mL |

Estrogen and progesterone receptor
assays, tissue

| | |
|---|---|
| Negative | <3 fmol/mg cytosol protein |
| Borderline | 3–9 fmol/mg cytosol protein |
| Positive | ≥ 10 fmol/mg cytosol protein |

Follicle-stimulating hormone (FSH), serum

| | Males (IU/L) | Females (IU/L) |
|---|---|---|
| Prepubertal | <2 | <2 |
| Adult | | |
| Follicular | | 1–10 |
| Midcycle | | 6–30 |
| Luteal | | 1–8 |
| Postmenopausal | | 20–100 |

FSH, urine

| | Males (IU/24 hrs) | Females (IU/24 hrs) |
|---|---|---|
| Prepubertal | <0.5 | <0.7 |
| Adult | | 7–10 |
| Nonmidcycle | | 0.7–10 |

| | | |
|---|---|---|
| Postmenopausal | | >10 |
| Gastrin, serum | | ≤ 200 pg/mL |
| Growth hormone, serum | | |
| Males | | ≤ 5 ng/mL |
| Females | | ≤ 10 ng/mL |
| Homovanillic acid (HVA), urine | | |
| <1 yr | | <35 μg/mg creatinine |
| >1 yr | | <23 μg/mg creatinine |
| 2–4 yrs | | <13.5 μg/mg creatinine |
| 5–9 yrs | | <9 μg/mg creatinine |
| 10–14 yrs | | <12 μg/mg creatinine |
| Adults | | <8 mg/24 hrs |
| 5-Hydroxyindoleacetic acid (HIAA), urine | | ≤ 6 mg/24 hrs |
| 17-Hydroxyprogesterone, serum | | |
| Males | | <220 ng/dL |
| Prepubertal | | <110 ng/dL |
| Females | | |
| Follicular phase | | <80 ng/dL |
| Luteal phase | | <285 ng/dL |
| Postmenopausal | | <51 ng/dL |
| Prepubertal | | <100 ng/dL |
| Newborns | | <630 ng/dL |
| Insulin, serum | | <20 μU/mL |
| Borderline | | 21–25 μU/mL |
| 17-Ketogenic steroids, urine | | |
| Adults | | |
| Males | | 4–14 mg/24 hrs |
| Females | | 2–12 mg/24 hrs |
| Children | | |
| 0–10 yrs | | 0.1–4 mg/24 hrs |
| 11–14 yrs | | 2–9 mg/24 hrs |
| 17-Ketosteroids, urine | | |
| Adults | | |
| Males | | 6–21 mg/24 hrs |
| Females | | 4–17 mg/24 hrs |
| Children | | |
| 0–10 yrs | | 0.1–3 mg/24 hrs |
| 11–14 yrs | | 2–7 mg/24 hrs |
| Leutinizing hormone (LH), serum | | |
| Prepubertal males | | <0.5 IU/L |
| Adult males | | 1–10 IU/L |
| Prepubertal females | | <0.2 IU/L |
| Adult females | | |
| Follicular | | 1–20 IU/L |
| Midcycle | | 25–100 IU/L |
| Postmenopausal females | | 20–100 IU/L |
| LH, urine | | |
| Prepubertal males | | <0.8 IU/24 hrs |
| Adult males | | 0.2–5.0 IU/24 hrs |
| Prepubertal females | | <0.8 IU/24 hrs |
| Adult females, nonmidcycle | | 0.5–5.0 IU/24 hrs |
| Postmenopausal females | | >5.0 IU/24 hrs |
| Metanephrine, urine | | <1.3 mg/24 hrs |
| Parathyroid hormone (PTH), serum (Intact + N-terminal PTH) | | 1.0–5.0 pmol/L |

| Pregnanetriol, urine | Males (mg/24 hrs) | Females (mg/24 hrs) |
|---|---|---|
| 0–5 yrs | <0.1 | <0.1 |
| 6–9 yrs | <0.3 | <0.3 |
| 10–15 yrs | 0.2–0.6 | 0.1–0.6 |

|  | >16 yrs | 0.2–2.0 | 0.0–1.4 |
|---|---|---|---|

Progesterone, serum

| | | Males (ng/mL) | Females (ng/mL) |
|---|---|---|---|
| | 0–1 yr | 0.87–3.37 | 0.87–3.37 |
| | 2–9 yrs | 0.12–0.14 | 0.20–0.24 |
| | Postpuberty | <1.0 | Increasing values |
| | Follicular phase | | ≤ 0.7 |
| | Luteal phase | | 2.0–20.0 |

Prolactin, serum

| | Males (ng/mL) | Females (ng/mL) |
|---|---|---|
| | 0–20 | 0–23 |

Renin activity (peripheral vein), plasma
   Na-depleted, upright

| | 18–39 yrs | 2.9–24.0 ng/mL/hr |
|---|---|---|
| | >40 yrs | 2.9–10.8 ng/mL/hr |

   Na-replete, upright

| | 18–39 yrs | ≤ 0.6–4.3 ng/mL/hr |
|---|---|---|
| | ≥ 40 yrs | ≤ 0.6–3.0 ng/mL/hr |

Sex hormone binding globulin (SHBG), serum

| Adult males (nmol/l) | Adult nonpregnant females (nmol/L) |
|---|---|
| 10–80 | 20–130 |

Somatomedin-C, plasma

| Age (yrs) | Males (ng/mL) | Females (ng/mL) |
|---|---|---|
| 0–5 | 0–103 | 0–112 |
| 6–8 | 2–118 | 5–128 |
| 9–10 | 15–148 | 24–158 |
| 11–13 | 55–216 | 65–226 |
| 14–15 | 114–232 | 124–242 |
| 16–17 | 84–221 | 94–231 |
| 18–19 | 56–177 | 66–186 |
| 20–24 | 75–142 | 64–131 |
| 25–29 | 65–131 | 55–121 |
| 30–34 | 58–122 | 47–112 |
| 35–39 | 51–115 | 40–104 |
| 40–44 | 46–109 | 35–98 |
| 45–49 | 43–104 | 32–93 |
| ≥ 50 | 40–100 | 29–90 |

Testosterone, serum

| | Total (ng/dL) | Free (ng/dL) | Percent |
|---|---|---|---|
| Males | 300–1200 | 9–30 | 2.0–4.8 |
| Females | 20–80 | 0.3–1.9 | 0.9–3.8 |

Thyroid microsomal and thyroglobulin
   antibodies             <1:100
(See Table 1-3.)

Vanillylmandelic acid (VMA), urine

| | <1 yr | <27 µg/mg creatinine |
|---|---|---|
| | 1 yr | <18 µg/mg creatinine |
| | 2–4 yrs | <13 µg/mg creatinine |
| | 5–9 yrs | <8.5 µg/mg creatinine |
| | 10–14 yrs | <7 µg/mg creatinine |
| | 15–18 yrs | <5 µg/mg creatinine |
| | Adults | <9 mg/24 hrs |

Vasoactive intestinal polypeptide (VIP),
   plasma             <75 pg/mL

## Normal Blood Antibody Levels

ACh
   Receptor-binding antibodies       ≤ 0.02 nmol/L

**Table 1-3.** Thyroid Function Indicators by Age (Serum Concentration)[a]

| Age | $T_4$ nmol/L | $FT_4$ pmol/L | TSH[b] mIU/L | TBG mg/L | $T_3$ nmol/L | $rT_3$ nmol/L | Thyroglobulin μg/L |
|---|---|---|---|---|---|---|---|
| 1–4 days | 142–277 | 28–68 | 1–39 | 22–42 | 1.5–11.4 | | 2–110 |
| 1–4 wks | 106–221 | 12–30 | 1.7–9.1 | | 1.6–5.3 | 0.4–4.5 | |
| 1–12 mos | 76–210 | 10–23 | 0.8–8.2 | 16–36 | 1.6–3.8 | 0.17–2.0 | |
| 1–5 yrs | 94–193 | 10–27 | 0.7–5.7 | 12–28 | 1.6–4.1 | 0.23–1.1 | 2–65 |
| 6–10 yrs | 82–171 | 13–27 | 0.7–5.7 | 12–28 | 1.4–3.7 | 0.26–1.2 | 2–65 |
| 11–15 yrs | 71–151 | 10–26 | 0.7–5.7 | 14–30 | 1.3–3.3 | 0.29–1.3 | 2–36 |
| 16–20 yrs | 54–152 | 10–26 | 0.7–5.7 | 14–30 | 1.2–3.2 | 0.39–1.2 | 2–36 |
| 21–80 yrs | 55–160 | 12–32 | 0.4–4.2 | 17–36 | | 0.46–1.2 | 2–25 |
| 21–50 yrs | | | | | 1.1–3.1 | | |
| 51–80 yrs | | | | | 0.6–2.8 | | |

[a]No clinically significant difference by gender or race.
[b]Diurnal variation of TSH ~50% between nadir (1500–1700 hrs) and peak (2300–2400 hrs).

| | |
|---|---|
| Receptor-blocking antibodies | <25% blockade of ACh receptors |
| Receptor-modulating antibodies | <20% loss of ACh receptors |
| Anti ds-DNA antibodies | |
|     Negative | <70 units |
|     Borderline | 70–200 units |
|     Positive | >200 units |
| Antiextractable nuclear antigens (anti-RNP, anti-Sm, anti-SSB, anti-SSA) | Negative |
| Antiglomerular basement membrane, antibody | Negative |
| Antimitochondrial antibodies | Negative |
| Antinuclear antibodies (ANA) | Negative |
| Antibodies to Scl 70 antigen | Negative |
| Antibodies to Jo 1 antigen | Negative |
| Antineutrophil cytoplasmic antibodies (c-ANCA and p-ANCA) | Negative |
| Granulocyte antibodies | Negative |
| Intrinsic factor blocking antibody | Negative |
| Parietal cell antibodies | Negative |
| Rheumatoid factor | |
|     Latex agglutination | Negative |
|     Rate nephelometry | |
|         Nonreactive | 0–39 IU/mL |
|         Weakly reactive | 40–79 IU/mL |
|         Reactive | ≥ 80 IU/mL |
| Smooth muscle antibody | Negative |
| Striated muscle antibodies | <1:60 |

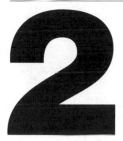

# Critical Values

These values may indicate the need for prompt clinical intervention. Any sudden changes may also be critical. Also called *action values* or *automatic call back values.*

Values will vary according to the laboratory performing the tests as well as patient age and other factors.

## Hematology

| | Low | High |
|---|---|---|
| WBC | <1500/cu mm | >15,000/cu mm |
| CSF | None | Increased |
| Packed cell volume (Hct) | <15 vol% | >60 vol% |
| Hb (adult) | <5 gm/dL | >18 gm/dL |
| Hb (infant) | <7 gm/dL | >21 gm/dL |
| Platelet count | <30,000/cu mm | >1,000,000/cu mm |
| Platelet count (pediatric) | <20,000/cu mm | >1,000,000/cu mm |
| PT | None | >40 secs or >3 × control level |
| aPTT | None | >90 secs |
| Positive test for fibrin split products, protamine sulfate, high heparin level | | |
| Fibrinogen | <80 mg/dL | >700 mg/dL |
| Presence of blast cells, sickle cells | | |
| New diagnosis of leukemia, sickle cell anemia, aplastic crisis | | |
| Blasts or malignant cells or organisms in CSF or any other body fluid | | |

## Blood Chemistry

| | Low | High |
|---|---|---|
| Total serum bilirubin (newborns) | None | >18 mg/dL |
| Serum calcium | <6 mg/dL | >14 mg/dL |
| Serum glucose | <40 mg/dL | >450 mg/dL |
| Newborn | <30 mg/dL | >300 mg/dL |
| Serum magnesium | <1.0 mg/dL | >5.0 mg/dL |
| Serum phosphorus | <1 mg/dL | None |
| Serum potassium | <2.5 mEq/L | >6.5 mEq/L |
| Newborn | <2.5 mEq/L | >8.0 mEq/L |
| Serum sodium | <120 mEq/L | >160 mEq/L |
| Serum chloride | <80 mEq/L | >115 mEq/L |
| Serum bicarbonate | <10 mEq/L | >40 mEq/L |
| Blood $pCO_2$ | <20 mm Hg | >70 mm Hg |
| Blood pH | <7.2 units | >7.6 units |
| Blood $pO_2$ | <40 mm Hg | None |

| Blood ammonia | None | >40 $\mu$mol/L |
|---|---|---|
| Serum CK | None | >3–5 × ULN |
| Serum CK-MB | None | >5% |
| Serum creatinine (except dialysis patients) | None | >7.5 mg/dL |
| BUN (except dialysis patients) | 2 mg/dL | >80 mg/dL |
| Serum amylase | None | >200 U/L |
| CSF total protein | None | >45 mg/dL |
| CSF glucose | <80% of blood level | |

## Microbiology

Positive blood culture
Positive CSF Gram's stain or culture or India ink preparation
Positive culture from body fluid (e.g., pleural, peritoneal, joint)
Positive acid-fast stain or culture
Positive culture or isolate for *Corynebacterium diphtheriae, Cryptococcus neoformans, Bordetella pertussis, Neisseria gonorrhoeae* (only nongenital sites), dimorphic fungi (histoplasma, *Coccidioides, Blastomyces brasiliensis*)
Presence of blood parasites (e.g., malaria, *Babesia*, microfilaria)
Positive rapid antigen detection for *Cryptococcus*, group B streptococci, *Haemophilus influenzae* B, *Neisseria meningitidis*, or *Streptococcus pneumoniae*
Stool culture positive for *Salmonella, Shigella, Campylobacter*, or *Vibrio*
Increased blood antibody levels for infectious agents (see Chapter 1)

## Urinalysis

Strongly positive test for glucose and ketone
Reducing sugars in infants
Presence of pathologic crystals (urate, cysteine, leucine, tyrosine)

## Serology

Incompatible cross match
Positive direct and indirect antiglobulin (Coombs') test on routine specimens
Positive direct antiglobulin (Coombs') test on cord blood
Titers of significant RBC alloantibodies during pregnancy
Transfusion reaction workup showing incompatible unit of transfused blood
Failure to call within 72 hrs for RhIG after possible or known exposure to Rh-positive RBCs
Positive test for hepatitis, syphilis, or AIDS

## Therapeutic Drugs

| | Blood Levels |
|---|---|
| Carbamazepine | >20 $\mu$g/mL |
| Digitoxin | >35 $\mu$g/mL |
| Digoxin | >2.5 ng/mL |
| Ethosuximide | >200 $\mu$g/mL |
| Lidocaine | >9 $\mu$g/mL |
| Lithium | >2 mEq/L |
| Phenobarbital | >60 $\mu$g/mL |
| Phenytoin | >40 $\mu$g/mL |
| Primidone | >24 $\mu$g/mL |
| Quinidine | >10 $\mu$g/mL |
| Theophylline | >25 $\mu$g/mL |
| Tobramycin | >12 $\mu$g/mL (peak) |
| Salicylate | >700 $\mu$g/mL |

See Chapter 19 in *Interpretation of Diagnostic Tests* (6th ed) for toxic levels of various therapeutic drugs and toxic substances.

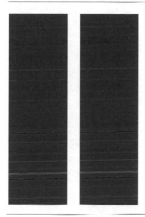

# Specific Laboratory Examinations

# Core Blood Chemical Analytes: Alterations by Diseases

## Alkaline Phosphatase (ALP)

### Use

Diagnosis of causes and monitor course of cholestasis (e.g., neoplasm, drugs)
Diagnosis of various bone disorders (e.g., Paget's disease, osteogenic sarcoma)

### Interferences

Intravenous injection of albumin
Decreased by collection of blood in ethylenediamine-tetraacetic acid (EDTA), fluoride, or oxalate anticoagulant
Increased (up to 30%) by standing at room or refrigerator temperature

### Increased in

Bone origin—increased deposition of calcium
- Hyperparathyroidism
- Paget's disease (osteitis deformans)
- *Increase in cases of metastases to bone is marked only in prostate carcinoma.*
- Osteoblastic bone tumors
- Osteogenesis imperfecta (due to healing fractures)
- Familial osteoectasia
- Osteomalacia, rickets
- Polyostotic fibrous dysplasia
- Late pregnancy
- Children
- Administration of ergosterol
- Hyperthyroidism
- Transient hyperphosphatasemia of infancy
- Hodgkin's disease

Liver disease—any obstruction of biliary system; is a sensitive indicator of intra- or extrahepatic cholestasis. *Whenever the ALP is elevated, a simultaneous elevation of 5'-N establishes biliary disease as the cause of the elevated ALP. If the 5'-N is not increased, the cause of the elevated ALP must be found elsewhere (e.g., bone disease).*
- Nodules in liver
- Liver infiltrates (e.g., amyloid, leukemia)
- Cholangiolar obstruction in hepatitis (e.g., infectious, toxic)
- Hepatic congestion due to heart disease
- Adverse reaction to therapeutic drug
- Increased synthesis of ALP in liver
  Diabetes mellitus—44% of diabetic patients have 40% increase of ALP
  Parenteral hyperalimentation of glucose
- Liver diseases with increased ALP
  2 times increase: acute hepatitis, acute fatty liver, cirrhosis
  5 times increase: infectious mononucleosis, postnecrotic cirrhosis

10 times increase: carcinoma of head of pancreas, choledocholithiasis, cholestatic hepatitis

15–20 times increase: primary biliary cirrhosis, primary or metastatic carcinoma

Chronic therapeutic use of anticonvulsant drugs (e.g., phenobarbital, phenytoin)

Hyperthyroidism

Hodgkin's disease

Placental origin—appears in weeks 16–20 of normal pregnancy; disappears 3–6 days after delivery of placenta

Intestinal origin—is a component in ~25% of normal sera

Benign familial hyperphosphatasemia

Ectopic production by neoplasm (Regan isoenzyme)

Vascular endothelium origin—some patients with myocardial, pulmonary, renal, or splenic infarction

Hyperphosphatasia (liver and bone isoenzymes)

Primary hypophosphatemia

ALP isoenzyme determinations are not widely used

Children—mostly bone; little or no liver or intestine

Adults—liver with little or no bone or intestine

### Decreased in

Excess vitamin D ingestion

Milk-alkali (Burnett's) syndrome

Congenital hypophosphatasia

Achondroplasia

Hypothyroidism, cretinism

Pernicious anemia in one-third of patients

Celiac disease

Malnutrition

Scurvy

Therapeutic agents (e.g., corticosteroids, trifluoperazine, antilipemic agents)

Cardiac surgery with cardiopulmonary bypass pump

## Ammonia

### Use

Should be measured in cases of unexplained lethargy and vomiting or encephalopathy and in any neonate with unexplained neurologic deterioration

Not useful to assess degree of dysfunction

### Increased in

Certain inborn errors of metabolism, especially ornithine carbamoyltransferase, citrullinemia, argininosuccinic aciduria

Transient hyperammonemia in newborn; unknown etiology

Moribund children without being diagnostic of a specific disease

May occur in any patient with severe liver disease. Increased in most cases of hepatic coma. *In cirrhosis, blood ammonia may be increased after portacaval anastomosis.*

GU tract infection with distention and stasis

Sodium valproate therapy

### Decreased in

Hyperornithinemia (deficiency of ornithine aminotransaminase activity)

## Aspartate Aminotransferase (AST; Serum Glutamic-Oxaloacetic Transaminase [SGOT])

### Use

Differential diagnosis of diseases of hepatobiliary system and pancreas

### Interferences

Increase due to hemolysis, lipemia
Increase due to calcium dust in air (e.g., due to construction in laboratory)
Increased (because enzymes are activated during test)
  • Therapy with oxacillin, ampicillin, opiates, erythromycin
Decreased (because of increased serum lactate–consuming enzyme)
  • Diabetic ketoacidosis
  • Beriberi
  • Severe liver disease
  • Chronic hemodialysis (reason unknown)
  • Uremia—proportional to BUN level (reason unknown)

### Increased in

Liver diseases
  • Active necrosis of parenchymal cells is suggested by extremely high levels.
  • Rapid rise and decline suggests extrahepatic biliary disease.
  • "Pseudomyocardial infarction" pattern. Administration of opiates to patients with diseased biliary tract or previous cholecystectomy.
  • Congestion (e.g., heart failure, cirrhosis, biliary obstruction, cancer).
  • Eclampsia.
  • Hepatotoxic drugs.
Musculoskeletal diseases, including trauma, surgery, and IM injections
  • Myoglobinuria
Acute myocardial infarction
Others
  • Acute pancreatitis
  • Intestinal injury (e.g., surgery, infarction)
  • Local irradiation injury
  • Pulmonary infarction
  • Cerebral infarction
  • Renal infarction
  • Drugs
  • Burns
  • Heat exhaustion
  • Lead poisoning
  • Hemolytic anemia

### Marked Increase (>3000 U/L) in

Acute hypotension (e.g., acute myocardial infarction, sepsis, post–cardiac surgery)
Toxic liver injury (e.g., drugs)
Viral hepatitis
Liver trauma
Liver metastases
Rhabdomyolysis

### Decreased in

Azotemia
Chronic renal dialysis
Pyridoxal phosphate deficiency states (e.g., malnutrition, pregnancy, alcoholic liver disease)
*Varies <10 U/day in the same person*

## Alanine Aminotransferase (ALT; Serum Glutamic-Pyruvic Transaminase [SGPT])

### Use

Differential diagnosis of diseases of hepatobiliary system and pancreas

Generally parallels but lower than AST in alcohol-related diseases

### Increased in

See AST (SGOT).
Obesity (AST not increased)
Severe preeclampsia (both)
Rapidly progressing acute lymphoblastic leukemia (both)

### Decreased in

GU tract infection
Malignancy
Pyridoxal phosphate deficiency states (e.g., malnutrition, pregnancy, alcoholic liver disease)

## AST:ALT (SGOT:SGPT) RATIO
**(normal = 0.7–1.4 depending on methodology)**

### Use

Differential diagnosis of diseases of hepatobiliary system and pancreas

### Increased in

Drug hepatotoxicity (>2.0)
Alcoholic hepatitis (>2.0 is highly suggestive; may be up to 6.0)
Cirrhosis (1.4–2.0)
Intrahepatic cholestasis (>1.5)
Hepatocellular carcinoma
Chronic hepatitis (slightly increased; 1.3)

### Decreased in

Acute hepatitis due to virus, drugs, toxins (with AST increased 3–10 times upper limit of normal, usually ≤ 0.65)
Extrahepatic cholestasis (normal or slightly decreased, 0.8)

## Bilirubin

### Use

Differential diagnosis of diseases of hepatobiliary system and pancreas and other causes of jaundice

### Interferences

Exposure to white or ultraviolet light decreases total and indirect bilirubin 2% to >20%.
Fasting for 48 hrs produces a mean increase of ~200%.

### Increased Direct (Conjugated) Bilirubin in

Hereditary disorders (e.g., Dubin-Johnson syndrome, Rotor's syndrome)
Hepatic cellular damage. *Increased conjugated bilirubin may be associated with normal total bilirubin in up to one-third of patients with liver diseases.*
Biliary duct obstruction
Infiltrations, space-occupying lesions
Direct bilirubin
  • 20–40% of total: more suggestive of hepatic than posthepatic jaundice
  • 40–60% of total: occurs in either hepatic or posthepatic jaundice
  • >50% of total: more suggestive of posthepatic than hepatic jaundice
Total serum bilirubin >40 mg/dL indicates hepatocellular rather than extrahepatic obstruction.

### Increased Unconjugated (Indirect) Bilirubin in (Conjugated <20% of Total)

Increased bilirubin production
- Hemolytic diseases
- Ineffective erythropoiesis (e.g., pernicious anemia)
- Blood transfusions
- Hematomas

Hereditary disorders (e.g., Gilbert's disease, Crigler-Najjar syndrome)
Drugs

### Decreased in

Ingestion of certain drugs (e.g., barbiturates)

## Urea Nitrogen (BUN)

### Use

Diagnosis of renal insufficiency
- *A BUN of 10–20 mg/dL almost always indicates normal glomerular function.*
- *A BUN of 50–150 mg/dL implies serious impairment of renal function.*
- *BUN equal to 150–250 mg/dL is virtually conclusive evidence of severely impaired glomerular function.*
- *In chronic renal disease, BUN correlates better with symptoms of uremia than does the serum creatinine.*

Evidence of hemorrhage into GI tract
Assess patients requiring nutritional support for excess catabolism (e.g., burns, cancer)

### Increased in

Impaired kidney function
Prerenal azotemia—any cause of reduced renal blood flow
- Congestive heart failure
- Salt and water depletion (vomiting, diarrhea, diuresis, sweating)
- Shock

Postrenal azotemia—any obstruction of urinary tract (increased BUN:creatinine ratio)
Increased protein catabolism (serum creatinine remains normal)
- Hemorrhage into GI tract
- AMI
- Stress

### Decreased in

Diuresis (e.g., with overhydration, often associated with low protein catabolism).
*BUN of 6–8 mg/dL is frequently associated with states of overhydration.*
Severe liver damage
- Drugs
- Poisoning
- Hepatitis

Increased use of protein for synthesis
- Late pregnancy
- Infancy
- Acromegaly
- Malnutrition
- Anabolic hormones

Diet
- Low protein and high carbohydrate
- IV feedings only

- Impaired absorption (celiac disease)
- Malnutrition
- Nephrotic syndrome

SIADH

Inherited hyperammonemias (urea is virtually absent in blood)

## Creatinine

### Use

Diagnosis of renal insufficiency. *Serum creatinine is a more specific and sensitive indicator of renal disease than BUN.*

### Increased in

Diet
- Ingestion of creatinine (roast meat)

Muscle disease
- Gigantism, acromegaly

Prerenal or postrenal azotemia

Impaired kidney function; 50% loss of renal function is needed to increase serum creatinine from 1.0 to 2.0 mg/dL; therefore, not sensitive to mild to moderate renal injury.

### Decreased in

Pregnancy—normal value is 0.4–0.6 mg/dL; *>0.8 mg/dL is abnormal and should alert clinician to further diagnostic evaluation.*

### Interferences (Depending on Methodology)

Artifactual decrease by
- Marked increase of serum bilirubin
- Enzymatic reaction (glucose >100 mg/dL)

Artifactual increase due to
- Reducing alkaline picrate (e.g., glucose, ascorbate, uric acid).
- Formation of colored complexes (e.g., acetoacetate, pyruvate, other ketoacids, certain cephalosporins). *Ketoacidosis may substantially increase serum creatinine results with alkaline picrate reaction.*
- Enzymatic reaction may increase serum creatinine (≤ 0.6 mg/dL).

## BUN:Creatinine Ratio

Normal range for a healthy person on a normal diet is 12–20; most individuals are 12–16. Should be used only as a rough guide.

### Use

Differentiate pre- and postrenal azotemia from renal azotemia

### Increased Ratio (>20:1) with Normal Creatinine in

Prerenal azotemia (BUN rises without increase in creatinine) due to decreased glomerular filtration rate

Catabolic states with increased tissue breakdown

GI hemorrhage

High protein intake

Impaired renal function plus
- Excess protein intake or production or tissue breakdown (e.g., GI bleeding, thyrotoxicosis, infection, surgery, burns, cachexia, high fever)
- Urine reabsorption (e.g., ureterocolostomy)
- Patients with reduced muscle mass

Certain drugs (e.g., tetracycline, glucocorticoids)

### Increased Ratio (>20:1) with Increased Creatinine in

Postrenal azotemia (BUN rises disproportionately more than creatinine) (e.g.,
   obstructive uropathy)
Prerenal azotemia superimposed on renal disease

### Decreased Ratio (<10:1) with Decreased BUN in

Acute tubular necrosis
Low-protein diet, starvation, severe liver disease, and other causes of decreased
   urea synthesis
Repeated dialysis (urea rather than creatinine diffuses out of extracellular fluid)
Inherited hyperammonemias (urea is virtually absent in blood)
SIADH (due to tubular secretion of urea)
Pregnancy

### Decreased Ratio (<10:1) with Increased Creatinine in

Phenacemide therapy (accelerates conversion of creatine to creatinine)
Rhabdomyolysis (releases muscle creatinine)
Muscular patients who develop renal failure

### Inappropriate Ratio

Diabetic ketoacidosis (acetoacetate causes artifactual increase in creatinine with
   certain methodologies, resulting in normal ratio when dehydration should produce an increased BUN:creatinine ratio)
Cephalosporin therapy (interferes with creatinine measurement)

## Total Calcium

### Use

Diagnosis of parathyroid dysfunction, hypercalcemia of malignancy

### Interferences

Increased by
   • Elevated serum protein
   • Dehydration
   • Venous stasis during blood collection by prolonged application of tourniquet
   • Use of cork-stoppered test tubes
   • Hyponatremia (<120 mEq/L)

### Decreased by

   • Hypomagnesemia (e.g., due to cisplatin cancer chemotherapy)
   • Hyperphosphatemia (e.g., laxatives, phosphate enemas, chemotherapy of
     leukemia or lymphoma, rhabdomyolysis)
   • Hypoalbuminemia
   • Hemodilution
*Total serum protein and albumin should always be measured simultaneously for
proper interpretation of serum calcium levels because 0.8 mg of calcium is
bound to 1.0 gm of albumin in serum. Correct by adding 0.8 mg/dL for every
1.0 gm/dL that serum albumin falls below 4.0 gm/dL. Binding to globulin only
affects total calcium if globulin >6 gm/dL.*

### Increased in

Hyperparathyroidism
   • Primary
   • Secondary
       Acute and chronic renal failure
       Postrenal transplant

Osteomalacia with malabsorption
Aluminum-associated osteomalacia
Malignant tumors (especially breast, lung, and kidney)
- Direct bone metastases (up to 30% of these patients)
- Osteoclastic activating factor (e.g., multiple myeloma, Burkitt's lymphoma; may be markedly increased in adult T-cell lymphoma)
- Humoral hypercalcemia of malignancy
- Ectopic production of 1,25-dihydroxyvitamin $D_3$ (e.g., lymphoma)

Effect of drugs
- Vitamin D intoxication
- Milk-alkali (Burnett's) syndrome
- Diuretics (thiazide and chlorthalidone rarely increase serum calcium >1.0 mg/dL)
- Therapeutic agents (e.g., estrogens, androgens, progestins, tamoxifen, lithium)
- Others (e.g., vitamin A intoxication, thyroid hormone, parenteral nutrition)

Chronic renal failure
Other endocrine conditions
- Hyperthyroidism
- Some patients with hypothyroidism, Cushing's syndrome, adrenal insufficiency, acromegaly, pheochromocytoma
- Multiple endocrine neoplasia

Granulomatous disease (1,25-dihydroxyvitamin D excess) (e.g., sarcoidosis, tuberculosis, mycoses, berylliosis)
Acute osteoporosis
Polyuric phase of acute renal failure
Miscellaneous
- Familial hypocalciuric hypercalcemia
- Rhabdomyolysis causing acute renal failure
- Porphyria
- Dehydration with hyperproteinemia
- Hypophosphatasia
- Idiopathic hypercalcemia of infancy

### Decreased in

Hypoparathyroidism
- Surgical
- Idiopathic
- Infiltration of parathyroids (e.g., sarcoid, amyloid, tumor)
- Congenital (DiGeorge syndrome)

Pseudohypoparathyroidism
Malabsorption of calcium and vitamin D
Obstructive jaundice
Chronic renal disease with uremia and phosphate retention; Fanconi's syndrome; renal tubular acidosis
Acute pancreatitis with extensive fat necrosis
Insufficient calcium, phosphorus, and vitamin D ingestion
- Bone disease (osteomalacia, rickets)
- Starvation
- Late pregnancy

Certain drugs
- Cancer chemotherapy drugs (e.g., cisplatin, mithramycin, cytosine)
- Fluoride intoxication
- Antibiotics (e.g., gentamicin, pentamidine, ketoconazole)
- Chronic use of anticonvulsant drugs (e.g., phenobarbital, phenytoin)
- Loop-active diuretics
- Calcitonin
- Multiple citrated blood transfusions

Neonates born of complicated pregnancies
- Hyperbilirubinemia
- Respiratory distress, asphyxia
- Cerebral injuries
- Infants of diabetic mothers
- Prematurity
- Maternal hypoparathyroidism

Hypomagnesemia
Malignant disease
Toxic shock syndrome
Rhabdomyolysis
Tumor lysis syndrome
*Concomitant hypokalemia is not infrequent in hypercalcemia.*
*Concomitant dehydration is almost always present.*

## Ionized Calcium

### Use

~50% of calcium is ionized, 40–45% is bound to albumin, and 5–10% is bound to
other anions. Total calcium values may be deceiving *(blood pH should always
be performed with ionized calcium, which is increased in acidosis and decreased
in alkalosis)*. In critically ill patients, elevated total serum calcium usually indicates ionized hypercalcemia.
Life-threatening complications are frequent when serum ionized calcium is <2 mg/dL.
With multiple blood transfusions, ionized calcium <3 mg/dL may be an indication to administer calcium.

### Interferences

Hypo- or hypermagnesemia; patients respond to serum magnesium that becomes
normal but not to calcium therapy. *Serum magnesium should always be mea-
sured in any patient with hypocalcemia.*
Increase of ions to which calcium is bound
- Phosphate (e.g., phosphorus administration in treatment of diabetic ketoaci-
dosis, chemotherapy causing tumor lysis syndrome, rhabdomyolysis)
- Bicarbonate
- Citrate (e.g., during blood transfusion)
- Radiographic contrast media containing calcium chelators

### Increased in

*Normal total serum calcium associated with hypoalbuminemia may indicate ion-
ized hypercalcemia.*
~25% of patients with hyperparathyroidism have normal total but increased ionized calcium levels.

### Decreased in

Hyperventilation (total serum calcium may be normal)
Administration of bicarbonate to control metabolic acidosis
Increased serum free fatty acids due to
- Certain drugs (e.g., heparin, IV lipids, epinephrine, norepinephrine, iso-
proterenol, alcohol)
- Severe stress (e.g., acute pancreatitis, diabetic ketoacidosis, sepsis, acute
myocardial infarction)
- Hemodialysis

Hypoparathyroidism
Vitamin D deficiency
Toxic shock syndrome
Fat embolism

*Hypokalemia protects patient from hypocalcemic tetany; correction of hypokalemia without correction of hypocalcemia may provoke tetany.*

## Chloride

### Use

With sodium, potassium, and $CO_2$ to assess electrolyte, acid-base, and water balance. Usually changes in same direction as sodium, except in metabolic acidosis with bicarbonate depletion and metabolic alkalosis with bicarbonate excess when serum sodium levels may be normal.

### Interferences

Hyperlipidemia (artifactual change)

### Increased in

Metabolic acidosis associated with prolonged diarrhea with loss of $NaHCO_3$
Renal tubular diseases with decreased excretion of $H^+$ and decreased reabsorption of $HCO_3^-$ ("hyperchloremic metabolic acidosis")
Respiratory alkalosis (e.g., hyperventilation, severe CNS damage)
Excessive administration of certain drugs (e.g., $NH_4Cl$, IV saline, steroids, salicylate intoxication; acetazolamide therapy; bromism)
Some cases of hyperparathyroidism
Diabetes insipidus, dehydration
Sodium loss > chloride loss (e.g., diarrhea, intestinal fistulas)
Ureterosigmoidostomy

### Decreased in

Prolonged vomiting or suction (loss of HCl)
Metabolic acidoses with accumulation of organic anions
Chronic respiratory acidosis
Salt-losing renal diseases
Adrenocortical insufficiency
Primary aldosteronism
Expansion of extracellular fluid (e.g., SIADH, hyponatremia, water intoxication, congestive heart failure)
Burns

## Creatine Kinase (CK)

### Use

Marker for injury to cardiac or voluntary muscle with good specificity

### Increased in

Necrosis or acute atrophy of cardiac muscle
- AMI
- Severe myocarditis

Necrosis or acute atrophy of striated muscle
- After thoracic/open heart surgery, values return to baseline in 24–48 hrs.
- Cardioversion may increase CK and CK-MB.
- Progressive muscular dystrophy.
- Amyotrophic lateral sclerosis.
- Polymyositis.
- Myotonic dystrophy.
- Thermal and electrical burns.
- Rhabdomyolysis.
- Severe or prolonged exercise.

- Status epilepticus.
- Chemical toxicity (benzene ring compounds).
- Parturition and frequently the last few weeks of pregnancy.
- Malignant hyperthermia; hypothermia.
- Endocrine myopathy.
   Hypothyroidism
   Acromegaly
   Hypoparathyroid myopathy
- Familial hypokalemic periodic paralysis.
- Cocaine use.

Extensive brain infarction
Some neoplasms

### Slight Increase Occasionally in

Variable increase after IM injection
Muscle spasms or convulsions in children
Moderate hemolysis

### Normal in

After cardiac catheterization and coronary arteriography unless myocardium has
   been injured by catheter
Exercise testing for coronary artery disease
*Increase* in angina pectoris or coronary insufficiency implies some necrosis of car-
   diac muscle even if a discrete infarct is not identified.
Pericarditis
Pulmonary infarction
Renal infarction
Liver disease
Biliary obstruction
Some muscle disorders
- Neurogenic muscle atrophy
- Thyrotoxicosis
- Steroid myopathy
Pernicious anemia
Most malignancies

### Decreased In

Untreated hyperthyroidism
Decreased muscle mass
RA
Pregnancy
Various drugs (e.g., phenothiazine, prednisone), toxins, and insecticides

## Creatine Kinase (CK) Isoenzymes

### Use

CK-MB is the most useful early marker for myocardial injury.

### CK-MB Isoenzyme May Be Increased in

Necrosis of cardiac muscle
- AMI
- Cardiac contusion
- Cardiac surgical procedures
- Cardioversion
- Percutaneous transluminal coronary angioplasty
- Pericarditis
- Myocarditis

- Prolonged supraventricular tachycardia
- Cardiomyopathies
- Collagen diseases involving the myocardium
- Congestive heart failure
- Coronary angiography

Noncardiac causes
- Skeletal muscle trauma.
- Extensive rhabdomyolysis.
- Myoglobinuria.
- Electrical and thermal burns and trauma.
- Malignant hyperthermia, hypothermia.
- Skeletal muscle diseases.
- Reye's syndrome.
- Peripartum period for first day beginning within 30 mins.
- Acute cholecystitis.
- Infections.
- Hypo- and hyperthyroidism and chronic renal failure may cause persistent increase although the proportion of CK-MB remains low.
- Acute exacerbation of obstructive lung disease.
- Diabetic ketoacidosis.
- Septic shock.
- Drugs (e.g., aspirin, tranquilizers).
- Carbon monoxide poisoning.
- Some neoplasms.

*CK-MB >15–20% should raise the possibility of an atypical macro CK-MB.*

### CK-MB Isoenzyme Is Not Increased in

Angina pectoris or coronary insufficiency. An *increase* implies some necrosis of cardiac muscle even if a discrete infarct is not identified.
Cardiac arrest or cardioversion not due to AMI
Cardiac pacemaker or catheterization
Cardiopulmonary bypass
IM injections
Seizures
Brain infarction or injury
Pulmonary embolism

## CK-BB Isoenzyme

### Use

Is rarely used clinically

### May Be Increased in

Malignant hyperthermia, uremia, brain infarction or anoxia, Reye's syndrome, necrosis of intestine, various neoplasms, biliary atresia

## Atypical Macro Isoenzyme
### (high-molecular-mass complex of a CK isoenzyme and immunoglobulin)

*May cause false CK-MB results resulting in an incorrect diagnosis of AMI.*
Discovered in <2% of all CK isoenzyme electrophoresis.

## Gamma-Glutamyl Transferase (GGT)

### Use

In liver disease, generally parallels changes in serum ALP

Sensitive indicator of occult alcoholism

Diagnosis of liver disease in presence of bone disease, pregnancy, or childhood, which increases serum ALP and LAP but not GGT

### Increased in

Liver disease. Parallels changes in serum ALP, but is more sensitive.
- Acute hepatitis. Increase is less marked than that of other liver enzymes.
- Chronic active hepatitis. More increased than AST and ALT.
- Alcoholic hepatitis.
- Cirrhosis. In inactive cases, average values are lower than those in chronic hepatitis cases. Increase >10–20 times in cirrhotic patients suggests superimposed primary carcinoma of the liver.
- Primary biliary cirrhosis.
- Fatty liver. Increase parallels that of AST and ALT but is greater.
- Obstructive jaundice. Increase is faster and greater than that of serum ALP and LAP.
- Liver metastases. Parallels ALP.
- Cholestasis.
- Children. Much more increased in biliary atresia than in neonatal hepatitis. Children with alpha$_1$-antitrypsin deficiency have higher levels than patients with biliary atresia.

Pancreatitis. Always elevated in acute pancreatitis.

AMI. Increased in 50% of the patients.

Heavy use of alcohol; *GGT is the most sensitive indicator and a good screening test for alcoholism.*

Various drugs (e.g., barbiturates, phenytoin [Dilantin], tricyclic antidepressants, acetaminophen)

Neoplasms, even in absence of liver metastases

### Normal in

Pregnancy (in contrast to serum ALP) and children older than 3 months of age; therefore, may aid in differential diagnosis of hepatobiliary disease occurring during pregnancy and childhood

Bone disease or patients with increased bone growth (children and adolescents); therefore, useful in distinguishing bone disease from liver disease as a cause of increased serum ALP

Renal failure

Strenuous exercise

## Glucose

### Use

Diagnosis of diabetes mellitus (defined by the World Health Organization as unequivocal increase of fasting serum [or plasma] glucose $\geq 140$ mg/dL on more than one occasion or any glucose $\geq 200$ mg/dL)

Control of diabetes mellitus

Diagnosis of hypoglycemia

### May Be Increased in

Diabetes mellitus, including
- Hemochromatosis
- Cushing's syndrome
- Acromegaly and gigantism

Increased circulating epinephrine
- Adrenalin injection
- Pheochromocytoma
- Stress (e.g., emotion, burns, shock, anesthesia)

Acute and chronic pancreatitis
Wernicke's encephalopathy
Some CNS lesions (e.g., subarachnoid hemorrhage, convulsive states)
Effect of drugs (e.g., corticosteroids, estrogens, alcohol, phenytoin)

## May Be Decreased in

Pancreatic disorders
- Islet cell tumor, hyperplasia
- Pancreatitis
- Glucagon deficiency

Extrapancreatic tumors
- Carcinoma of adrenal gland
- Carcinoma of stomach
- Fibrosarcoma

Hepatic disease
- Diffuse severe disease (e.g., poisoning, hepatitis, cirrhosis, tumor)

Endocrine disorders
- Hypopituitarism
- Addison's disease
- Hypothyroidism
- Adrenal medulla unresponsiveness
- Early diabetes mellitus

Functional disturbances
- Postgastrectomy
- Gastroenterostomy

Pediatric disorders
- Prematurity
- Infant of diabetic mother
- Ketotic hypoglycemia
- Spontaneous hypoglycemia in infants

Enzyme diseases
- von Gierke's disease
- Galactosemia
- Fructose intolerance
- Some amino acid and organic acid defects
- Some fatty acid metabolism defects

Other
- Exogenous insulin (factitious)
- Oral hypoglycemic medications (factitious)
- Malnutrition
- Hypothalamic lesions
- Alcoholism

## Interferences

*Blood samples in which serum is not separated from blood cells will show glucose values decreasing at a rate of 7 mg/dL/hr at room temperature.*

# Lactate Dehydrogenase (LD)

## Use

Is a very nonspecific test
Supports diagnosis of AMI after CK has returned to normal
Marker for hemolysis

## Increased in

Diseases of heart, liver, lung, kidney, muscle, hematologic system, malignant tumors, others

## Magnesium (Mg)

### Use

Diagnosis and monitor hypo- and hypermagnesemia, especially in renal failure or GI disorders

### Increased in

Iatrogenic (is usual cause; most often with renal failure)
Renal failure
Diabetic coma before treatment
Hypothyroidism
Adrenocortical insufficiency

### Decreased in
### (almost always due to GI or renal disturbance)

GI disease (malabsorption or abnormal loss of GI fluids)
Renal disease
Nutritional
Endocrine
Metabolic
*Mg deficiency frequently coexists with other electrolyte abnormalities.*

## Osmolality

### Use

Diagnosis of nonketotic hyperglycemic coma
Monitor fluid and electrolyte balance
• Evaluation of hyponatremia.
• *Urine and plasma osmolality are more useful to diagnose state of hydration than changes in Hct, serum proteins, and BUN.*

### Increased in

Hyperglycemia
Diabetic ketoacidosis
Nonketotic hyperglycemic coma
Hypernatremia
Alcohol ingestion is the most common cause of hyperosmolar state

### Decreased in
### (equivalent to hyponatremia)

Hyponatremia with hypovolemia (urine sodium is usually >20 mEq/L)
• Adrenal insufficiency
• Renal losses
• GI tract loss (e.g., vomiting, diarrhea)
• Other losses (e.g., burns, peritonitis, pancreatitis)
Hyponatremia with normal volume or hypervolemia (dilutional syndromes)
• Congestive heart failure, cirrhosis, nephrotic syndrome
• SIADH
Formulas for *calculation* or *prediction* of serum osmolality:

$$\text{mOsm/L} = (1.86 \times \text{serum Na}) + \frac{\text{serum glucose}}{18} + \frac{\text{BUN}}{2.8} + 9 \ (in \ mg/dL)$$

or

in SI units = $(1.86 \times \text{serum Na})$ + serum glucose (mmol/L) + BUN (mmol/L) + 9

Osmolal gap is the difference between measured and calculated values; is <10 in healthy persons.

### Use

*Osmolal gap has been used to estimate the blood alcohol. Since serum osmolality increases 22 mOsm/kg for every 100 mg/dL of ethanol:*

$$\text{Estimated blood alcohol (mg/dL)} = \text{osmolal gap} \times \frac{100}{22}$$

### Osmolal Gap >10 Due to

Decreased serum water content
- Hyperlipidemia
- Hyperproteinemia (total protein >10 gm/dL)

Additional low-molecular-weight substances are in serum (measured osmolality will be >300 mOsm/kg water):
- Ethanol. (An especially large osmolal gap with only moderately elevated ethanol level should raise the possibility of another low-molecular-weight toxin [e.g., methanol].)
- Methanol.
- Isopropyl alcohol.
- Mannitol. (Osmolal gap can be used to detect accumulation of infused mannitol in serum.)
- Ethylene glycol, acetone, paraldehyde result in relatively small osmolal gaps even at lethal levels.

Severely ill patients, especially those in shock; lactic acidosis; renal failure
Laboratory analytic error

## Phosphorus

### Use

Monitor blood phosphorus level in renal and GI disorders, effect of drugs

### Increased in

See Fig. 3-1.
Most causes of hypocalcemia except vitamin D deficiency, in which phosphorous is usually decreased
Acute or chronic renal failure (most common cause) with decreased glomerular filtration rate
Increased tubular reabsorption of phosphate
- Hypoparathyroidism
- Secondary hyperparathyroidism (renal rickets)
- Pseudohypoparathyroidism
- Addison's disease
- Acromegaly
- Hyperthyroidism
- Sickle cell anemia

Increased cellular release of phosphate
- Neoplasms (e.g., myelogenous leukemia)
- Excessive breakdown of tissue (e.g., chemotherapy for neoplasms)
- Bone disease
  Healing fractures
  Multiple myeloma
  Paget's disease
  Osteolytic metastatic tumor in bone
- Childhood

Increased phosphate load
- Exogenous phosphate
  Phosphate enemas, laxatives, or infusions
  Excess vitamin D intake
  IV therapy for hypophosphatemia or hypercalcemia
  Milk-alkali syndrome

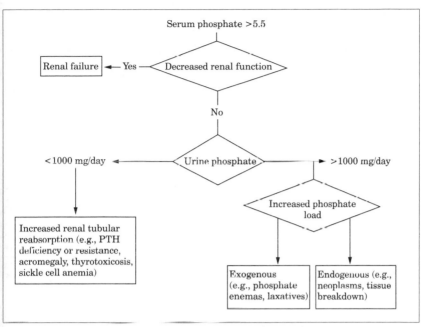

**Fig. 3-1.** Algorithm for hyperphosphatemia.

Massive blood transfusions
Hemolysis of blood
Miscellaneous
- High intestinal obstruction
- Sarcoidosis

### Decreased in

Renal or intestinal loss
- Administration of diuretics
- Renal tubular defects (e.g., Fanconi's syndrome; isolated hypophosphatemia due to drugs, neoplasia, X-linked)
- Primary hyperparathyroidism
- Idiopathic hypercalciuria
- Hypokalemia
- Hypomagnesemia
- Dialysis
- Primary hypophosphatemia
- Idiopathic hypercalciuria
- Acute gout
Decreased intestinal absorption
- Malabsorption
- Vitamin D deficiency and/or resistance, osteomalacia
- Malnutrition, vomiting, diarrhea
- Administration of phosphate-binding antacids
Intracellular shift of phosphate
- Alcoholism*
- Diabetes mellitus*
- Acidosis (especially diabetic ketoacidosis)
- Hyperalimentation*
- Nutritional recovery syndrome (rapid refeeding after prolonged starvation)*

- Administration of IV glucose (e.g., recovery after severe burns)
- Alkalosis, respiratory (e.g., gram-negative bacteremia) or metabolic
- Salicylate poisoning
- Administration of anabolic steroids, androgens, epinephrine, glucagon, insulin
- Cushing's syndrome
- Prolonged hypothermia

*Indicates conditions that may be associated with serum phosphate <1 mg/dL.

Often, more than one mechanism is operative, usually associated with prior phosphorus depletion.

## Potassium

See Figs. 3-2 and 3-3.

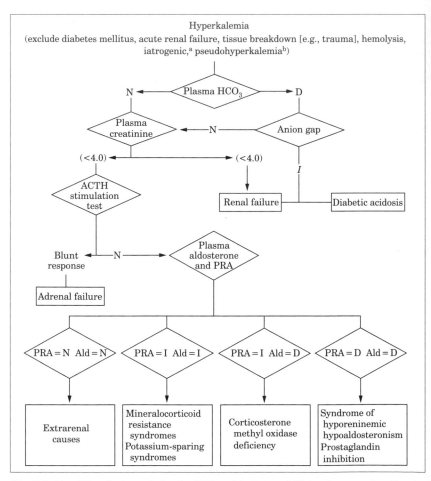

**Fig. 3-2.** Algorithm for hyperkalemia. (Ald = aldosterone.) [a]Potassium-sparing diuretics, administration of potassium (e.g., blood transfusions, salt substitutes, potassium penicillin). [b]Pseudohyperkalemia = WBC >100,000/cu mm or platelet count >1,000,000/cu mm (serum potassium > plasma potassium).

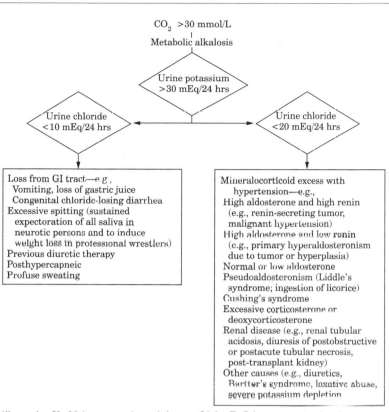

Change in pH of 0.1 causes reciprocal change of 0.6 mEq/L in serum potassium in hyperchloremic acidosis, but <0.4 mEq/L in other acid-base disturbances.

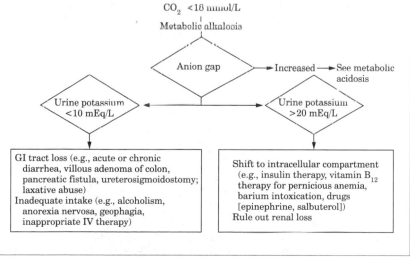

**Fig. 3-3.** Algorithm for hypokalemia.

## Use

Diagnosis and monitoring hyper- and hypokalemia in various conditions (e.g., treatment of diabetic coma, renal failure, severe fluid and electrolyte loss, effect of certain diuretics). Diagnosis of familial hyperkalemic periodic paralysis and hypokalemic paralysis.

### Increased in

### Potassium Retention

Glomerular filtration rate <3–5 mL/min
- Oliguria due to any condition (e.g., renal failure)
- Chronic nonoliguric renal failure associated with dehydration, obstruction, trauma, or excess potassium

Glomerular filtration rate >20 mL/min
- Decreased aldosterone activity
  Addison's disease
  Hypofunction of renin-angiotensin-aldosterone system
    Hyporeninemic hypoaldosteronism with renal insufficiency
    Various drugs (e.g., nonsteroidal anti-inflammatory drugs, angiotensin-converting enzyme inhibitors, cyclosporine, pentamidine)
    Decreased aldosterone production
    Pseudohypoaldosteronism
    Aldosterone antagonist drugs (e.g., spironolactone, captopril)
- Inhibition of tubular secretion of potassium
  Drugs (e.g., spironolactone, triamterene, amiloride)
  Hyperkalemic type of distal renal tubular acidosis (e.g., sickle-cell disease, obstructive uropathy)
- Mineralocorticoid-resistant syndromes. (Increased renin and aldosterone may be low in those marked with *.)
  Primary tubular disorders
    Hereditary
    Acquired (e.g., SLE, amyloidosis, sickle cell nephropathy,* obstructive uropathy,* renal allograft transplant, chloride shift)

### Potassium Redistribution

Familial hyperkalemic periodic paralysis (e.g., Gamstorp's disease, adynamia episodica hereditaria)

Acute acidosis (e.g., diabetic ketoacidosis, lactic acidosis, acute renal failure, acute respiratory acidosis) (especially hyperchloremic metabolic acidosis; less with respiratory; little with metabolic acidosis due to organic acids)
- Decreased insulin
- Beta-adrenergic blockade
- Drugs (e.g., succinylcholine)
- Use of hypertonic solutions (e.g., saline, mannitol)
- Intravascular hemolysis
- Rapid cellular release (e.g., crush injury, chemotherapy for leukemia or lymphoma, burns, major surgery)

### Increased Supply of Potassium

Laboratory artifacts (e.g., hemolysis during venipuncture, thrombocytosis [>1,000,000/cu mm] or leukocytosis [>100,000/cu mm], incomplete separation of serum and clot)

Prolonged tourniquet use and hand exercise when drawing blood

Excess dietary intake or rapid potassium infusion

### Urinary Diversion

Ureteral implants into jejunum

### In Neonates

Dehydration, hemolysis (e.g., cephalohematoma, intracranial hemorrhage, bruising, exchange transfusion), acute renal failure, congenital adrenal hyperplasia, adrenocortical insufficiency

## Decreased in

*(Each 1 mEq/L decrease of serum potassium reflects a total deficit of <200–400 mEq; serum potassium <2 mEq/L may reflect total deficit >1000 mEq.)*

### Excess Renal Excretion

Osmotic diuresis of hyperglycemia (e.g., uncontrolled diabetes)
Nephropathies
- Renal tubular acidosis (proximal or distal)
- Bartter's syndrome
- Liddle's syndrome
- Magnesium depletion

Endocrine
- Hyperaldosteronism
- Cushing's syndrome
- Congenital adrenal hyperplasia

Drugs
- Loop or thiazide diuretics
- Mineralocorticoids (e.g., aldosterone, corticosterone, Cushing's syndrome especially due to ectopic adrenocorticotropic hormone production; renal vascular disease, malignant hypertension, renin-producing tumors) by excess administration or production by tumor
- Antibiotics (e.g., carbenicillin, ticarcillin, amphotericin B, gentamicin)
- Glycyrrhizic acid (licorice)

### Nonrenal Causes of Excess Potassium Loss

GI
- Vomiting
- Diarrhea
- Neoplasms (e.g., villous adenoma of colon; pancreatic islet cell tumor that produces vasoactive intestinal polypeptide >200 pg/mL)
- Excessive spitting
- Excessive sweating
- Cystic fibrosis
- Extensive burns
- Draining wounds

Cellular shifts
- Respiratory alkalosis
- Insulin
- Adrenergic activity (e.g., epinephrine)
- Barium chloride poisoning
- Treatment of megaloblastic anemia with vitamin $B_{12}$ or folic acid
- Classic periodic paralysis
- Physiologic—e.g., highly trained athletes

Diet
- Severe eating disorders (e.g., anorexia nervosa, bulimia)
- Dietary deficiency

### In Neonates

Asphyxia, alkalosis, renal tubular acidosis, iatrogenic (glucose and insulin), diuretics

# Protein—Total

## Use

Screening for nutritional deficiencies and gammopathies

## Increased in

Hypergammaglobulinemias (mono- or polyclonal; see following sections)
Hypovolemic states

### Decreased in

Nutritional deficiency
Decreased or ineffective protein synthesis
- Severe liver disease
- Agammaglobulinemia

Increased loss
- Renal
- GI disease (e.g., protein-losing enteropathies, surgical resection)
- Severe skin disease (e.g., burns, pemphigus vulgaris)
- Blood loss, plasmapheresis

Increased catabolism
- Fever
- Inflammation
- Hyperthyroidism
- Malignancy
- Chronic diseases

Dilutional
- IV fluids
- SIADH

## Protein—Albumin
**(generally parallels total protein except when total protein changes are due to gamma globulins)**

### Use

Marker of disorders of protein metabolism (e.g., nutritional, decreased synthesis, increased loss)

### Increased in

Dehydration (relative increase)
IV albumin infusions

### Decreased in

Inadequate intake
Decreased absorption
Increased need
Impaired synthesis (e.g., liver diseases, chronic infection)
Increased breakdown (e.g., neoplasms, infection, trauma)
Increased loss (e.g., edema, ascites, burns, hemorrhage, nephrotic syndrome, protein-losing enteropathy)
Dilutional (e.g., IV fluids, SIADH, psychogenic diabetes/water intoxication)
Congenital deficiency

## Protein—Separation (Immunofixation, Electrophoresis)

### Use

Diagnosis of specific diseases
- Multiple myeloma
- Waldenström's macroglobulinemia
- Hypogammaglobulinemia
- Agammaglobulinemia
- Agamma-A-globulinemia
- Analbuminemia
- Bisalbuminemia
- Afibrinogenemia
- Atransferrinemia
- Alpha$_1$-antitrypsin variant

- Cirrhosis
- Acute phase reactant

### Other Changes

Nonspecific changes in serum proteins
Protein pattern changes in urine, cerebrospinal fluid, peritoneal fluid, etc.

## Protein—Gammopathies

### Monoclonal Increase in

Various monoclonal gammopathies with or without BJ protein (see Chapter 11)

### Polyclonal Gammopathy with Hyperproteinemia

Collagen diseases (e.g., SLE, RA, scleroderma)
Liver disease (e.g., chronic hepatitis, cirrhosis)
Chronic infection (e.g., bronchiectasis, lung abscess, TB, osteomyelitis, subacute
  bacterial endocarditis)
Miscellaneous (e.g., sarcoidosis, malignant lymphoma, acute leukemia, diabetes
  mellitus)

## Protein—Immunoglobulin G (IgG)

### Increased in

Sarcoidosis
Chronic liver disease (e.g., cirrhosis)
Autoimmune diseases
Parasitic diseases
Chronic infection

### Decreased in

Protein-losing syndromes
Pregnancy
Non-IgG myeloma
Waldenström's macroglobulinemia

## Protein—Immunoglobulin M (IgM)

### Increased in

Liver disease
Chronic infections

### Decreased in

Protein-losing syndromes
Non-IgM myeloma
Infancy, early childhood

## Protein—Immunoglobulin A (IgA)

### Increased in
*(in relation to other immunoglobulins)*

Gamma-A myeloma (M component)
Cirrhosis of liver
Chronic infections
RA with high titers of RF
SLE

Sarcoidosis
Wiskott-Aldrich syndrome

### Decreased in
### (alone)

Hereditary telangiectasia
Type III dysgammaglobulinemia
Malabsorption
Non-IgA myeloma
Waldenström's macroglobulinemia
Acquired immunodeficiency

### Decreased in
### (combined with other immunoglobulin decreases)

Agammaglobulinemia
Hereditary thymic aplasia
Dysgammaglobulinemias
Infancy, early childhood

## Protein—Immunoglobulin E (IgE)

### Increased in

Atopic diseases
  • Exogenous asthma
  • Hay fever
  • Atopic eczema
Parasitic diseases
E-myeloma

### Decreased in

Hereditary deficiencies
Acquired immunodeficiency
Ataxia-telangiectasia
Non-IgE myeloma

## Apolipoproteins

### Apolipoprotein A-I

### Use
Decreased level is associated with increased risk of coronary heart disease
  (CHD)
### Increased in
Familial hyperalphalipoproteinemia
Pregnancy
Estrogen therapy
Alcohol consumption
Exercise
### Decreased in
Tangier disease
Fish-eye disease
Familial hypoalphalipoproteinemia
Familial lecithin-cholesterol acyltransferase deficiency
Type I and V hyperlipoproteinemia
Diabetes mellitus
Cholestasis
Hemodialysis
Infection

Drugs (e.g., diuretics, beta-blockers, androgenic steroids, glucocorticoids)

### Apolipoprotein A-II

**Increased in**
Alcohol consumption
**Decreased in**
Tangier disease
Cholestasis
Cigarette smoking

### Apolipoprotein A-IV

**Increased in**
Postprandial lipemia
**Decreased in**
Abetalipoproteinemia
Chronic pancreatitis
Malabsorption
Obstructive jaundice
Acute hepatitis

### Apolipoprotein (a)

**Use**
Increased risk of CHD with serum levels >0.03 gm/L
**Increased in**
Pregnancy
Patients who have had AMI
**Decreased in**
Drugs (e.g., nicotinic acid, neomycin, anabolic steroids)

### Apolipoprotein B-48

Normally absent during fasting
**Increased in**
Hyperlipoproteinemia (types I, V)
Apo E deficiency
**Decreased in**
Liver disease
Hypo- and abetalipoproteinemia
Malabsorption

### Apolipoprotein B-100

**Use**
Increased levels are associated with increased risk of CHD
**Increased in**
Hyperlipoproteinemia (types IIa, IIb, IV, V)
Familial hyperapobetalipoproteinemia
Nephrotic syndrome
Pregnancy
Biliary obstruction
Hemodialysis
Cigarette smoking
Drugs (e.g., diuretics, beta-blockers, cyclosporine, glucocorticoids)
**Decreased in**
Hypo- and abetalipoproteinemia
Type I hyperlipoproteinemia (hyperchylomicronemia)
Liver disease
Exercise
Infections
Drugs (e.g., cholesterol-lowering drugs, estrogens)

### Apolipoprotein C-1

**Increased in**
Hyperlipoproteinemia (types I, III, IV, V)
**Decreased in**
Tangier disease

### Apolipoprotein C-II

**Increased in**
Hyperlipoproteinemia (types I, III, IV, V)
**Decreased in**
Tangier disease
Hypoalphalipoproteinemia
Apo C-II deficiency
Nephrotic syndrome

### Apolipoprotein C-III

**Use**
With combined hereditary apo A-I and apo C-III deficiency increased risk of premature CHD
**Increased in**
Hyperlipoproteinemia (types III, IV, V)
**Decreased in**
Tangier disease
Combined with hereditary deficiency apo A-1

### Apolipoprotein E

**Increased In**
Hyperlipoproteinemia (types I, III, IV, V)
Pregnancy
Cholestasis
Multiple sclerosis in remission
Drugs (e.g., dexamethasone)
**Decreased in**
Drugs (e.g., adrenocorticotropic hormone)

## Sodium

See Chapter 13.

### Use

Diagnosis and treatment of dehydration and overhydration. *Changes in serum sodium most often reflect changes in water balance rather than sodium balance.* Determinations of blood sodium and potassium levels are performed to monitor changes in sodium and potassium during therapy.

### Interference

Hyperglycemia—serum sodium decreases 1.7 mEq/L for every increase of serum glucose of 100 mg/dL.
Hyperlipidemia and hyperproteinemia cause spurious results with flame photometric but not with specific ion electrode techniques for measuring sodium.

## Uric Acid

Values are very labile and show day-to-day and seasonal variation in the same person; also increased by stress, total fasting, and increased body weight.

## Use

Monitor treatment of gout
Monitor chemotherapeutic treatment of neoplasms to avoid renal deposition

## Increased in

Renal failure (does not correlate with severity of kidney damage)
Gout
25% of relatives of patients with gout
Asymptomatic hyperuricemia
Increased destruction of nucleoproteins
- Leukemia, multiple myeloma
- Polycythemia
- Lymphoma, especially postirradiation
- Other disseminated neoplasms
- Cancer chemotherapy
- Hemolytic anemia
- Sickle cell anemia
- Resolving pneumonia
- Toxemia of pregnancy
- Psoriasis

Some drugs, intoxications (e.g., barbiturates, methyl alcohol, ammonia, carbon monoxide; some patients with alcoholism)
Metabolic acidosis
Diet
- High-protein weight reduction diet
- Excess nucleoprotein (e.g., sweetbreads, liver)
- Alcohol consumption

Miscellaneous
- von Gierke's disease
- Lead poisoning
- Lesch-Nyhan syndrome
- Maple syrup urine disease
- Down syndrome
- Polycystic kidneys
- Calcinosis universalis and circumscripta
- Hypoparathyroidism
- Primary hyperparathyroidism
- Hypothyroidism
- Sarcoidosis

## Decreased in

Drugs
- ACTH
- Uricosuric drugs (e.g., high doses of salicylates, probenecid, cortisone, allopurinol, coumarin)
- Various other drugs (x-ray contrast agents, glyceryl guaiacolate, estrogens, phenothiazine)

Wilson's disease
Fanconi's syndrome
Acromegaly
Pernicious anemia in relapse
Xanthinuria
Neoplasms
Healthy adults with isolated defect in tubular transport of uric acid
Decreased in ~5% of hospitalized patients; most common causes are postoperative state, diabetes mellitus, various drugs, SIADH with hyponatremia

*Unchanged in*

Colchicine administration

## Vitamin D

*Use*

Diagnosis of rickets and vitamin D toxicity
Differential diagnosis of hypercalcemias

*Increased*

- 1,25-dihydroxyvitamin D
  Hyperparathyroidism
  Sarcoidosis
  Idiopathic calcium nephrolithiasis
- 25-hydroxyvitamin D
  Vitamin D toxicity

*Decreased*

- 1,25-dihydroxyvitamin D
  Hypoparathyroidism
  Chronic renal failure
- 25-hydroxyvitamin D
  Vitamin D deficiency
  Inadequate exposure to ultraviolet light
  Malabsorption syndromes
  Hepatocellular disease
  Nephrotic syndrome
  Drugs (e.g., high-dosage glucocorticoid or anticonvulsant therapy)

## Other Tests

### Acute Inflammatory Reactants

C-reactive protein, alpha$_1$-antitrypsin, haptoglobin, ferritin, ceruloplasmin, alpha$_1$-acid glycoprotein, serum complement, total WBC, neutrophils and bands, ESR
It is important to recognize this cause of increase when they are used in testing for other conditions (e.g., ceruloplasmin).

### Antistreptococcal Antibody Titers (ASOT)

**Use**
A high or 4 *times* increase in titer is indicative of current or recent streptococcal infection (scarlet fever, erysipelas, pharyngitis, tonsillitis; rheumatic fever, glomerulonephritis).

### Cold Autohemagglutination

**Use**
Diagnosis of *Mycoplasma* pneumonia. Titer $\geq$ 1:14–1:224. See Table 3-1.

### Complement

**Decreased in (Acquired)**
Certain diseases associated with arthritis, vasculitis, nephritis
**Use of Individual Complement Levels**
CH50 measures functional activity of C1–C9. Normal result indicates classic complement pathway is functionally intact. Detects all inborn and most acquired complement deficiencies.

**Table 3-1.** Immunologic Tests

| Antibody Test | Interpretation |
| --- | --- |
| Anti–acetylcholine receptor | Result <1 unit makes the diagnosis of myasthenia gravis. May be negative in ocular myasthenia, Eaton-Lambert syndrome, and treated or inactive generalized myasthenia gravis. |
| Anti-adrenal | High titers are characteristic of autoimmune hypoadrenalism (70%); rarely found in Addison's disease due to tuberculosis. |
| Anti–glomerular basement membrane | See Rapidly Progressive Nonstreptococcal Glomerulonephritis in Chapter 14. |
| Anti–intrinsic factor | Antibodies indicate overt or latent pernicious anemia; present in ~75% of cases. |
| Anti-mitochondrial | Strongly positive in >90% of patients with primary biliary cirrhosis but almost never in extrahepatic biliary obstruction; therefore, are useful in differentiating these two conditions. May also be found in 5% of chronic hepatitis. See Chapter 8. |
| Anti-reticulin | Presence supports the diagnosis of gluten-sensitive enteropathy. Especially useful in childhood, in which positive in 80% of cases. |
| Anti-skin, dermal-epidermal | Positive in >80% of bullous pemphigus cases. Absence does not exclude that diagnosis. Some correlation of titer and severity. Low sensitivity; high specificity. |
| Anti-skin, inter-epithelial | Positive test confirms diagnosis of pemphigus and is helpful in evaluating bullous diseases. Positive in >90% of pemphigus cases; absence largely excludes that diagnosis. Rise and fall of titer may indicate impending relapse or effective control of disease. High sensitivity; lower specificity. |
| Anti–smooth muscle (antiactin) | Titer ≥ 1:160 in >95% of patients with autoimmune chronic active hepatitis. Less often in other liver and viral diseases. |
| Anti-striational | Found in >80% of cases of myasthenia gravis with thymoma; ≤ 25% of thymoma without myasthenia gravis; 30% of patients with myasthenia gravis alone. In 25% of drug reactions due to penicillamine. |
| Anti-thyroglobulin and antithyroid microsome antibodies | Absence of both antibodies is strong evidence against autoimmune thyroiditis. |
| Neutrophil antibodies | |
| Cytoplasmic (c-ANCA) | Wegener's granulomatosis |
| Perinuclear (p-ANCA) | Vasculitis, Churg-Strauss syndrome, microscopic polyarteritis nodosa, ulcerative colitis |
| Parietal cell antibodies | See Chapter 11. |
| RF | See Rheumatoid Arthritis in Chapter 10. |
| TSI | Elevated TSI occurs only in Graves' disease. Failure of TSI to fall after antithyroid therapy predicts relapse. Elevated TSI in a patient who is HLA-DR3 positive predicts poor response to antithyroid therapy and suggests need for alternate mode of treatment. |

C3 is useful for screening for classic and activation of alternate complement pathway. May be increased in subacute inflammation, biliary obstruction, nephrotic syndrome, corticosteroid therapy. May be decreased in immune complex disease (especially lupus nephritis), acute poststreptococcal glomerulonephritis, hypercatabolism (especially C3b inactivator deficiency), massive necrosis and tissue injury, sepsis, viremia, hereditary deficiency, infancy.

C4 may be decreased in immune complex disease (especially lupus nephritis), hereditary angioneurotic edema, hereditary deficiency, acute glomerulonephritis, infancy, or when classic pathway is activated.

Decreased C3 and C4 indicate initiation of classic activation pathway and activation of functional unit (e.g., active viral hepatitis, immune complex formation).

Normal C3 with decreased C4 suggests C4 deficiency (e.g., hereditary angioedema, malaria, some SLE patients).

Normal C4 and decreased C3 suggests congenital C3 deficiency or deficiency of C3b inactivator, or activation of functional unit by alternate pathway (e.g., gram-negative toxemia).

Normal C3 and C4 with decreased CH50 indicates isolated deficiency of another complement component and further testing is indicated.

C2 may be decreased in immune complex disease (especially lupus nephritis), hereditary angioedema, hereditary deficiency, infancy.

C1 esterase inhibitor deficiency is characteristic of hereditary angioedema.

C1q can be very low in acquired angioedema, severe combined immunodeficiency, and X-linked hypogammaglobulinemia. May be decreased in SLE, infancy.

Absence of, or marked decrease, in any of the components of complement will cause absence of or marked decrease in the total hemolytic complement assay, but mild to moderate decrease of an individual component of complement may not alter this total.

### Erythrocyte Sedimentation Rate (ESR)

See Table 3-2.

### Use

*Indicates presence and intensity of an inflammatory process; never diagnostic of a specific disease. Changes are more significant than a single value.*

Screening for occult disease, but a normal ESR does not exclude serious disease.

Monitor the course or response to treatment.

Confirm or exclude certain diagnoses (a normal ESR virtually excludes diagnosis of temporal arteritis or polymyalgia rheumatica).

### Pregnancy Test
*(immunoassay detection of human chorionic gonadotropin [hCG] in blood)*

See also Urinary Chorionic Gonadotropins in Chapter 13 and Serum Human Chorionic Gonadotropin in Chapter 16.

### Use—Positive in

Pregnancy. Test becomes positive as early as 4 days after expected date of menstruation; it is reliable by day 10–14. An increase in hCG <66% in 48 hrs indicates ectopic pregnancy or abnormal intrauterine pregnancy.

Hydatidiform mole, choriocarcinoma. Quantitative titers should be used.

**Table 3-2.** Changes in ESR*

| Disease | Increased In | Not Increased In |
|---|---|---|
| Infectious | TB (especially)<br>Acute hepatitis<br>Many bacterial infections | Typhoid fever<br>Undulant fever<br>Malarial paroxysm<br>Infectious mononucleosis<br>Uncomplicated viral diseases |
| Cardiac | AMI<br>Active rheumatic fever<br><br>After open heart surgery | Angina pectoris<br>Active renal failure with<br>   heart failure |
| Abdominal | Acute pelvic inflammatory disease<br><br>Ruptured ectopic pregnancy<br>Pregnancy—third month to<br>   about 3 wks postpartum<br>Menstruation | Acute appendicitis (first<br>   24 hrs)<br>Unruptured ectopic pregnancy<br>Early pregnancy |
| Joint | RA<br>Pyogenic arthritis | Degenerative arthritis |
| Miscellaneous | Significant tissue necrosis,<br>   especially neoplasms (most<br>   frequently malignant lymphoma<br>   cancer of colon and breast)<br>Increased serum globulins (e.g.,<br>   myeloma, cryoglobulinemia,<br>   macroglobulinemia)<br>Decreased serum albumin<br>Hypothyroidism<br>Hyperthyroidism<br>Acute hemorrhage<br>Nephrosis, renal disease with<br>   azotemia<br>Arsenic and lead intoxication<br>Dextran and polyvinyl compounds<br>   in blood<br>Temporal arteritis<br>Polymyalgia rheumatica | Peptic ulcer<br>Acute allergy |

*Extreme increase of ESR is found particularly in association with malignancy (most frequently malignant lymphoma, carcinomas of colon and breast), hematologic diseases (most frequently myeloma), collagen diseases (e.g., SLE, RA), renal diseases (especially azotemia), infections, drug fever, and other conditions (e.g., cirrhosis). Westergren method is more accurate. Wintrobe method is more convenient.

# 4

## Urine

## Normal Values

| | |
|---|---|
| Addis count (no longer performed) | |
| Amylase | Depends on methodology |
| Calcium | <150 mg/24 hrs on low-calcium (Bauer-Aub) diet |
| Chloride | 140–250 mEq/L |
| Coproporphyrin | 50–300 $\mu$g/24 hrs; 0–75 $\mu$g/24 hrs in children weighing <80 pounds |
| Creatine | <100 mg/24 hrs (<6% of creatinine); higher in children (<1 yr: may equal creatinine; older children: ≤ 30% of creatine) and during pregnancy (≤ 12% of creatinine) |
| Creatinine | |
|     Males | 19–26 mg/kg of body weight/24 hrs |
|     Females | 14–21 mg/kg of body weight/24 hrs |
| Cystine or cysteine | 0 |
| Delta-aminolevulinic acid | 1.5–7.5 mg/24 hrs |
| Glucose | Qualitative = 0 |
| | ≤ 0.3 gm/24 hrs |
| Hb and myoglobin | 0 |
| Homogentisic acid | 0 |
| Ketones | Qualitative = 0 |
| Lead | <0.08 $\mu$g/mL or 120 gm/24 hrs |
| Microscopic examination | ≤ 1–2 RBC, WBC, epithelial cells/HPF; occasional hyaline cast/LPF |
| Osmolality | 500–1200 mOsm/L |
| Oxalate | |
|     Males | ≤ 55 mg/24 hrs |
|     Females | ≤ 50 mg/24 hrs |
| pH | 4.6–8.0 depending on diet; >9 indicates old specimen |
| Phenylpyruvic acid | 0 |
| Phosphorus | 1 gm/24 hrs (average), depending on diet |
| Porphobilinogen | 0–2 mg/24 hrs |
| Protein | Qualitative = 0 |
| | 0–0.1 gm/24 hrs |
| Specific gravity | 1.003–1.030 |
| Total solids | 30–70 gm/L. To estimate, multiply last two figures of specific gravity by 2.66. |
| Uric acid | ≤ 750 mg/24 hrs |
| Urobilinogen | 0–4 mg/24 hrs |
| Uroporphyrin | 0 |

Volume
    Adults                                 600–2500 mL/24 hrs

Night volume usually <700 mL with specific gravity <1.018 or osmolality >825 mOsm/kg of body weight in children. Ratio of night to day volume in adults 1:2–1:4.

Infants
| | |
|---|---|
| Premature | 1–3 mL/kg/hr |
| Full-term | 15–60 mL/24 hrs |
| 2 weeks | 250–400 mL/24 hrs |
| 8 weeks | 250–400 mL/24 hrs |
| 1 year | 500–600 mL/24 hrs |

# Calcium

## Use

Diagnosis of idiopathic hypercalciuria causes of renal calculi

## Increased in

Hyperparathyroidism
Idiopathic hypercalciuria
High-calcium diet
Excess milk intake
Immobilization
Lytic bone lesions
  • Metastatic tumor
  • Multiple myeloma
  • Osteoporosis (primary or secondary to hyperthyroidism, acromegaly)
Excess vitamin D ingestion
Drug therapy
  • Mercurial diuretics
  • Ammonium chloride
Fanconi's syndrome
Renal tubular acidosis
Sarcoidosis
Glucocorticoid excess due to any cause
Rapidly progressive osteoporosis
Paget's disease

## Decreased in

Hypoparathyroidism
Rickets, osteomalacia
Familial hypocalciuric (benign) hypercalcemia
Steatorrhea
Renal failure
Metastatic carcinoma of prostate
**Hypercalciuria without Hypercalcemia**
Idiopathic hypercalciuria
Sarcoidosis
Glucocorticoid excess due to any cause
Hyperthyroidism
Rapidly progressive bone diseases, Paget's disease, malignant tumors
Renal tubular acidosis
Medullary sponge kidney
Furosemide administration

## Chyluria

### Use

Diagnosis of injury or obstruction of lymphochylous system of chest or abdomen

### Due to

Obstruction of the lymphochylous system, usually filariasis
Trauma to chest or abdomen
Abdominal tumors or lymph node enlargement
Milky urine is due to chylomicrons recognized as fat globules by microscopy.
    Protein is normal or low. Hematuria is common.
A test meal of milk and cream may cause chyluria in 1–4 hrs.

## Color

Red ("red" often includes colors from pink to red-brown)
- No specific test (chlorzoxazone, ethoxazene, oxamniquine, phenothiazines, rifampin)
- Acid urine only (phenolphthalein)

Red-orange
- No specific test (butazopyridine, chlorzoxazone, ethoxazene, mannose, oxamniquine, phenothiazines, rifampin)
- Alkaline urine only (phenindione)
- Acid urine only (phenolphthalein)

Red or pink
- No specific test (aminopyrine, aniline dyes, antipyrine, doxorubicin, fuscin, ibuprofen, phenacetin, phenothiazines, phensuximide, phenytoin)
- Acid urine only (beets, blackberries, anisindione)
- Alkaline urine only (anthraquinone laxatives, rhubarb, santonin, phenolsulfonphthalein, sulfobromophthalein sodium [Bromsulphalein]; eosin produces green fluorescence)
- Darkens on standing (porphyrins)
- Presence of urates and bile
- On contact with hypochlorite bleach (toilet bowl cleaner) (aminosalicylic acid)
- Centrifuged specimen shows RBC in base (blood)

Purple
- Alkaline urine only (phenolphthalein)
- Darkens on standing (porphyrins; fluoresces with ultraviolet light)
- No specific test (chlorzoxazone)

Red-brown (see Fig. 4-1)
- Acid urine only (methemoglobin, metronidazole, anisindione)
- Alkaline urine only (anthraquinone laxatives, levodopa, methyldopa, parahydroxyphenylpyruvic acid, phenazopyridine)
- Positive *o*-toluidine test for blood
    Centrifuged urine shows RBC in base if blood; centrifuged blood shows pink supernatant plasma if Hb but clear plasma if myoglobin
- Green in reflected light (antipyrine)
- Orange with addition of HCl (phenazopyridine)
- No specific test (chloroquine, deferoxamine, ethoxazene, ibuprofen, iron sorbitex, pamaquine, phenacetin, phenothiazines, phensuximide, phenytoin, trinitrophenol)

Brown-black
- Darkens on standing (homogentisic acid, melanin, melanogen, nitrobenzene, parahydroxyphenyl pyruvic acid [alkaline urine only], phenol, cresol, naphthol)
- Does not darken on standing
    Ferric chloride test

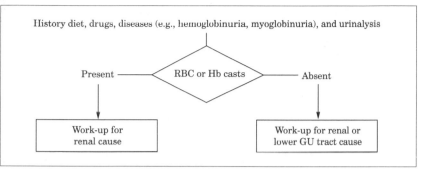

**Fig. 4-1.** Algorithm for red or brown urine.

Color fades (Argyrol)
Blue-green (homogentisic acid)
Black (melanin or melanogen)
    Nitroprusside test is red with melanin, black with melanogen
Yellow-brown
- Darkens on standing in acid urine (anthraquinone laxatives, rhubarb)
- Positive test for bile (bilirubin, urobilin)
- No specific test (niridazole, nitrofurantoin, pamaquine, primaquine, sulfamethoxazole)
Yellow
- Acid urine only (quinacrine, santonin)
- Alkaline urine only (beets)
- Positive test for bile (bilirubin, urobilin)
- No specific test (fluorescein dye, phenacetin, riboflavin, trinitrophenol)
Yellow-orange
- Alkaline urine only (anisindione, sulfasalazine)
- Positive test for bile (bilirubin, urobilin)
- Color increases with HCl (phenazopyridine)
- Ether soluble (carrots, vitamin A)
- High specific gravity (dehydration)
- No specific test (aminopyrine, warfarin)
Yellow-green or brown-green
- Darkens on standing (cresol, phenol [Chloraseptic], methocarbamol [Robaxin], resorcinol)
- Positive test for bile (biliverdin)
Blue-green
- Darkens on standing (methocarbamol, resorcinol).
- Blue fluorescence in acid urine (triamterene).
- Bacteriuria, pyuria (*Pseudomonas* infection [rare]).
- Decolorizes with alkali (indigo-carmine dye).
- Obermayer's test (indican).
- No specific test (chlorophyll breath mints [Clorets], Evans blue dye, guaiacol, magnesium salicylate [Doan's Pills], methylene blue, thymol [Listerine]).
- Biliverdin due to oxidation of bilirubin in poorly preserved specimens. Gives negative diazo tests for bilirubin (Ictotest), but oxidative tests (Harrison spot test) may still be positive.
Milky
- Lipuria, chyluria (ether soluble)
- Many PMN leukocytes (microscopic examination)

White cloud is due to excessive oxalic acid and glycolic acid in urine; occurs in oxalosis (primary hyperoxaluria).

Colorless
* Specific gravity
* High (diabetes mellitus with glycosuria; positive test for glucose)
* Low (diabetes insipidus, recent fluid intake)
* Variable (diuretics, ethyl alcohol, hypercalcemia)

Clear to deep yellow
* Normal (due to urochrome pigment)

Blue diaper syndrome results from indigo blue in urine due to familial metabolic defect in tryptophan absorption associated with idiopathic hypercalcemia and nephrocalcinosis.

Red diaper syndrome is due to a nonpathogenic chromobacterium (*Serratia marcescens*) that produces a red pigment when grown aerobically at 25–30°C.

Darkening of urine on standing, alkalinization, or oxygenation is nonspecific and may be due to
* Melanogen, Hb, indican, urobilinogen, porphyrins, phenols, salicylate metabolites (e.g., gentisic acid), homogentisic acid (due to alkaptonuria); administration of metronidazole (Flagyl). In acid pH, urine may not darken for hours (e.g., tyrosinosis).
* Sickle cell (SC) crises produce a characteristic dark-brown color independent of volume or specific gravity that becomes darker on standing or on exposure to sunlight due to increase in porphyrins.

## Creatine

### *Increased in*

### Physiologic states
* Growing children
* Pregnancy
* Puerperium (2 wks)
* Starvation
* Raw meat diet

### Increased formation
* Myopathy
  Amyotonia congenita
  Muscular dystrophy
  Poliomyelitis
  Myasthenia gravis
  Crush injury
  Acute paroxysmal myoglobinuria
* Endocrine diseases
  Hyperthyroidism
  Addison's disease
  Cushing's syndrome
  Acromegaly
  Diabetes mellitus
  Eunuchoidism
  Therapy with ACTH, cortisone, or desoxycorticosterone acetate

### Increased Breakdown
* Infections
* Burns
* Fractures
* Leukemia
* SLE

### *Decreased in*

Hypothyroidism

## Crystalluria

| Disorder | Substance |
|---|---|
| Massive hepatic necrosis (acute yellow atrophy), tyrosinemia, tyrosinosis | Tyrosine |
| Cystinuria, cystinosis | Cystine |
| Fanconi's syndrome | Leucine |
| Hyperoxaluria, oxalosis | Calcium oxalate |
| Lesch-Nyhan syndrome | Uric acid |
| Orotic aciduria | Orotic acid |
| Xanthinuria | Xanthine |

## Cytology

### Use

Screen persons exposed to urothelial or bladder carcinogens

Detect urothelial dysplasia and carcinomas

Monitor effects of radiation or chemotherapy

Detect nonbacterial infections

Characterize cells with inclusions

Flow cytometry and DNA analysis are used for diagnosis, prognosis, and to monitor therapy but not for screening.

## Electrolytes

### Use

Diagnosis of causes of hyponatremia and hypokalemia

Suspected disorders of adrenal cortex

Aid diagnosis of causes of acute renal failure

### Interferences

Value may be limited due to failure to obtain 24-hr excretion levels rather than random samples or administration of diuretics.

## Ferric Chloride Test
### (primarily used as screening test for phenylketonuria)

| Positive In | Phenistix Color |
|---|---|
| Phenylketonuria (unreliable for diagnosis) | Gray-green |
| Tyrosinuria (transient elevation in newborns) | Green |
| Maple syrup urine disease | Negative |
| Alkaptonuria | Negative |
| Histidinemia | Blue-gray to green |
| Tyrosinosis | Green (fades quickly) |
| Oasthouse urine disease | — |
| Bilirubin | — |
| Lactic acidosis | Gray |
| Melanin | — |
| Methionine malabsorption | — |
| Pyruvic acid | Yellow |
| Xanthurenic acid | Negative |
| Acetoacetic acid | Negative |
| Drugs | |
| Para-aminosalicylic acid | Purple |
| Phenothiazines | Purple |
| Salicylates | Purple |

*A positive test should always be followed by other tests (e.g., chromatography of blood and urine) to rule out genetic metabolic disorders.*

## Gonadotropins, Chorionic

See also Pregnancy Test and Serum Human Chorionic Gonadotropin in Chapter 3.

### Increased in

Normal pregnancy. Becomes positive as early as 4 days after expected date of menstruation; it is >95% reliable by day 10–14. hCG increases to peak within days 60–70, then drops progressively.
Hydatidiform mole, choriocarcinoma. Serum is preferred test.

### Interferences

False negative
  • Dilute urine
  • Missed abortion
  • Dead fetus syndrome
  • Ectopic pregnancy
False positive
  • Bacterial contamination
  • Protein or blood in urine
  • Methadone therapy

### Normal in

Nonpregnant state
Fetal death

## Gonadotropins, Pituitary

### Increased in

Menopause
Male climacteric
Primary hypogonadism
Early hyperpituitarism

### Decreased in

Secondary hypogonadism
Simmonds' disease
Late hyperpituitarism

## Hematuria

### Use

Screening and diagnosis of disorders of GU tract
Screening for excess anticoagulation medication

### Interpretation

<3% of normal persons have ≥ 3 RBCs/HPF or >1000 RBCs/cu mL (no easy conversion formula between these two methods). Abnormal is >3 RBCs/HPF.
Dipsticks (orthotolidine or peroxidase) detect heme peroxidase activity in RBCs, Hb, or myoglobin; may miss 10% of patients with microscopic hematuria.
Hematuria found in 18% of persons after very strenuous exercise.
In microscopic hematuria, number of RBCs is not related to the significance of the causative lesion. See Fig. 4-2.
Presence of blood clots virtually rules out glomerular origin of blood. Large thick clots suggest bladder origin; small stringy clots suggest upper tract origin.
Wright's stain or phase microscopy in urine sediment is said to show distortion with crenation and uneven Hb distribution of RBCs of glomerular origin; if

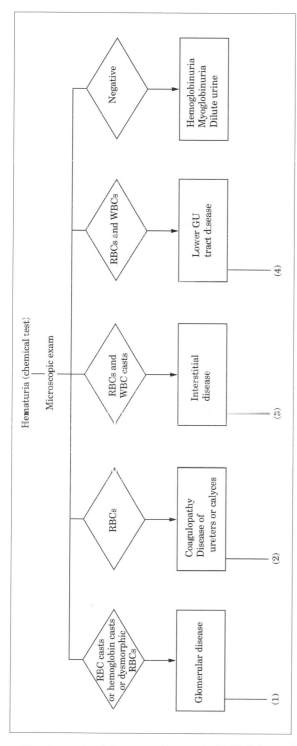

**Fig. 4-2.** Algorithm for diagnosis of microhematuria (1) Hypertension, diabetes mellitus, glomerulonephritis, immune-complex or postinfectious glomerular disease, drug reaction, endocarditis, embolic diseases. Tests: Antistreptolysin O titer, ANAs, $C_3$, HBsAg, renal biopsy. (2) Calculi, papillary necrosis, polycystic disease, sickle cell disease, GU tract trauma, neoplasm, or parasites. Tests: Cytology, CT scan, ultrasound, IV pyelogram. (3) Pyelonephritis, TB, sarcoidosis, drug reaction. Tests: Urine cultures, lymph node biopsy. (4) GU tract infection (e.g., prostatitis, urethritis, vaginitis), reflux, GU tract carcinoma. Tests: Urine cultures, cytology, cytoscopy, ultrasound.

>80% are similar to RBCs in peripheral blood, the source is likely to be distal to glomeruli.

RBC casts or Hb casts indicate blood is of glomerular origin, but their absence does not rule out glomerular disease. Gross hematuria that is initial suggests origin in urethra distal to urogenital diaphragm; terminal suggests origin in bladder neck or prostatic urethra; total suggests origin in bladder proper or upper urinary tract.

Proteinuria may occur with gross hematuria. In nonglomerular hematuria, sufficient proteinuria to produce 2+ dipstick requires equivalent of 25 mL of blood/L urine (if Hct is normal), which would cause gross hematuria; in glomerular hematuria, proteins filter through glomerulus out of proportion to RBCs. Therefore, microscopic hematuria with 2+ protein on dipstick favors glomerular origin; one exception is papillary necrosis, which may show 2+ proteinuria with nonglomerular type of RBCs.

Pyuria or WBC casts suggest inflammation or infection of GU tract.

Persistent or intermittent hematuria should always be evaluated; one episode of microscopic hematuria usually does not require full evaluation (may be due to viral infection, mild trauma, exercise).

### Interferences

### False Positive
- Vaginal bleeding
- Factitious
- Bacteriuria (due to catalase production by gram-negative bacteria)
- Red diaper syndrome
- Drugs (e.g., rifampin, phenolphthalein)
- Foods (e.g., beets, blackberries, rhubarb)
- Pigmenturia (porphyria, hemoglobinuria, myoglobinuria)
- Oxidizing contaminants (e.g., bacterial peroxidases, povidone, hypochlorite)

### False Negative
- Reducing agents (e.g., ascorbic acid)
- pH <5.1

### Nonglomerular Hematuria Due to

Trauma
Hemoglobinopathies (especially SC trait and Hb SC disease)
Hypercalciuria
Polycystic disease
GU tract tumors, infections

## Hemoglobinuria

Renal threshold is 100–140 mg/dL plasma.

### Use

Confirms hemolyzed blood in urine from GU tract or intravascular cause

### Due to

Hematuria with hemolysis in urine
Infarction of kidney
Intravascular hemolysis due to
- Parasites (e.g., malaria)
- Infection (e.g., clostridial, *Escherichia coli* bacteremia due to transfused blood)
- Antibodies (e.g., transfusion reactions, acquired hemolytic anemia, paroxysmal cold hemoglobinuria, paroxysmal nocturnal hemoglobinuria)
- Disseminated intravascular coagulation

- Inherited hemolytic disorders (e.g., SC disease, thalassemias, G6PD deficiency, pyruvate kinase deficiency, hereditary spherocytosis)
- Fava bean sensitivity
- Mechanical (e.g., prosthetic heart valve)
- Hypotonicity (e.g., transurethral prostatectomy with irrigation of bladder with water, hemodialysis accidents)
- Chemicals (e.g., naphthalene, sulfonamides)
- Thermal burns injuring RBCs
- Strenuous exercise and march hemoglobinuria

## Hemosiderin

Centrifuged specimen of random urine incubated for 10 minutes with Prussian blue stain shows blue granules.
Normal—absent

### Use

Present in intravascular hemolysis even when hemoglobinuria is absent (e.g., paroxysmal nocturnal hemoglobinuria)

## Ketonuria
**(ketone bodies [acetone, beta-hydroxybutyric acid, acetoacetic acid] appear in urine)**

### Use

Screening for ketoacidosis, especially in diabetes mellitus when blood is not immediately available.
Confirm fasting in testing for insulinoma.

### Occurs in

### Metabolic Conditions
- Diabetes mellitus
- Renal glycosuria
- Glycogen storage disease

### Dietary Conditions
- Starvation
- High fat diets

### Increased Metabolic Requirements
- Hyperthyroidism
- Fever
- Pregnancy and lactation

## Melanogenuria

### Use

In some patients with malignant melanoma, when the urine is exposed to air for several hours urine becomes deep brown and later black; occurs in 25% of patients.
Is also said to occur in some patients with Addison's disease or hemochromatosis and in intestinal obstruction in black persons

### Confirmatory Tests
- Ferric chloride test
- Thormählen's test
- Ehrlich's test

*None of these is consistently more reliable or sensitive than observation of urine for darkening.*

### Interferences

*Beware of false-positive red-brown or purple suspension due to salicylates.*

## Myoglobinuria

Renal threshold is 20 mg/dL plasma.

### Use

Indicates recent necrosis of skeletal or cardiac muscle

### Interpretation

Diagnosis based on
- Positive benzidine or *o*-toluidine test of urine that contains few or no RBCs when urine is red or brown. Tests may be positive even when urine is normal in color.
- Serum is clear (not pink) unless renal failure is present in contrast to hemoglobinemia.
- Serum haptoglobin is normal (in contrast to hemoglobinemia).
- Serum enzymes of muscle origin are increased.
- Identification of myoglobin in urine by various means (e.g., immunodiffusion).

Hereditary
- Phosphorylase deficiency (McArdle syndrome)
- Metabolic defects (e.g., associated with muscular dystrophy)

Sporadic
- Ischemic (e.g., arterial occlusion)
- Crush syndrome
- Exertional (e.g., exercise, some cases of march hemoglobinuria, electric shock, convulsions, and seizures)
- Metabolic myoglobinuria (e.g., alcoholism, carbon monoxide poisoning, diabetic acidosis, hypokalemia, systemic infection, barbiturate poisoning)
- In up to 50% of patients with progressive muscle disease (e.g., polymyositis, SLE) in active stage
- Various drugs and chemicals, especially illicit (e.g., cocaine, heroin, methadone, amphetamines, diazepam)

## Odors

### Use

Clue to various metabolic disorders

| Condition | Odor |
|---|---|
| Maple syrup urine disease | Maple syrup, burned sugar |
| Oasthouse disease, methionine malabsorption | Brewery, oasthouse |
| Methylmalonic, propionic, isovaleric and butyric/hexanoic acidemia | Sweaty feet |
| Tyrosinemia | Cabbagelike, fishy |
| Trimethylaminuria | Stale fish |
| Hypermethioninemia | Rancid butter, rotten cabbage |
| Phenylketonuria | Musty, mousy |
| Ketosis | Sweet |
| Cystinuria, homocystinuria | Sulfurous |

## Porphyrinuria
**(due mainly to coproporphyrin)**

### *Use*

Porphyrias
Lead poisoning
Cirrhosis
Infectious hepatitis
Passive in newborn of mother with porphyria; lasts for several days

## Proteinuria

See Fig. 4-3.

### *Use*

Detection of various renal disorders and BJ proteinuria

### *Interpretation*

Refers to protein excretion >150 mg/day in adults; >100 mg/day in children <10 yrs; or >140 mg/m$^2$/day. Significant proteinuria is >300 mg/day in adults. >1000 mg/day makes a diagnosis of renal parenchymal disease very likely. >2000 mg/day in adults or >40 mg/m$^2$ in children usually indicates glomerular etiology. >3500 mg/day or protein:creatinine ratio >3.5 points to a nephrotic syndrome.

A spot urine for urine protein:creatinine ratio often correlates well. Normal <0.2. Low-grade proteinuria = 0.2–1.0. Moderate proteinuria = 1.0–5.0. >5 is typical of nephrosis.

Dipstick is sensitive to ~30 mg/dL of protein; 1+ = 100 mg/dL; 2+ = 300 mg/dL; 4+ = 1000 mg/dL; may be falsely negative with predominantly low-molecular-weight or nonalbumin proteins, with very alkaline or dilute urine. May be falsely positive due to certain drugs. Positive dipstick should always be followed by sulfosalicylic acid test. When sulfosalicylic acid test shows a significantly higher concentration than the dipstick in an adult, BJ proteinuria should be ruled out. Association with hematuria indicates high likelihood of disease.

Urine electrophoresis
• Glomerular
  Selective: primarily albumin (>80%) and transferrin
  Nonselective: pattern resembles serum. Primary and secondary glomerulonephropathies
• Tubular: principally alpha$_1$, alpha$_2$, beta, and gamma globulins; albumin is not marked. Most often seen in chronic pyelonephritis, interstitial tubular nephritis, congenital tubular nephropathies, polycystic kidneys.
• Dysglobulinemias (multiple myeloma, macroglobulinemia, heavy chain diseases)

### *Due to*

Orthostatic (postural)
• First morning urine before arising shows high specific gravity but no protein (protein:creatinine ratio <0.1). Protein only appears after person is upright; usually <1.5 gm/day (protein:creatinine ratio usually 0.1–1.3).
• Urine microscopy is normal.
• Progressive renal insufficiency does not occur.
• Renal biopsy, electron microscopy, and immunofluorescent stains show pathologic changes in some patients.
Transient
• Commonly found in routine initial urinalysis of asymptomatic healthy children and young adults.

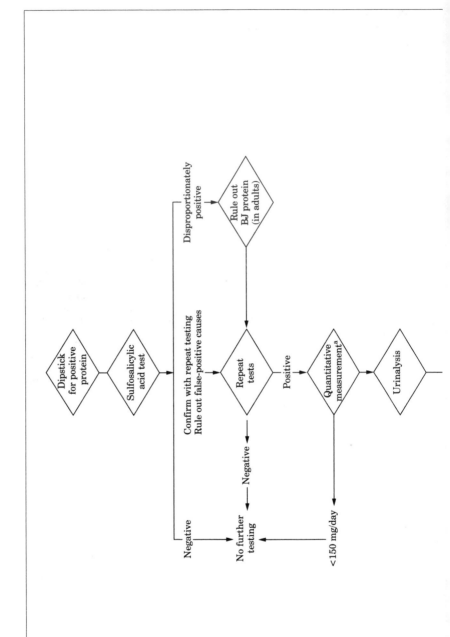

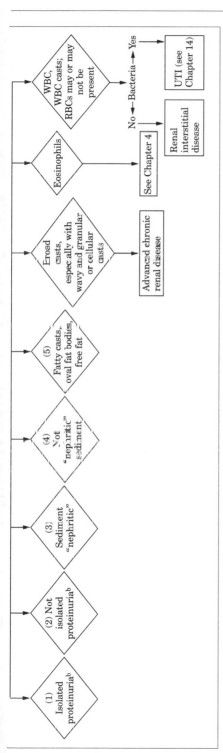

**Fig. 4-3.** Algorithm for diagnosis of proteinuria. Additional studies may include blood and throat cultures; blood chemistries, serum complement, antistreptolysin O titer, ANAs, cryoglobulins, BJ protein, renal biopsy; ultrasound for obstruction or cystic renal disease, nephrologist consultation. (1) Isolated proteinuria: Follow for orthostatic, nonorthostatic, functional proteinuria, or possible early renal disease. IV pyelogram, periodic renal function tests, and urinalysis. (2) Not isolated proteinuria <2 gm/day may occur in some glomerular diseases where there is marked hypoalbuminemia or marked impairment of glomerular filtration or overflow proteinuria (e.g., BJ proteinuria) or tubular proteinuria (e.g., hereditary, metabolic inflammatory conditions). Also acute tubular necrosis. (3) "Nephritic" sediment = RBCs or RBC casts; other casts and WBCs may or may not be present. May occur in various types of glomerulonephritis, SLE, subacute bacterial endocarditis, mixed cryoglobulinemia, hereditary nephritis, IgA nephropathy. (4) Proteinuria >2 gm/day without "nephritic" sediment may occur in preeclampsia, some infections (hepatitis B virus, syphilis, malaria), drugs, and disorders listed in (5). (5) Proteinuria ≥ 3.5 gm/day may occur in primary glomerular disease (minimal change disease, focal segmental glomerulosclerosis, membranous glomerulonephropathy, membranoproliferative glomerulonephritis) or multisystem disease (diabetic glomerulosclerosis, amyloidosis, SLE, cryoglobulinemia). [a]Check creatinine to assure 24-hr sample collection. [b]Isolated proteinuria = no findings of GU tract abnormalities, renal manifestations of systemic disease, hypertension, decreased renal function, or abnormal renal sediment.

- Progressive renal disease is not present.
- Functional occurs in 10% of hospital medical patients; associated with high fever, congestive heart failure, hypertension, stress, exposure to cold, strenuous exercise, seizures. Usually <2 gm/day; disappears with recovery from precipitating cause.

Persistent
- Glomerular (composed of large proteins [e.g., albumin, alpha$_1$-antitrypsin, transferrin])

 Idiopathic

 Secondary

 Infection (e.g., poststreptococcal, hepatitis B, bacterial endocarditis, pyelonephritis)

 Vascular (e.g., thrombosis of inferior vena cava or renal vein, renal artery stenosis)

 Drugs (e.g., nonsteroidal anti-inflammatory drugs, heroin, gold, captopril, penicillamine)

 Autoimmune (e.g., SLE, RA, polyarteritis, Goodpasture's syndrome, Henoch-Schönlein purpura)

 Neoplasia

 Hereditary and metabolic (e.g., polycystic kidney disease, diabetes mellitus)
- Decreased tubular reabsorption (composed of low-molecular-weight proteins [e.g., alpha and beta microglobulins, free Ig light chains, retinol-binding protein, lysozyme; usually <1.5 gm/day])

 Acquired

 Drugs (e.g., phenacetin, aminoglycoside, cephalosporins, cyclosporine, high-dose analgesics, lithium, methicillin)

 Heavy metal (e.g., lead, mercury, cadmium)

 Sarcoidosis

 Acute tubular necrosis

 Interstitial nephritis

 Renal tubular acidosis

 Acute and chronic pyelonephritis

 Renal graft rejection

 Balkan nephropathy

 Congenital (e.g., Fanconi's syndrome)

 Hereditary (e.g., Wilson's disease, SC disease, medullary cystic disease, oxalosis, cystinosis)
- Increased plasma levels of normal or abnormal proteins (e.g., BJ proteins, myoglobin)

Some common causes of low-grade proteinuria (<1 gm/24 hrs)
- Idiopathic low-grade proteinuria—normal history and physical examination, renal function and urine sediment with no hematuria
- Nephrosclerosis
- Polycystic kidney disease
- Medullary cystic disease
- Chronic obstruction of urinary tract
- Chronic interstitial nephritis (e.g., analgesic abuse, uric acid, oxalate, hypercalcemia, hypokalemia, lead, cadmium)

*Interferences*

**False Positive**
See also Chapter 18.

|  | Dipstick | Sulfosalicylic Acid |
|---|---|---|
| Gross hematuria* | + | + |
| Highly concentrated urine | + | + |
| Highly alkaline urine (pH >8) (e.g., GU tract infection with urea-splitting bacteria | + | − |

| | | |
|---|---|---|
| Antiseptic contamination (e.g., benzal-konium, chlorhexidine) | + | − |
| Phenazopyridine | + | − |
| Radiopaque contrast media | − | + |
| Tolbutamide metabolites | − | + |
| High levels of cephalosporin or penicillin analogs | − | + |
| Sulfonamide metabolites | − | + |

*Protein excretion > 500 mg/m$^2$/day is significant. With microscopic hematuria, any amount more than an occasional trace of protein is abnormal.

**False Negative**

Very dilute urine

## Proteinuria Predominantly Globulin Rather Than Albumin

Multiple myeloma
Macroglobulinemia
Primary amyloidosis
Adult Fanconi's syndrome

## Bence Jones (BJ) Proteinuria

*Use*

Detection of various gammopathies
80% of tests are true positive due to
- Myeloma (70% of all positive tests)
- Cryoglobulinemia
- Waldenstrom's macroglobulinemia
- Primary amyloidosis
- Adult Fanconi's syndrome
- Hyperparathyroidism
- Benign monoclonal gammopathy

20% of tests will be false positive (i.e., urine electrophoresis does not show a spike, and immunoelectrophoresis does not show a monoclonal light chain) due to
- Connective tissue disease (e.g., RA, SLE, polymyositis)
- Chronic renal insufficiency
- Lymphoma and leukemia
- Metastatic carcinoma of lung, GI, or GU tracts
- High doses of penicillin and aminosalicylic acid
- Presence of x-ray contrast media

*Positive test for BJ proteinuria by heat test should always be confirmed by elec-trophoresis and immunoelectrophoresis of concentrated urine. Heat test is not reliable and should not be used for diagnosis.*
*"Dipstick" test for albumin does not detect BJ protein.*

## Postrenal Proteinuria

Primarily associated with epithelial tumors of bladder or renal pelvis
Degree of proteinuria related to size and invasiveness; generally < 1 gm/day (sim-ilar to pyelonephritis) and includes IgM

## Reducing Substances (Benedict Reactions)

*Use*

Screening for diabetes mellitus (not recommended as primary screening modal-ity due to poor sensitivity)

### Interferences

False-negative tests for glucose may occur in presence of ascorbic acid using glucose oxidase paper test (Labstix); found in >1% of routine urine analyses in hospital.

Dipsticks exposed to air (uncapped bottles) for a week or more may give false-positive results for glucose.

### Due to

Glycosuria
- Hyperglycemia
  Endocrine (e.g., diabetes mellitus, pituitary, adrenal, thyroid disease)
  Nonendocrine (e.g., liver, CNS diseases)
  Due to administration of hormones (e.g., ACTH, corticosteroids, thyroid, epinephrine) or drugs (e.g., morphine, anesthetic drugs, tranquilizers)
- Renal
  Tubular origin (serum glucose <180 mg/dL; oral and IV glucose tolerance tests are normal; ketosis is absent)
  Fanconi's syndrome
  Toxic renal tubular disease (e.g., lead, mercury, degraded tetracycline)
  Inflammatory renal disease (e.g., acute glomerulonephritis, nephrosis)
- Glomerular due to increased glomerular filtration rate without tubular damage
- Idiopathic

Melituria (5% of cases of melituria in the general population are due to renal glycosuria, pentosuria, essential fructosuria)
- Hereditary (e.g., galactose, fructose, pentose, lactose)
  Galactose (classic and variant forms of galactosemia). *Galactosuria (in galactosemia) shows a positive urine reaction with Clinitest (Miles, Inc., Elkhart, IN) but negative with Clinistix.*
  Fructose (fructosemia, essential fructosuria, hereditary fructose intolerance)
  Lactose (lactase deficiency, lactose intolerance)
  Phenolic compounds (phenylketonuria, tyrosinosis)
  Xylulose (pentosuria)
- Neonatal (e.g., physiologic lactosuria, sepsis, gastroenteritis, hepatitis)
- Lactosuria during lactation
- Xylose (excessive ingestion of fruit)

Non–sugar-reducing substances (e.g., ascorbic acid, glucuronic acid, homogentisic acid, salicylates)

## Specific Gravity

### Increased by

Temperature
Proteinuria
Glucosuria
Sucrosuria
Radiographic contrast medium (frequently 1.040–1.050)
Mannitol
Dextran
Diuretics
Antibiotics
Detergent

Urinometer readings should be corrected for temperature, protein, and glucose.

*Decreased volume of concentrated urine (specific gravity >1.030 and osmolality >500 mOsm/kg) is diagnostic of prerenal azotemia.*

Urine:plasma osmolality ratio is more accurate than urine osmolality or specific gravity to distinguish prerenal azotemia (with increased ratio) from acute tubular necrosis (with decreased ratio that is rarely >1.5).

## Uric Acid:Creatinine Ratio

Ratio >1.0 in most patients with acute renal failure due to hyperuricemia but lower in other causes of acute renal failure.

## Urobilinogen

### Use

Rarely useful instead of serum direct and indirect bilirubin.

## Volume

### Anuria
*(excretion <100 mL/24 hrs)*

**Due to**
Bilateral complete urinary tract obstruction
Acute cortical necrosis
Necrotizing glomerulonephritis
Certain causes of acute tubular necrosis

### Oliguria
*(excretion usually <500 mL/24 hrs or ~20 mL/hr; <15–20 mL/kg/24 hrs in children)*

**Due to**
Prerenal causes
Postrenal causes
Renal causes
 • Glomerular: urine protein >2+ (>1.5 gm/24 hrs), RBCs, RBC casts
 • Tubulointerstitial: urine protein ≤ 2+ (≤ 1.5 gm/24 hrs), WBCs, WBC casts

### Polyuria
*(normal or increased urine excretion in presence of increasing serum creatinine and BUN)*

**Due to**
Diabetic ketoacidosis
Partial obstruction of urinary tract with impaired urinary concentration
Some types of acute tubular necrosis (e.g., due to aminoglycosides)

# Diseases of
# Organ Systems

# Cardiovascular Diseases

## Bacterial Endocarditis

Blood culture is positive in 80–90% of patients. *Streptococcus viridans* causes 40–50% of cases, *Staphylococcus aureus* 15–20%, *Streptococcus pneumoniae* 5%, and enterococcus 5–10%. Other causes may be gram-negative bacteria (~10% of cases) and fungi.

In drug addicts, *S. aureus* causes 50–60% of cases and ~80% of tricuspid infections; gram-negative bacteria cause 10–15% of cases; polymicrobial and unusual organisms appear to be increasing. ≤ 75% may be HIV positive.

*Proper blood cultures require adequate volume of blood, at least five cultures taken during a period of several days with temperature 101°F or higher (preferably when highest), anaerobic as well as aerobic growth, variety of enriched media, prompt incubation, prolonged observation (growth is usual in 1–4 days but may require 2–3 wks).* Negative culture may be due to recent antibiotic therapy or endocarditis due to *Rickettsia burnetii*. Transient bacteremia after dental procedures, tonsillectomy, etc. does not represent bacterial endocarditis.

Positive blood cultures may be more difficult to obtain in prosthetic valve endocarditis (due to unusual and fastidious organisms), right-side endocarditis, uremia, and long-standing infection. Aside from these exceptions, diagnosis should be based on ≥ 2 cultures positive for the same organism. A single positive culture must be interpreted with extreme caution.

Serum bactericidal test measures ability of patient's serum to sterilize a standardized inoculum of the infecting organisms; may be useful to demonstrate inadequate antibiotic levels or to avoid unnecessary drug toxicity.

Progressive normochromic normocytic anemia is a characteristic feature.

WBC is normal in ~50% of patients or increased < 15,000/cu mm, with 65–86% neutrophils. Higher WBC indicates presence of a complication. Occasionally, there is leukopenia. Monocytosis may be pronounced.

Increased ESR may correlate with course and severity of disease.

Increased serum gamma globulin, cryoglobulins, RF, etc. may be found.

Hematuria (usually microscopic) occurs at some stage in many patients. Albuminuria is almost invariable.

*Endocarditis occurs in ≤ 4% of patients with prosthetic valves.*

## Coronary Heart Disease (CHD)

Increased risk factors
* Increased serum total and LDL cholesterol, decreased HDL cholesterol and various ratios.
* Apolipoprotein (Apo) A-1 and Apo B may be better discriminators of CHD than cholesterol levels and low ratio of Apo A-1/Apo B may be best predictor.
* Atherogenic index.

$$\text{(combination of ratio of LDL to HDL with ratio of Apo B to Apo A-1)} = \frac{\text{(total cholesterol minus HDL)} \times \text{Apo B}}{\text{(Apo A-1} \times \text{HDL)}}$$

- Increased serum homocysteine >15.9 $\mu$mol/L (normal = 5–15 $\mu$mol/L) triples risk of myocardial infarction (MI). Increase may be due to vitamin B deficiency or genetic deficiency of methylene-tetrahydrofolate reductase enzyme.
- Increased serum triglycerides is not considered an independent risk factor.
- Clinical evidence of CHD or atherosclerosis in patient <age 40, family history of premature CHD, hypertension, males, smokers, lipoprotein electrophoresis. See Table 12-3.

Perform lab tests to rule out diabetes mellitus, liver disease, nephrotic syndrome, dysproteinemias, hypothyroidism.

## Congestive Heart Failure

No diagnostic laboratory findings.

## Myocardial Infarction, Acute

See Figs. 5-1 through 5-4 and Table 5-1.

### Diagnostic Criteria

Two of these three findings:
- History of ischemic chest discomfort for $\geq$ 30 mins
- Characteristic evolution of ECG changes
- Typical rise and fall of cardiac enzymes

### Use

Especially when ECG changes are inconclusive
For differential diagnosis of chest pain
To follow the course of the patient
To estimate prognosis
For noninvasive assessment of coronary reperfusion after thrombolytic therapy
Blood should be drawn promptly after onset of symptoms. Repeat determinations should be performed at appropriate intervals (see Fig. 5-2) and if symptoms recur or new signs or symptoms develop.

### Specific Findings

Serum total CK is valuable because it
- Allows early diagnosis.
- Is a sensitive indicator.
- Is not increased by some diseases often associated with AMI.
- Returns to normal by day 3. Reinfarction is indicated by an elevated level after day 5 that had previously returned to normal.

Serial CK-MB has become the gold standard for diagnosis within 24 hrs of onset of symptoms. Diagnosis of MI should not be based on only a single enzyme value. Increased CK-MB usually is evident at 4–8 hrs and peaks at 15–24 hrs. Sampling every 6 hrs is more likely to identify a peak value. CK-MB should be reported in units as well as percentage, because if there is injury of both cardiac and skeletal muscle, CK-MB percentage may not appear increased.

In a "classic" protocol, the criteria for MI are an increasing (above reference range) and then decreasing total CK and CK-MB in serial specimens drawn on admission and at intervals; no blood need be collected after 48 hrs in patients with uneventful course.

New CK-MB immunoassays at 0, 3, and 6 hrs can measure small but significant early changes that may still be within the normal range.

Thrombolytic agents alter the enzyme patterns. >2 times increase in CK-MB occurs within 90 mins of reperfusion and peak CK-MB occurs in ~6–10 hrs.

Total CK and CK-MB are also increased after cardiac surgery, when diagnostic value of enzymes is diminished. Significant increases in CK, CK-MB, and myoglobin are also common after coronary angioplasty. Cardiac trauma and contusions, elec-

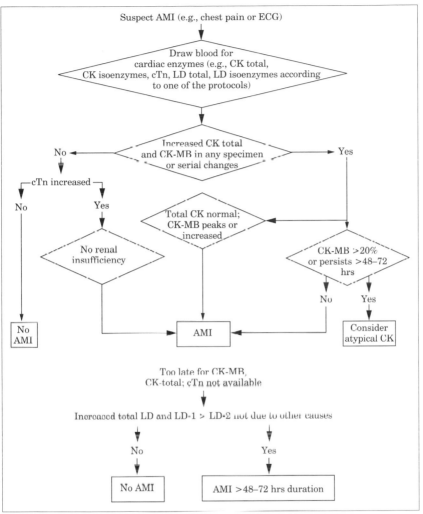

**Fig. 5-1.** Algorithm for laboratory diagnosis of AMI. Details of interpretation according to text. (cTn = cardiac troponin.)

trical injury, and inflammatory myocarditis may produce enzyme changes that cannot be distinguished from MI. No significant increase after pacemaker implantation. Other causes of CK and CK-MB changes are given in Chapter 3.

*Cardiac troponin T (cTnT)* is as sensitive as CK-MB during the first 48 hrs after MI and for up to 5–7 days but not sensitive from 0 to 4 hrs (similar to CK-MB). Is sensitive marker for minor myocardial injury in unstable angina. May be increased in chronic muscle disease, trauma, and chronic renal disease. Useful in diagnosis of perioperative MI when CK-MB may be increased by skeletal muscle injury.

*Cardiac troponin I (cTnI)* sensitivity and specificity is ≥ CK-MB in first 6–8 hrs; not increased by skeletal muscle injury, pulmonary or orthopedic surgery, or chronic renal disease; can remain increased 5–9 days after MI. Serial mea-

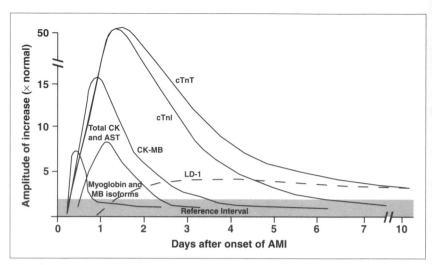

**Fig. 5-2.** Comparison of sequential changes in cTnT, cTnI, serum total CK-MB, CK isoforms, myoglobin, AST, and LD days after AMI. Cardiac serum markers showing relative concentrations versus time after onset of AMI.

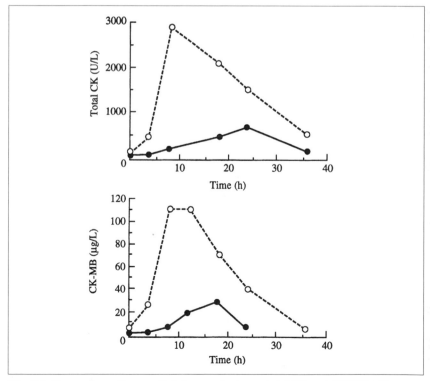

**Fig. 5-3.** Comparison of sequential changes in serum total CK and CK-MB with successful thrombolytic therapy (open circles) and without thrombolytic therapy (closed circles) hours after AMI.

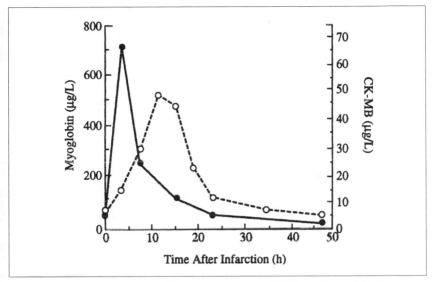

**Fig. 5-4.** Comparison of sequential changes in serum CK-MB and myoglobin hours after AMI.

surements are useful to assess reperfusion. Additional studies of cTnT and cTnI are under way.

*Serum myoglobin* becomes increased within 2–6 hrs in >85% of AMI patients, peaks in ~8–12 hrs, and becomes normal in ~24–36 hrs. Precedes release of CK-MB by 2–5 hrs. May also be increased in renal failure, shock, open heart surgery, skeletal muscle damage or exhaustive exercise, patients and carriers of progressive muscular dystrophy but not by cardioversion, cardiac catheterization, or congestive heart failure.

Combination of *serum CK-MB, cardiac troponin, and myoglobin* has superseded all other laboratory tests.

*Serum LD* is almost always increased, beginning in 10–12 hrs, reaching a peak in 48–72 hrs, and remaining increased for 10–14 days. Increased serum LD with an LD-1:LD-2 ratio >1 ("flipped" LD) usually appears in 12–24 hrs and peaks at 55–60 hrs in AMI. May also occur in acute renal infarction, hemolysis, some muscle disorders, pregnancy, and some neoplasms. LD-1:total LD >0.4 or LD-1 >90 U/L have also been used instead of flipped ratio.

*Serum CK-MM and CK-MB isoforms, and cardiac myosin light chains and glycogen phosphorylase BB* are not widely used.

Leukocytosis (12,000–15,000 with 75–90% neutrophils) is almost invariable; commonly detected by day 2 but as early as 2 hrs.

ESR is increased, usually by day 2 or 3; peaks in 4–5 days; persists for 2–6 months.

### Differential Diagnosis

Serum cardiac enzymes are not increased in angina pectoris; increased values mean myocardial necrosis or another condition.

Serum cardiac enzymes usually show little increase in inflammatory myocardial lesions (e.g., rheumatic fever [RF]) unless disease is severe.

Little or no change occurs in chronic heart failure.

## Myocarditis, Viral

Serologic tests for viral antigen, IgM antibody, or changed titer using acute and convalescent paired sera

**Table 5-1.** Summary of Increased Serum Marker Levels After AMI

| Serum Marker | Earliest Increase (hrs)[a] | Peak (hrs)[a] | Return to Normal (days)[a] | Amplitude of Increase (× Normal) | Specificity (%)[b] | Sensitivity (%)[b] |
|---|---|---|---|---|---|---|
| Total CK | 3–6 | 24–36 | 3 | 6–12 | 57–88% | 93–100% |
| CK-MB | 4–8 | 15–24 | 3–4 | 16 | 93–100% | 94–100% |
| CK-MB-2/MB-1 | 2 | 4–6 | ~2 | | 94% | 95% |
| CK-MM-3/MM-1 | 6 | 10 | ~2 | | | |
| Troponin T | 4–6 | 10–24 | 10–15 | | 80% | >98% |
| Troponin I | 4–6 | 10–24 | 10–15 | | 95% | >98% |
| Total LD | 10–12 | 48–72 | 11 | 3 | 88% | 87% |
| LD-1 | 8–12 | 72–144 | 8–14 | | 85% | 40–90% |
| LD-1/LD-2 | >6 | | >3 | | 94–99% | 61–90% |
| Myoglobin | 2–3 | 6–9 | Often >12 hrs | 10 | 70% | 75–95% |
| Myosin light chain | 3–8 | 24–35 | 10–15 | | | |
| ECG | | | | | 100% | 63–84% |
| AST[c] | 6–8 | 24–48 | 4–6 | 5 | 48–88% | 89–97% |
| ALT[c] | Usually normal unless liver damage is present (e.g., congestive heart failure) | | | | | |

Note: Range of reported values because different studies used different time periods after onset of symptoms, benchmarks for establishing the diagnosis, patient populations, etc.

[a]Time periods represent average reported values.
[b]Depends on time after onset of AMI.
[c]Not used for diagnosis of AMI.

Endomyocardial biopsy of right ventricular muscle has become a major diagnostic tool to establish diagnosis of myocarditis and rule out other lesions.
Increased serum cardiac enzymes is common only in early stages.
Increased ESR, CRP
Mild to moderate leukocytosis

## Pericarditis, Acute

### *Laboratory Findings Due to Primary Disease*

- Active RF (40% of patients).
- Bacterial infection (20% of patients).
- Other infections (e.g., viral, rickettsial, parasites, mycobacteria, fungi). Viruses are the most common infectious causes.
- Uremia (11% of patients).
- Benign nonspecific pericarditis (10% of patients).
- Neoplasms (3.5% of patients).
- Collagen disease (e.g., SLE, polyarteritis nodosa) (2% of patients).
- AMI, postcardiac injury syndrome
- Trauma.
- Myxedema.

WBC is usually increased in proportion to fever; normal or low in viral disease and tuberculous pericarditis; markedly increased in suppurative bacterial pericarditis.
Examination of aspirated pericardial fluid

## Phlebothrombosis of Leg Veins

Laboratory tests indicate recent extensive clotting of any origin (e.g., postoperative status); are often not helpful.
- Staphylococcal clumping test measures breakdown products of fibrin in serum; these indicate the presence of a clot that has begun to dissolve.
- Serial dilution protamine sulfate test measures the presence of a fibrin monomer that is one of the polymerization products of fibrinogen. It is less sensitive than the staphylococcal clumping test but indicates clotting earlier.

## Renovascular Hypertension

See Chapter 14.

## Rheumatic Fever, Acute

Increased titer of antistreptococcal antibodies, positive throat culture for group A streptococcus, and recent scarlet fever are supporting evidence for acute RF.
Acute phase reactants (ESR, CRP, increased WBC) are minor manifestations.
ESR increase is a sensitive test of rheumatic activity; returns to normal with adequate treatment with ACTH or salicylates.
CRP parallels ESR.
WBC is usually increased (10,000–16,000/cu mm) with shift to the left; may persist for weeks after fever subsides. May decrease with therapy.
Serologic titers: One of these is elevated in 95% of patients with acute RF. If all are normal, a diagnosis of RF is less likely.
- ASOT increase indicates recent group A streptococcus pharyngitis within the last 2 months. Increased titer develops only after week 2 and reaches a peak in 4–6 wks. Usually >250 units; more significant if >400–500 units. A normal titer helps to rule out clinically doubtful RF.
- Anti-DNase-B assay should also be performed because >15% of patients with acute RF will not have an increased ASOT.

- Antihyaluronidase titer of 1000–1500 follows recent streptococcus A disease; ≤ 4000 with RF.
- Antifibrinolysin (antistreptokinase) titer is increased in RF and in recent hemolytic streptococcus infections.

Decreased serum albumin and increased alpha$_2$ and gamma globulins. (*Streptococcus A infections do not increase alpha$_2$ globulin.*)

Fibrinogen is increased.

Anemia (hemoglobin 8–12 gm/dL) is common; gradually improves as activity subsides.

There is a slight febrile albuminuria. Protein, casts, RBCs, WBCs indicate mild focal nephritis.

Blood cultures are negative.

Throat culture is often negative for group A streptococci.

To determine clinical activity—follow ESR, CRP, and WBC. Return to normal is seen in 6–12 wks in 80–90% of patients; it may take ≤ 6 months. Normal findings do not prove inactivity if patient is receiving hormone therapy.

## Valvular Heart Disease

No diagnostic laboratory findings.

# Respiratory Diseases

# Laboratory Tests for Respiratory System Disease

## Bronchoscopy and Bronchoalveolar Lavage (BAL)

### Use

For biopsy of endobronchial tumor
To obtain bronchial washings for
- Cytologic diagnosis of tumors
- Diagnosis of pulmonary infection

Giemsa stain
- Normal persons show <3% neutrophils, 8–18% lymphocytes, 80–89% alveolar macrophages.
- >10% neutrophils: acute inflammation.
- >1% squamous epithelial cells: indicates that a positive culture may reflect saliva contamination.
- >80% macrophages: common in pulmonary hemorrhage. Occurs in aspergillosis infection and in >10% of patients with hematologic malignancies.
- >30% lymphocytes: may indicate hypersensitivity pneumonitis.
- >10% neutrophils and >3% eosinophils are characteristic of idiopathic pulmonary fibrosis; alveolar macrophages predominate.
- >$10^5$ colony-forming bacteria/mL indicates bacterial infection if <1% squamous epithelial cells are present on Giemsa stain.

Gram's stain
- Many bacteria suggests bacterial infection if there are <1% squamous epithelial cells, especially if culture shows >$10^4$ bacteria/mL.
- No bacteria suggests bacterial infection is unlikely but should rule out *Legionella* with DFA if Giemsa stain shows increased neutrophils.
- Combined with methenamine silver or Papanicolaou's (Pap) stain for diagnosis of *Pneumocystis* infection.

Acid-fast stain—for *Mycobacterium tuberculosis* or *Mycobacterium avium-intracellulare*
Toluidine blue stain may show *Pneumocystis carinii* cysts in pneumocystis pneumonia or *Aspergillus* hyphae.
Prussian blue–nuclear red stain strongly positive indicates severe alveolar hemorrhage; moderate positive indicates some hemorrhage; absent indicates no evidence of alveolar hemorrhage.
DFA stain for *Legionella*, herpes simplex I and II, and cytomegalovirus may indicate infection with corresponding organism.
Pap stain: for cytology
Oil red O stain in some patients with fat embolism due to bone fractures

## Pleura, Needle Biopsy of (Closed Chest)

Positive for tumor in ~6% of malignant mesothelioma and ~60% of other cases
of malignancy

Positive for tubercles in two-thirds of cases on first biopsy with increased yield
on second and third biopsies. Can also culture material.

## Pleural Effusion, Causes

See Table 6-1 and Fig. 6-1.

The underlying cause of an effusion is best determined by first classifying fluid
as an exudate or a transudate. A transudate may not require additional testing but *exudates always do.*

### Transudate

Congestive heart failure (causes 15% of cases)
Cirrhosis with ascites (pleural effusion in ~5% of cases)
Nephrotic syndrome
Early (acute) atelectasis
Pulmonary embolism (some cases)
Superior vena cava obstruction
Hypoalbuminemia
Peritoneal dialysis
Early mediastinal malignancy
Misplaced subclavian catheter
Myxedema (rare cause)

### Exudate

Pneumonia, malignancy, pulmonary embolism, and GI conditions (especially pan-
creatitis and abdominal surgery, which cause 90% of all exudates)
Infection (causes 25% of cases)
  • Parapneumonic effusion (empyema)
  • Tuberculous empyema
  • Viral, mycoplasmal, rickettsial
  • Parasitic (amoeba, hydatid cyst, filaria)
  • Fungal effusion
Pulmonary embolism/infarction
Neoplasms (cause ~40% of cases)
Meigs' syndrome (protein and specific gravity are often at transudate-exudate
  border but usually not transudate)
Trauma
  • Hemothorax, chylothorax, empyema, associated with rupture of diaphragm
Immunologic mechanisms
  • RA (5% of cases).
  • SLE.
  • Other collagen vascular diseases occasionally cause effusions (e.g., Wegener's
    granulomatosis, Sjögren's syndrome).
  • After myocardial infarction or cardiac surgery.
  • Vasculitis.
  • Hepatitis.
Drug reaction (e.g., nitrofurantoin hypersensitivity, methysergide)
Chemical mechanisms
  • Uremic
  • Pancreatic
  • Esophageal rupture
  • Subphrenic abscess
Lymphatic abnormality
  • Irradiation

**Table 6-1.** Pleural Fluid Findings in Various Clinical Conditions

| Disease | Appearance | Total WBC (1000/cu mm) | Predominant Type WBC | Total RBC (1000/cu mm) | pH | Glucose mg/dL | Glucose PF:S | Protein PF:S | LD PF:S | LD IU/L | Amylase PF:S | Comments |
|---|---|---|---|---|---|---|---|---|---|---|---|---|
| **Transudates** | | | | | | | | | | | | |
| Congestive heart failure | Clear, straw | <1 | M | 0–1 | >7.4 | >60 | 1 | <0.5 | <0.6 | <200 | ≤1 | If right side not involved, rule out pulmonary infarct. |
| Cirrhosis | Clear, straw | <0.5 | M | <1 | >7.4 | >60 | 1 | <0.5 | <0.6 | <200 | ≤1 | Occurs in 5% of cirrhotics with clinical ascites. |
| Pulmonary embolus; atelectasis | Clear, straw | 5–15 | M | <5 | >7.3 | >60 | 1 | <0.5 | <0.6 | | ≤1 | |
| **Exudates** | | | | | | | | | | | | |
| Pulmonary embolus: infarction | Turbid to hemorrhagic. Small volume | 5–15 | P  May show many mesothelial cells | Bloody in one-third to two-thirds of patients | >7.3 | >60 | 1 | >0.5 | >0.6 | | ≤1 | Occurs in 15% of patients; often no characteristic findings. |
| Pneumonia[a] | Turbid | 5–40 | P | <5 | ≥7.3 | >60 | 1 | >0.5 | >0.6 | | ≤1 | Occurs in 50% of bacterial pneumonias and Legionnaires' disease, 5–20% of viral and mycoplasma pneumonias. |
| Empyema[b] | Turbid to purulent | 25–100 | P | <5 | 5.50–7.29 | <60 | <0.5 | >0.5 | >0.6 | May be >1000/L | ≤1 | Most commonly due to anaero- |

**Table 6-1.** (continued)

| Disease | Appearance | Total WBC (1000/cu mm) | Predominant Type WBC | Total RBC (1000/cu mm) | pH | Glucose mg/dL | PF:S | Protein PF:S | LD PF:S | LD IU/L | Amylase PF:S | Comments |
|---|---|---|---|---|---|---|---|---|---|---|---|---|
| | | | | | | | | | | | | bic bacteria, *Staphylococcus aureus*, gram-negative aerobic bacteria. |
| TB | Straw; serosanguineous in 15% | 5–10 | M | <10 | <7.3 in 20% | 30–60 in 20% | 1 | >0.5 | >0.6 | | ≤1 | AFB stain positive in 15–20% and culture of fluid positive in 30% of cases. Biopsy for histologic examination and culture of pleura are diagnostic in 75–85% of cases. Often presents as effusion; pulmonary disease may be absent. |
| Malignancy[c] | Straw to turbid to bloody | <10 | M | 1 to >100 | <7.3 in 30% | <60 in 30% | 1 | >0.5 | >0.6 | | ≤1 | |
| RA effusion[d] | Turbid or green or yellow | 1–20 | P in acute M in chronic | <1 | <7.3; usually ~7.0 | <30 in 95% | | >0.5 | >0.6 | Often >1000/L | ≤1 | Biopsy is useful, especially in men with rheumatoid nodules and high RF titer. |

| | | | | | | | | | |
|---|---|---|---|---|---|---|---|---|---|
| SLE | Straw to turbid | | P in acute M in chronic | <7.3 in 30% | <60 in 30% | | >0.5 | >0.6 | >2 | PF may show LE cells, ANA titer, and low complement. Usually found only when lupus is active. |
| Rupture of esophagus | Purulent | 1–10 | P | 6.0 | N or D | 1 | >0.5 | >0.6 | >2 | Salivary type |
| Pancreatitis | Serous to turbid to serosanguineous | 5–20 | P | >7.3 | >60 | 1 | >0.5 | >0.6 | >2 | Occurs in 15% of acute cases. Left-sided in 70% of cases. |

Note: Blood specimens should always be drawn at the same time as serous fluid for determination of glucose, protein, LD, amylase, pH, etc. Pleural fluid for pH should be collected in the same way as arterial blood samples (i.e., heparinized syringe, maintained anaerobically on ice, analyzed promptly). Pleural fluid pH should normally be at least 0.15 greater than arterial blood pH. Normal pH is alkaline and may approach 7.6.

PF:S = ratio of pleural fluid to serum; M = mononuclear cells; P = polynuclear leukocytes; PF = pleural fluid.

[a]Parapneumonic effusions (exudate type of effusion associated with lung abscess, bronchiectasis; ~5% of bacterial pneumonias). Aerobic gram-negative organisms (Klebsiella, Escherichia coli, Pseudomonas) are associated with a high incidence of exudates (with 5000–40,000/cu mm, high protein, normal glucose, normal pH) and resolve with antibiotic therapy.

Nonpurulent fluid with positive Gram's stain, positive blood culture or low pH suggests that effusion will become or behave like empyema.

Streptococcus pneumoniae causes parapneumonic effusions in 50% of cases, especially with positive blood culture.

Staphylococcus aureus has effusion in 90% of infants, 50% of adults.

Streptococcus pyogenes in 90% of cases; massive effusion, greenish color

Haemophilus influenzae has effusion in 50–75% of cases.

[b]pH <7.0 and glucose <40 mg/dL indicate need for closed chest tube drainage even without grossly purulent fluid.

pH of 7.0–7.2 is a questionable indication and should be repeated in 24 hrs, but tube drainage is favored if pleural fluid LD >1000 IU/L. Tube drainage is also indicated if there is grossly purulent fluid or positive Gram's stain or culture.

In Proteus mirabilis empyema, high ammonia level may cause a pH ~8.

[c]Usually is large; frequently hemorrhagic (50% have RBC >10,000/cu mm).

Cytology plus biopsy is diagnostic in about 90% of cases. Cytology establishes the diagnosis in approximately 50% of patients. Lung and breast cancer and lymphoma cause 75% of malignant effusions; in 3%, no primary tumor is found. Pleural or ascitic effusion occurs in 20–30% of patients with malignant lymphoma. In some instances of suspected lymphoma with negative conventional test results, flow cytometry of pleural fluid showing a monoclonal lymphocyte population can establish the diagnosis.

Mucopolysaccharide level may be increased in mesothelioma.

[d]Decreased glucose is the most useful finding clinically; may be 0. RA cells may be present but may also be found in other effusions (e.g., TB, cancer, bacterial pneumonia). Needle biopsy usually may show characteristic rheumatoid nodule. Protein level is >3 gm/dL.

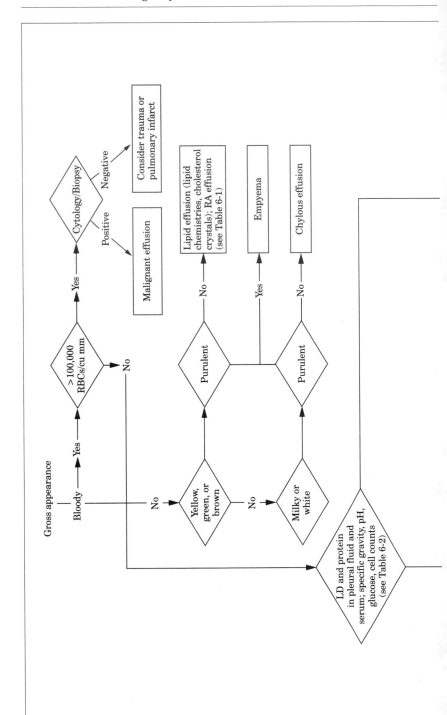

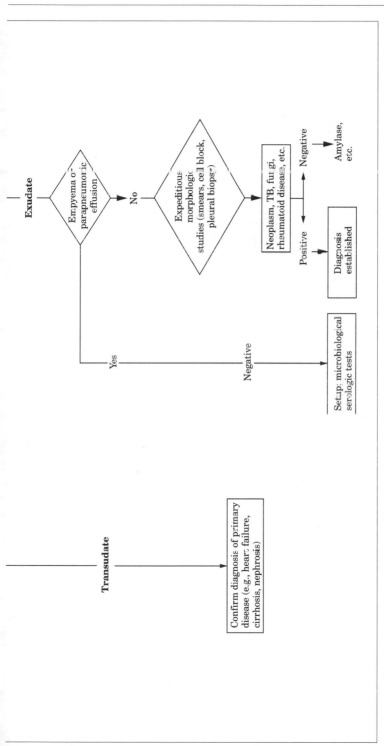

**Fig. 6-1.** Algorithm for pleural effusion.

Injury
  • Asbestosis
Altered pleural mechanics
  • Late (chronic) atelectasis
  • Trapped lung
Unknown (~15% of all exudates)
*Cirrhosis, pulmonary infarct, trauma, and connective tissue diseases compose ~9% of all cases.*
Pleural fluid analysis results in definitive diagnosis in ~20% of patients and a probable diagnosis in 50%; may help to rule out a suspected diagnosis in 30%.

### Gross Appearance

Clear, straw-colored fluid is typical of transudate.
Cloudy, opaque appearance indicates more cell components.
Bloody fluid suggests malignancy, pulmonary infarct, trauma, postcardiotomy syndrome. Bloody fluid from traumatic thoracentesis should clot within several minutes; blood present more than several hours has become defibrinated and does not form a good clot. Nonuniform color during aspiration and absence of hemosiderin-laden macrophages and some crenated RBCs also suggest traumatic aspiration.
Chylous (milky) appearance is usually due to trauma but may be obstruction of duct (e.g., lymphoma, metastatic carcinoma, granulomas). Pleural fluid triglyceride >110 mg/dL or triglyceride pleural fluid:serum >2 occurs only in chylous effusion. Triglyceride <30 mg/dL in nonchylous effusions.
"Pseudochylous" in chronic inflammatory conditions (e.g., RA) due to either cholesterol crystals or lipid-containing inclusions in leukocytes.
White fluid suggests chylothorax, cholesterol effusion, or empyema.
Black fluid suggests *Aspergillus niger* infection.
Greenish fluid suggests biliopleural fistula.
Purulent fluid indicates infection.
Anchovy (dark red-brown) color is seen in amebiasis.
Turbid and greenish yellow fluid is classic for rheumatoid effusion.
Turbidity may be due to lipids or increased WBCs; after centrifugation, a clear supernatant indicates WBCs as cause; white supernatant is due to chylomicrons.
Very viscous (clear or bloody)—characteristic of mesothelioma
Debris in fluid suggests rheumatoid pleurisy; food particles indicate esophageal rupture.
Foul odor suggests anaerobic empyema.

### Protein, Albumin, Lactase Dehydrogenase

See Table 6-2.

### Glucose

Same concentration as serum in transudate
Usually normal, but 30–55 mg/dL or pleural fluid:serum ratio <0.5 and pH <7.30 may be found in TB, malignancy, SLE, and esophageal rupture; lowest levels occur in empyema and RA. Therefore, only helpful if very low level (e.g., <30). 0–10 mg/dL highly suspicious for RA.

### pH

  • Low pH (<7.30) always means exudate, especially empyema, malignancy, rheumatoid pleurisy, SLE, TB, esophageal rupture.
  • Esophageal rupture is only cause of pH close to 6.0.
  • Collagen vascular disease is only other cause besides esophageal rupture of pH <7.0.
  • pH <7.10 in parapneumonic effusion indicates need for tube drainage.

**Table 6-2.** Comparison of "Typical"[a] Findings in Transudates and Exudates[b]

| Findings | Transudates | Exudates |
|---|---|---|
| Specific gravity[c] | <1.016 | >1.016 |
| Protein (gm/dL)[d] | <3.0 | >3.0 |
| Pleural fluid:serum ratio[e] | <0.5 | >0.5 |
| LD[f] | | |
| IU | <200 | >200 |
| Pleural fluid:serum ratio[e] | <0.6 | >0.6 |
| Ratio pleural fluid:upper limit normal serum[e] | <2:3 | >2:3 |
| WBC count | <1000/cu mm | >1000/cu mm |
| | Mainly lymphocytes | May be grossly purulent |
| RBCs | Few | Variable; few or may be grossly bloody |
| Glucose | Equivalent to serum | May be decreased because of bacteria or many WBCs |
| Cholesterol (mg/dL) | <55 | Usually >55 |
| Pleural fluid:serum ratio | <0.32 | >0.32 |
| pH | Usually 7.4–7.5 | Usually 7.35–7.45 |
| Appearance | Clear | Usually cloudy |
| Color | Pale yellow | Variable |

[a]"Typical" means 67–75% of patients.
[b]Isoenzymes not useful for differentiating.
[c]Long-standing transudates, however, can produce a high specific gravity.
[d]Protein level of 3.0 gm/dL misclassifies ~15% of effusions if it is the only criterion.
[e]Each of these three criteria has been used to define pleural fluid exudate and transudate. *All three* constitute the best differential of exudate and transudate. Transudate meets none of these criteria, and exudate meets at least one criterion. Unequivocal criteria of transudate precludes the need for pleural biopsy in most cases unless two mechanisms are suspected (e.g., nephrotic syndrome with miliary TB, congestive heart failure with malignancy). It would be uncommon for use of diuretics in congestive heart failure to change characteristics of transudate to that of exudate.
[f]If nonhemolyzed, nonbloody effusion.

### Amylase

Increased in acute pancreatitis, perforated peptic ulcer, necrosis of small intestine, pancreatic pseudocyst, 10% of cases of metastatic cancer (ovary, lung), esophageal rupture, salivary gland tumor. Pleural fluid:serum ratio >1 strongly favors pancreatitis (normal ratio = 1); may be >5.

### Other Chemical Determinations

Cholesterol <55 mg/dL is said to be found in transudates and >55 mg/dL in exudates.
CEA >10 ng/mL may be due to cancer of lung, breast, GI tract, or mucinous ovarian carcinoma.
CA-125 suggests nonmucinous carcinoma of ovary, fallopian tube, or endometrium.
Combined CEA and CA-125 may indicate primary site when the source is unknown or cytology is negative.
Immune complexes (e.g., measured by Raji cell, C1q component of C, radioimmunoassay) are often found in exudates due to collagen vascular diseases (SLE, RA). RA tests show frequent false positives and should not be ordered.

### Cell Count
*(performed in counting chamber)*

Total WBC count is almost never diagnostic.
* >10,000/cu mm indicates inflammation, most commonly with pneumonia, pulmonary infarct, pancreatitis, and postcardiotomy syndrome.
* >50,000/cu mm is typical only in parapneumonic effusions, usually empyema.
* Malignancy and TB are usually <5000/cu mm.
* Transudates are usually <1000/cu mm.

5000–6000 RBCs/cu mm needed to give red appearance to pleural fluid
* Can be caused by needle trauma that causes 2 mL of blood/1000 mL of pleural fluid

>100,000 RBCs/cu mm is grossly hemorrhagic and suggests malignancy, pulmonary infarct, or trauma but occasionally seen in congestive heart failure alone.

Hemothorax (pleural fluid Hct ≥ 50% venous Hct) suggests trauma, bleeding from a vessel, bleeding disorder, or malignancy.

### Smears

Wright's stain differentiates PMNs from mononuclear cells.

Mononuclear cells predominate in transudates, early effusions, and chronic exudates (lymphoma, carcinoma, TB, rheumatoid, uremia). >50% is seen in two-thirds of cases due to cancer. >85–90% suggests TB, lymphoma, sarcoidosis, or rheumatoid causes.

PMNs predominate in early inflammatory effusions (e.g., pneumonia, pulmonary infarct, pancreatitis, subphrenic abscess).

After several days, mesothelial cells, macrophages, and lymphocytes may predominate.

Eosinophils in pleural fluid (>10% of total WBCs) is not diagnostically significant. May mean blood or air in pleural space or infection. Is also said to be associated with asbestosis, pulmonary infarction, polyarteritis nodosa, parasitic or fungal disease, and drug-related (e.g., nitrofurantoin or dantrolene) and idiopathic effusion but is not unusual with malignant effusions and rules out TB.

Gram's stain for early diagnosis of bacterial infection

Acid-fast smears are positive in 20% of tuberculous pleurisy.

### Culture

Is often positive in empyema but not in parapneumonic effusions

### Bacterial Antigen Assay

May detect *Haemophilus influenzae* type b, *Streptococcus pneumoniae*, and several types of *Neisseria meningitidis*. May be useful when viable organisms cannot be recovered.

### Cytology

Positive in 60% of malignancies on first tap, 80% by third tap. Is more sensitive than needle biopsy.

Rheumatoid effusions: giant multinucleated macrophages and necrotic background material with characteristically low glucose is said to be pathognomonic.

Assay for DNA aneuploidy and staining with monoclonal antibodies (e.g., CEA, cytokeratin) can distinguish malignant mesothelioma, metastatic tumor, and reactive mesothelial cells.

## Pleural Fluid

### Normal Values

| | |
|---|---|
| Specific gravity | 1.010–1.026 |
| TP | |
| Albumin | 0.3–4.1 gm/dL |

Globulin             50–70%
Fibrinogen           30–45%
pH                   6.8–7.6

## Scalene Lymph Node Biopsy

Positive in 15% of bronchogenic carcinoma. May also show various granulomatous diseases (e.g., TB, sarcoidosis, pneumoconiosis).

## Sputum

| Color | Condition |
|---|---|
| Rusty | Lobar pneumonia |
| Anchovy-paste (dark brown) | Amebic liver abscess rupture into bronchus |
| Red-currant jelly | *Klebsiella pneumoniae* |
| Red (pigment, not blood) | *Serratia marcescens*; rifampin overdose |
| Black | *Bacteroides melaninogenicus* pneumonia; anthracosilicosis |
| Green (with WBCs, sweet odor) | *Pseudomonas* infection |
| Milky | Bronchioalveolar carcinoma |
| Yellow (without WBCs) | Jaundice |

### Smears and Cultures

For infections; monobacterial population if due to bacterial infection; acute inflammation without a definite bacterial pattern may be due to *Legionella* or respiratory syncytial or influenza viruses. For possible anaerobic aspiration, fine-needle aspiration or alveolar lavage is needed.

### Cytology

For malignant cells

## Thoracoscopy/Open Lung Biopsy

### Use

Diagnosis of pleural malignancy
Diagnosis of pulmonary infection or neoplasm

# Respiratory Diseases

## Bronchial Asthma

Sputum is white and mucoid without blood or pus (unless infection is present).
• Eosinophils, crystals (Curschmann's spirals), and mucus casts of bronchioles may be found.
Eosinophilia may be present.
Blood $p(a)O_2$ decreases early before $p(a)O_2$ increases.
With severe episode, hyperventilation causes decreased $p(a)O_2$ in early stages (may be <35 mm Hg). Rapid deterioration of patient's condition may be associated with precipitous fall in $p(a)O_2$ and rise in $p(a)O_2$ (>40 mm Hg).
• $p(a)O_2$ <60 mm Hg may indicate severe attack or presence of complication.
Mixed metabolic and respiratory acidosis occurs.
When patient requires hospitalization, arterial blood gases should be measured frequently to assess status.

## Bronchogenic Carcinoma

Cytologic examination of sputum for malignant cells—positive in 40% of patients on first sample, 70% with three samples, 85% with five samples
Biopsy of scalene lymph nodes for diagnosis is positive in 15% of patients.
Biopsy of bronchus, pleura, lung, metastatic sites in appropriate cases
Cytology of pleural effusion
Needle biopsy of pleura is positive in 58% of cases with malignant effusion.
Transthoracic needle aspiration provides definitive cytologic diagnosis of cancer in 80–90% of cases.
Cancer cells may be found in bone marrow and rarely in peripheral blood.
Syndromes due to metastases (e.g., Addison's disease, diabetes insipidus, liver metastases with functional hepatic changes)
Findings due to secretion of active hormone substances (e.g., SIADH, Cushing's syndrome, hypercalcemia, serotonin production by carcinoid of bronchus)
Biochemical tumor markers
- Serum carcinoembryonic antigen is increased in one-third to two-thirds of patients with all four types of lung cancer.
- Serum neuron-specific enolase may be increased in ≤ 87% of patients with small cell lung cancer (SCLC) and in 10% of non-SCLC and nonmalignant lung diseases.

## Goodpasture's Syndrome
(malignant hypertension associated with pulmonary hemorrhages)

Proteinuria, RBCs, and RBC casts in urine
Renal function may deteriorate rapidly.
Renal biopsy may show characteristic linear immunofluorescent deposits and focal or diffuse proliferative glomerulonephritis.
Serum may show anti–glomerular basement membrane antibodies, which may be found in cases without pulmonary hemorrhage.
Eosinophilia absent and iron-deficiency anemia more marked compared to idiopathic pulmonary hemosiderosis.

## Legionnaires' Disease
(due to *Legionella pneumophila*—facultative intracellular pathogen)

Gram's stain of sputum shows few to moderate number of PMNs.
Special culture techniques may show growth in 3–7 days.
Serologic tests
- Direct immunofluorescent microscopy on sputum, pleural fluid, lung, or other tissue is extremely useful for rapid, specific diagnosis; may be negative with few organisms present, especially after erythromycin therapy. PCR and gene probes will become useful.
- Antibody titers show 4-fold increase to 1:128; most useful for retrospective diagnosis or epidemiologic study.
- Single immunofluorescent assay titer of 1:256 is strong presumptive evidence.
- Urine antigen assay can detect infection.
Increased WBC (10,000–20,000/cu mm) in 75% of cases; leukopenia is a bad prognostic sign.
Mild to moderate increase of serum AST, ALP, LD, or bilirubin in ~50% of patients. Hypoalbuminemia <2.5 gm/dL.
Pleural effusion in ≤ 50% of patients may be bilateral; are usually small exudates; organism can be isolated.

## Lung Abscess

Sputum
- Marked increase in amount; abundant, foul, purulent.

- Gram's stain is diagnostic—sheets of PMN leukocytes with a bewildering variety of organisms.
- Bacterial cultures—including for tubercle bacilli; anaerobic as well as aerobic; rule out amebas, parasites.
- Cytologic examination for malignant cells to rule out underlying cancer may be bloody; contains elastic fibers.

Blood culture may be positive in acute stage.
Increased WBC in acute stages (15,000–30,000/cu mm)
Normochromic normocytic anemia in chronic stage

## Pneumoconiosis

Biopsy of lung, scalene lymph node—histologic, chemical, spectrographic, and x-ray diffraction studies (e.g., silicosis, berylliosis; also metastatic tumor, sarcoidosis, TB, fungus infection)
Asbestos bodies sometimes in sputum after exposure to asbestos dust even without clinical disease
Acute beryllium disease may show occasional transient hypergammaglobulinemia
Chronic beryllium disease
- Secondary polycythemia
- Increased serum gamma globulin
- Increased urine calcium
- Increased beryllium in urine long after beryllium exposure has ended

Bacterial smears and cultures of sputum (especially for tubercle bacilli)
Cytologic examination of sputum and bronchoscopic secretions for malignant cells, especially carcinoma of bronchus and mesothelioma of pleura

## Pneumonia

### Due to

*S. pneumoniae*—blood culture positive in 25% of untreated cases during first 3–4 days
*Staphylococcus* causes bacteremia in <20% of patients.
*H. influenzae* is important in 0- to 24-month age group; rare in adults except for middle-aged men with chronic lung disease and/or alcoholism and patients with immunodeficiency.
Gram-negative bacilli are common causes of hospital-acquired but not community-acquired pneumonia.
*Mycoplasma pneumoniae*—is most common in the young adult male population (e.g., armed forces camps).

| Underlying Condition | Organism |
| --- | --- |
| Obstructive cancer | *S. pneumoniae, H. influenzae, Moraxella catarrhalis*, anaerobes |
| Alcoholism | *S. pneumoniae, H. influenzae, Klebsiella* sp., *Legionella* sp., anaerobes, *Mycobacterium tuberculosis* |
| HIV infection | *S. pneumoniae, H. influenzae, Staphylococcus aureus*, gram-negative bacilli, *Pneumocystis carinii, Mycobacterium tuberculosis, Mycobacterium avium-intracellulare, Toxoplasma gondii*, cryptococcus, *Nocardia*, CMV, histoplasmosis coccidioidomycosis, *Legionella, M. catarrhalis, Rhodococcus equi* |
| Atypical pneumonia | *M. pneumoniae, Chlamydia psittaci, Chlamydia pneumoniae, Coxiella burnetii, Francisella tularensis*, many viruses |

### Laboratory Findings

Respiratory pathogens isolated from blood, lung tissue, pleural fluid, or transtracheal aspirate (except patients with chronic bronchitis), or identified by bacterial antigen in urine may be considered the definite etiologic agent.

Blood and sputum cultures and smear for Gram's stain should be performed before antibiotic therapy is started.

Sputum shows abundant organisms in bacterial pneumonias. *Sputum that contains many organisms and WBCs on smear but no pathogens on aerobic culture may indicate aspiration pneumonia. Sputum is not appropriate for anaerobic culture.*

Transtracheal aspiration generally yields a faster, more accurate diagnosis.

Protected brush bronchoscopy and bronchoalveolar lavage have high sensitivity.

Open lung biopsy is gold standard.

Pleural effusions that are aspirated should also have Gram's stain and culture performed.

Urine for capsular antigen from *S. pneumoniae* or *H. influenzae* type b may be helpful; is positive in ~90% of bacteremic pneumococcal and 40% of nonbacteremic pneumonias. May be useful when antibiotic therapy has already begun.

Acute-phase serum should be stored at onset. If etiologic diagnosis is not established, a convalescent-phase serum should be taken.

## Pulmonary Embolism and Infarction

No laboratory test is diagnostic. *Findings depend on the size and duration of the infarction.*

Arterial blood gases (when patient is breathing room air) are the most sensitive and specific laboratory tests.

- $pO_2$ <80 mm Hg in 88% of cases but normal value does not rule out pulmonary embolus. In appropriate clinical setting, $pO_2$ <88 mm Hg (even with a normal chest x-ray) is indication for lung scans and search for deep vein thromboses. $pO_2$ >90 mm Hg with a normal chest x-ray suggests a different diagnosis.
- Hypocapnia and slightly elevated pH. Increased WBC in 50% of patients is rarely >15,000/cu mm.

Serum enzymes

- To differentiate from AMI.
- Increased LD (due to isoenzymes 2 and 3) in 80% of patients rises on day 1, peaks on day 2, normal by day 10.
- Increased ALP and GGT 4–10 days after onset.

Serum bilirubin is increased (as early as day 4) to ~5 mg/dL in 20% of cases.

Fibrin degradation products and soluble fibrin complexes are higher in blood of patients with thromboembolism. Chief value is that plasma D-dimer <500 ng/mL obviates need for pulmonary angiography. Increased D-dimer is also found in DIC with fibrinolysis and thrombolytic therapy.

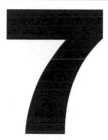

# Gastrointestinal Diseases

# Laboratory Tests of Gastrointestinal Diseases

## Bentiromide

Bentiromide is acted on by pancreatic chymotrypsin, releasing para-aminoben-zoic acid, which is measured in a 6-hr urine sample (normal value is >50%) and (sometimes) a 1- to 2-hr serum sample.

### Use

Initial test gauges pancreatic exocrine activity to rule out pancreatic disease in patients with chronic diarrhea, weight loss, or steatorrhea.
In conjunction with D-xylose tolerance test for differentiation of pancreatic exocrine insufficiency from intestinal mucosal disease.

### Interference

False negatives may occur due to drugs (e.g., thiazides, chloramphenicol, sulfonamides, acetaminophen, phenacetin, sunscreens, procaine anesthetics).
Abnormal kidney function, gastric emptying, or gut function.

## Breath Test

Radiolabeled material administered orally is absorbed in bowel, excreted by lungs, and measured in expired breath.

### Interpretation

Increased in
- Bacterial overgrowth
- Disease or resection of terminal ileum

## Carotene Tolerance Test

Measure serum carotene after oral loading of carotene for 3–7 days.

### Use

Low values for serum carotene levels are usually associated with steatorrhea.

### Normal

Increase of serum carotene by $>35\ \mu g/dL$ indicates previously low dietary intake of carotene and/or fat.

### Decreased in

Steatorrhea

### Interference

Mineral oil interferes with carotene absorption.
Only 10% is absorbed in patients on a fat-free diet.

## Gastric Analysis

### Use

Determine status of acid secretion in hypergastrinemia patients being treated
for gastrinoma.
Determine if patients who have undergone surgery for ulcer disease and who
have complications are secreting acid.

| Finding | Interpretation |
| --- | --- |
| 1-hr basal acid | |
| <2 mEq | Normal gastric ulcer or carcinoma |
| 2–5 mEq | Normal gastric or duodenal ulcer |
| >5 mEq | Duodenal ulcer |
| >20 mEq | Z-E syndrome |
| 1 hr after stimulation by pentagastrin | |
| 0 mEq | Achlorhydria, gastritis, gastric carcinoma |
| 1–20 mEq | Normal gastric ulcer or carcinoma |
| 20–35 mEq | Duodenal ulcer |
| 35–60 mEq | Duodenal ulcer, high normal, Z-E syndrome |
| >60 mEq | Z-E syndrome |
| Ratio of basal acid to post-stimulation outputs | |
| 20% | Normal gastric ulcer or carcinoma |
| 20–40% | Gastric or duodenal ulcer |
| 40–60% | Duodenal ulcer, Z-E syndrome |
| >60% | Z-E syndrome |

### Achlorhydria

| | |
| --- | --- |
| Chronic atrophic gastritis (serum gastrin is frequently increased) | |
| Pernicious anemia | 100% of patients |
| Gastric carcinoma (even after histamine or betazole stimulation) | 50% |
| Gastric ulcer | Common |
| Adenomatous polyps of stomach | 85% of patients |
| Ménétrier's disease | 75% |
| Iatrogenic | |
| Postvagotomy, postantrectomy | >90% |
| Medical (e.g., potent $H_2$-receptor antagonists, substituted benzimidazoles) | >80% |

Normal persons: 4% of children, increasing to 30% of adults older than age 60
*True achlorhydria excludes duodenal ulcer.*

### Hyperchlorhydria and Hypersecretion

| | |
| --- | --- |
| Duodenal ulcer | 40–45% |
| Z-E syndrome | |
| 12-Hr night secretion shows acid of >100 mEq/L and volume >1500 mL. | |
| Basal secretion is >60% of secretion caused by histamine or betazole stimulation. | 100% |
| Hyperplasia/hyperfunction of antral gastrin cells | >90% |

| Hypertrophic hypersecretory gastropathy | 100% |
| Massive resection of small intestine (transient) | 50% |

When basal serum gastrin level is equivocal, serum gastrin level should be measured after stimulation with infusion of secretin or calcium.

## Gastrin, Serum

Normal values: 0 to ≤ 200 pg gastrin/mL serum
Elevated values: >500 pg/mL
Secretin infusion: Normal patients and patients with duodenal ulcer show no increase in serum gastrin. Patients with Z-E syndrome show increased serum gastrin that usually peaks in 45–60 mins (usually >400 pg/mL). Secretin test is preferred first test. With other causes of hypergastrinemia associated with hyperchlorhydria, serum gastrin is unchanged or decreases.
Calcium infusion: Normal patients show minimal serum gastrin response to calcium. Patients with Z-E syndrome show excessive increase in serum gastrin in 2–3 hrs. Positive in one-third of patients with a negative secretin test. Recommended when secretin test is negative in patients suspicious for Z-E syndrome.
Indications for measurement of serum gastrin and gastric analysis include
- Atypical peptic ulcer of stomach, duodenum, or proximal jejunum, especially if multiple, unusual location, or poorly responsive to therapy, or rapid or severe recurrence after adequate therapy
- Unexplained chronic diarrhea with or without peptic ulcer
- Peptic ulcer disease with associated endocrine conditions
Serum gastrin levels are indicated with any of the following:
- Basal acid secretion >10 mEq/hr in patients with intact stomachs
- Ratio of basal to poststimulation output >40% in patients with intact stomachs
- All patients with recurrent ulceration after surgery for duodenal ulcer
- All patients with duodenal ulcer for whom elective gastric surgery is planned

### Increased Serum Gastrin without Gastric Acid Hypersecretion

Atrophic gastritis, especially when associated with circulating parietal cell antibodies
Pernicious anemia in ~75% of patients
Some patients have carcinoma of body of stomach, a reflection of the atrophic gastritis that is present.
Chronic renal failure

### Increased Serum Gastrin with Gastric Acid Hypersecretion

Z-E syndrome
Hyperplasia of antral gastrin cells
Isolated retained antrum
Pyloric obstruction with gastric distention
Short-bowel syndrome

## Oleic Acid [131]I Absorption Test

Normal values are the same as for the triolein absorption test.

### Interpretation

An abnormal result indicates a defect in small-bowel mucosal absorption function. Abnormal pancreatic function does not affect the test.

## Polyvinylpyrrolidone (PVP-$^{131}$I)

### Interpretation

Normal: <2% of 15–25 $\mu$Ci of PVP-$^{131}$I is excreted in feces when the mucosa of
the GI tract is intact. In protein-losing enteropathy, >2% of administered
radioactivity appears in the stool.

## Triolein $^{131}$I Absorption Test

### Use

Screening patients with steatorrhea

### Interpretation

Normal: ≥ 10% of administered 15–20 $\mu$Ci of triolein $^{131}$I radioactivity appears in
the blood within 6 hrs; <5% appears in the feces. Normal values indicate that
digestion of fat in the small bowel and absorption of fat in the small bowel are
normal.
If results are abnormal, perform an oleic acid $^{131}$I absorption test.

## Laboratory Examination of Stool

### Normal Values

| | |
|---|---|
| Bulk | 100–200 gm |
| Water | Up to 75% |
| Total osmolality | 200–250 mOsm |
| pH | 7.0–7.5 (may be acid with high lactose intake) |
| Nitrogen | <2.5 gm/day |
| Potassium | 5–20 mEq/kg |
| Sodium | 10–20 mEq/kg |
| Magnesium | <200 mEq/kg |
| Coproporphyrin | 400–1000 mg/24 hrs |
| Trypsin | 20–950 U/gm |
| Urobilinogen | 50–300 mg/24 hrs |

### Color

Brown: normally
Clay color (gray-white): biliary obstruction
Tarry: if >100 mL of blood in upper GI tract
Red: blood in large intestine or undigested beets or tomatoes
Black: blood or iron or bismuth medication
Various colors: depending on diet

## Fecal Leukocytes

Agglutination test kit detects a marker protein for fecal leukocytes.
High positive and negative predictive values compared to microscopy.

## Occult Blood

### Use

Screening for asymptomatic ulcerated lesions of GI tract, especially carcinoma
of the colon. High false-negative rate; poor specificity.

### Interpretation

Kits (e.g., Hemoccult cards [SmithKline Diagnostics, Sunnyvale, CA]) use guaiac;
detect blood losses of ~20 mL/day; "normal" amount of blood lost in stool daily is

<2 mL/day or 2 mg Hb/gm of stool. Poor sensitivity of Hemoccult and HemoQuant (SmithKline BioSciences, Van Nuys, CA) for colorectal cancer and polyps.

Benzidine reaction is too sensitive; guaiac test yields too many false-negative results. Quantitative HemoQuant test kit doubles sensitivity of guaiac tests; may be affected by red meat and aspirin (for up to 4 days) but not by certain foods and drugs that affect the benzidine reaction (normal <2 mg/gm; >4 mg/gm is increased; 2–4 mg/gm is borderline).

Immunochemical tests (e.g., HemeSelect [SmithKline Diagnostics, Sunnyvale, CA]) specifically detect human Hb, do not require restrictions; detect ~0.3 mg Hb/gm of stool.

### Osmotic Gap
*(= measured osmolality –2 × [Na + K])*

### Increased in

Osmotic diarrhea
• Saline laxatives.
• Surreptitious addition of water to fecal specimen causes stool osmolality to be considerably lower than plasma osmolality.

## Qualitative Screening Test for Fecal Fat

### Use

Screening for steatorrhea (malabsorption)

### Interpretation

≥ 2 random stool samples are collected on diet of >80 gm of fat daily. Microscopic examination after staining for fat has high sensitivity with moderate/severe fat malabsorption.

### Interference

Neutral fat
• Mineral and castor oil ingestion
• Dietetic, low-calorie mayonnaise ingestion
• Rectal suppository use

## Quantitative Determination of Fecal Fat

### Use

Is gold standard test to establish the diagnosis of malabsorption

Normal is <7 gm/24 hrs when a 3-day pooled stool sample is collected on diet of 80–100 gm of fat daily. <5 gm/24 hrs (or <4% of measured fat intake) on diet of <50 gm of fat/day for a 3-day period.

### Increased in

Chronic pancreatic disease (>9.5 gm/24 hrs)
May also be increased in
• High fiber diet (>100 gm/24 hrs)
• When dietary fat is ingested in solid form (e.g., whole peanuts)
• Neonatal period

## Urobilinogen
**(Normal = 50–300 mg/24 hrs; 100–400 Ehrlich units/100 gm)**

### Increased in

Hemolytic anemias

### Decreased in

Complete biliary obstruction
Severe liver disease
Oral antibiotic therapy altering intestinal bacterial flora
Decreased Hb turnover (e.g., aplastic anemia, cachexia)

## Other Procedures

Alkalinization of stool to pH 10 turns blue due to phenolphthalein in certain laxatives. Useful in cases of laxative abuse.
Examination for ova and parasites
Trypsin digestion

# Diseases of the Gastrointestinal Tract

## Acute Appendicitis

Increased WBC (12,000–14,000/cu mm) with shift to the left; higher and more rapid rise with suppuration or perforation.
ESR may be normal during first 24 hrs.
It has been reported that a CRP <2.5 mg/dL 12 hrs after onset of symptoms excludes acute appendicitis.

## Acute Diverticulitis

Increased WBC and ESR
Occult blood in stool

## Carcinoma of Esophagus

Cytologic examination of esophageal washings confirmed by biopsy of tumor.

## Carcinoma of Stomach

Exfoliative cytology positive in 80% of patients.
Biopsy of lesions confirms diagnosis.
Lymph node biopsy for metastases; needle biopsy of liver, bone marrow, etc.
Tumor markers are not useful for early detection. May be useful for postoperative monitoring for recurrence or to estimate tumor burden.
Occult blood in stool
*Carcinoma of the stomach should be searched for in high-risk patients (e.g., patients with pernicious anemia, gastric atrophy, gastric polyps).*

## Celiac Disease (Gluten-Sensitive Enteropathy, Nontropical Sprue)

See Fig. 7-1.
Steatorrhea
Xylose tolerance test distinguishes malabsorption due to impaired transport across diseased mucosa from impaired digestion in lumen.
Biopsy of small intestine shows characteristic, although not specific, mucosal lesions. Is essential to establish the diagnosis; patients should not be committed to gluten-free diet without first assessing mucosal histology.
Firm diagnosis requires definite clinical response to gluten-free diet, preferably with histologic documentation that mucosa has reverted to normal by repeat biopsy in 6–12 months. If patient fails to respond to rigid dietary control, GI lymphoma should be ruled out.

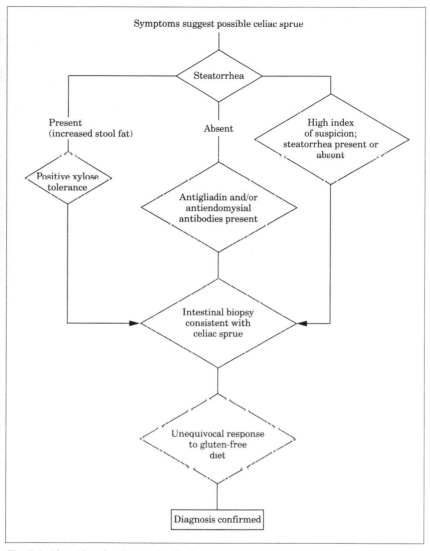

**Fig. 7-1.** Algorithm for diagnosis of celiac sprue.

Gluten challenge is performed if diagnosis is uncertain and not documented by biopsy before gluten withdrawal to determine if symptoms recur and mucosal changes occur.

Antigliadin antibodies and antiendomysial antibodies in serum of untreated patients

## Chronic Duodenal Ulcer

*Helicobacter pylori*–associated gastritis is present in ~95% of all patients with duodenal ulcer except those with Z-E syndrome.

## Chronic Gastritis

Diagnosis depends on biopsy of gastric mucosa.

Fasting serum gastrin is greatly increased in chronic gastritis with achlorhydria and relative sparing of antral mucosa but may be normal with severe antral involvement even with achlorhydria.

Parietal cell antibodies and intrinsic factor antibodies help define the autoimmune type of chronic gastritis and those patients prone to pernicious anemia.

Chronic antral gastritis is consistently present in patients with benign gastric ulcer.

*H. pylori* is detectable in ~80% of patients with peptic ulcer and chronic gastritis.

## Disaccharide Malabsorption

See Fig. 7-2.

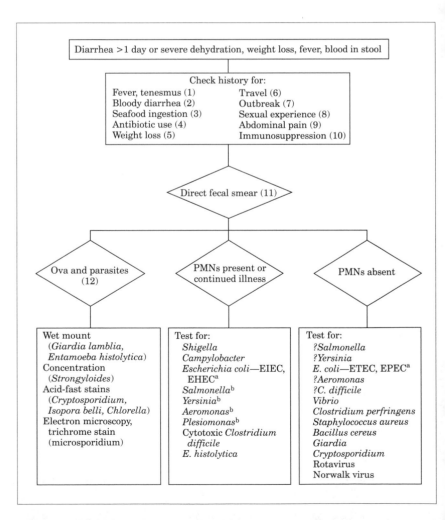

### Due to

Primary malabsorption due to absence of specific disaccharidase in brush border
of small intestine mucosa
- Isolated lactase deficiency
- Sucrose-isomaltose malabsorption
  - Oral sucrose tolerance curve is flat, but glucose plus fructose tolerance
    test is normal.
- Glucose-galactose malabsorption
  - Oral glucose or galactose tolerance curve is flat, but IV tolerance curves
    are normal.
  - Glucosuria is common. Normal fructose tolerance.

Secondary malabsorption
- Resection of >50% of disaccharidase activity.
- Diffuse intestinal disease—especially celiac disease in which activity of all
  disaccharidases may be decreased, with increase as intestine becomes normal
  on gluten-free diet; also cystic fibrosis of pancreas, severe malnutrition, ulcerative colitis, severe *Giardia* infestation, blind-loop syndrome, beta-lipoprotein
  deficiency, effect of drugs (e.g., colchicine, neomycin, birth control pills)

◀**Fig 7-2** Algorithm for etiology of infectious diarrhea. Bacteria cause the severest
forms of infectious diarrhea; viruses (e.g., rotaviruses, Norwalk viruses) are most
common causes. (1) Fever or tenesmus suggests inflammatory proctocolitis. (2)
Diarrhea with blood, especially without fecal WBCs, suggests EHEC *Escherichia coli*
0157 or amebiasis in which WBCs are destroyed by parasite. (3) Eating inadequately
cooked seafood suggests *Vibrio* or Norwalk-like viruses. (4) Stop antibiotics if possible;
consider cytotoxigenic *Clostridium difficile*; may also predispose to other infections
(e.g., salmonellosis). (5) Diarrhea >10 days with weight loss suggests giardiasis or
cryptosporidiosis. (6) Travel to tropical regions: consider ETEC *E. coli*, viral
(Norwalk-like or rotaviral), parasitic (*Giardia, Entamoeba, Strongyloides,
Cryptosporidium*), or invasive bacterial infections. (7) Outbreaks suggest anisakiasis,
infection with *Staphylococcus aureus, Bacillus cereus* (incubation period <6 hrs),
*Clostridium perfringens*, ETEC *E. coli*, *Vibrio*, *Salmonella*, *Campylobacter*, *Shigella*,
EIEC *E. coli*. (8) Sigmoidoscopy in symptomatic gay men should distinguish proctitis
in distal 15 cm (due to herpes simplex virus, gonococcal, *Chlamydia*, syphilitic infections) from colitis (*Campylobacter, Shigella, C. difficile, Chlamydia* infections) or noninflammatory diarrhea (giardiasis). (9) Appendicitis-like syndrome or persistent
abdominal pain and fever suggest culture for *Yersinia enterocolitica* with cold enrich-
ment. (10) In immunocompromised hosts, consider many viral (CMV, herpes simplex
virus, coxsackievirus, rotavirus), bacterial (*Salmonella, Mycobacterium avium-intracellulare*), or parasitic (*Cryptosporidium isospora, Strongyloides, Entamoeba,
Giardia*) causes. (11) Some inflammatory pathogens (e.g., cytotoxigenic *C. difficile,
Entamoeba histolytica*) may destroy fecal WBC morphology. (12) Especially if diarrhea
>10 days or recurrent. [a]*Special* tests (*E. coli* samples for serotyping and testing for
heat-labile and heat-stable toxin, invasiveness, adherence). Stools and paired serum
samples for Norwalk-like virus or toxin testing. [b]Rare. (EIEC = enteroinvasive;
EHEC = enterohemorrhagic; ETEC = enterotoxigenic; EPEC = enteropathogenic.)

### Oral Tolerance Tests (Especially Lactose)

Are frequently abnormal, with later return to normal with gluten-free diet. Tolerance tests with monosaccharides may also be abnormal because of defect in absorption as well as digestion.

### Laboratory Tests for Lactase Deficiency

(Similar tests can be performed for other disaccharide deficiencies.)

Oral lactose tolerance curve is flat but is normal using constituent monosaccharides (glucose and galactose), indicating isolated lactase deficiency rather than general mucosal absorptive defect.

Stool examination: After ingestion of lactose, frothy diarrheal stools show low pH, high osmolality, positive test for reducing substances; found in children but rarely in adults. Chromatography detects specific carbohydrates.

Hydrogen breath test

Endoscopic biopsy for histology and enzyme assay is now considered obsolete.

## Inflammatory Disorders of the Intestine

Idiopathic—ulcerative colitis, regional enteritis, colitis of indeterminate type (e.g., collagenous colitis)

Infectious
- Bacteria
- Tubercle bacilli
- Chlamydiae
- Viruses (e.g., rotavirus, CMV, herpes)
- Parasites (*Entamoeba histolyticum, Giardia lamblia*)
- Fungi (e.g., *Cryptosporidium*)

Motility disorders—diverticulitis, solitary rectal ulcer syndrome

Circulatory disorders—ischemic colitis, associated with obstruction of colon

Iatrogenic
- Enemas, laxatives, drugs
- Radiation
- After small intestinal bypass and diversion of fecal stream
- Graft versus host disease

Specific disease association
- Chronic granulomatous disease of childhood
- Immunodeficiency syndromes
- Hemolytic uremic syndrome
- Behçet's disease

Miscellaneous
- Collagenous colitis
- Eosinophilic colitis and allergic proctitis
- Necrotizing enterocolitis
- Idiopathic ulcer of colon

## Malabsorption

See Fig. 7-3.

### Due to

Inadequate mixing of food with bile salts and lipase (e.g., pyloroplasty, gastrectomy, gastrojejunostomy)

Inadequate lipolysis due to lack of lipase (pancreatic diseases, vagotomy)

Inadequate emulsification of fat due to lack of bile salts (e.g., obstructive jaundice, severe liver disease, bacterial overgrowth of small intestine, disorders of terminal ileum)

Primary absorptive defect in small bowel

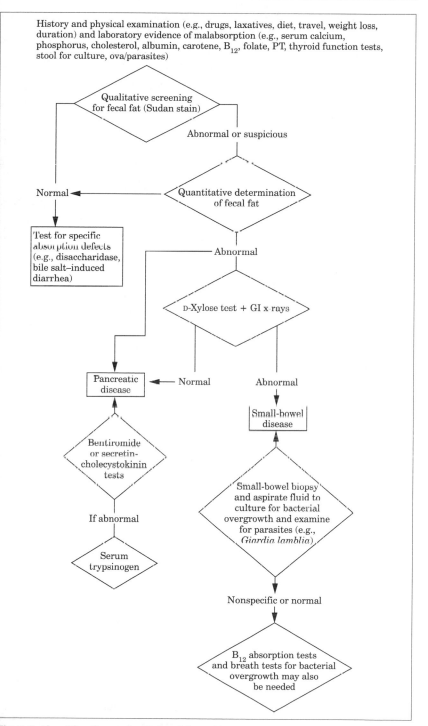

**Fig. 7-3.** Algorithm for work-up of malabsorption.

Inadequate absorptive surface due to extensive mucosal disease (e.g., regional enteritis, tumors, amyloid disease, scleroderma, irradiation)

Biochemical dysfunction of mucosal cells (e.g., celiac sprue syndrome, severe starvation, intestinal infections, infestations, or certain drugs)

Obstruction of mesenteric lymphatics (e.g., by lymphoma, carcinoma, Whipple's disease, intestinal TB)

Inadequate length of normal absorptive surface (e.g., surgical resection, fistula, shunt)

Miscellaneous (e.g., "blind loops" of intestine, diverticula, Z-E syndrome, agammaglobulinemia, endocrine and metabolic disorders)

Chronic infection

### Direct Stool Examination

- Gross—oil droplets, egg particles, buttery materials.
- Sudan III stain for qualitative screening for fecal fat.
- Quantitative test for fecal fat is gold standard to establish diagnosis. Increased in chronic pancreatic disease >9.5 gm/24 hrs.
- Weight—much heavier (>300 gm/24 hrs) than normal.
- $Na_2CO_3$ and Nile blue dye give blue color to stool proportional to the concentration of oleates.

Indirect indices of fat absorption lack sensitivity and specificity for routine screening.
- Serum cholesterol may be decreased.
- PT may be prolonged due to malabsorption of vitamin K.
- Serum carotene is always abnormal in steatorrhea unless therapy is successful. Normal is 70–290 $\mu$g/dL. 30–70 $\mu$g/dL indicates mild depletion; <30 indicates severe depletion.
- Vitamin A tolerance test (for screening steatorrhea).
    Flat curve in liver disease.
    Flat curve also occurs in both pancreatic disease and intestinal mucosal abnormalities; when water-soluble forms of vitamin A are used, the curve becomes normal in patients with pancreatic disease but remains flat in intestinal mucosal abnormalities.
- Triolein [131]I and oleic acid [131]I absorption.

Carbohydrate absorption indices
- Oral glucose tolerance test—limited value.
- D-Xylose tolerance test of carbohydrate absorption; accurate in distinguishing normal levels in pancreatic disease from decreased levels in intestinal mucosal disease and intestinal bacterial overgrowth, but opinions vary on usefulness.

Protein absorption indices
- Normal fecal nitrogen is <2 gm/day. There is marked increase in sprue and severe pancreatic deficiency.
- Measure plasma glycine or urinary hydroxyproline after gelatin meal. Plasma glycine increases 5 times in 2 hrs in normal persons. In cystic fibrosis of the pancreas, the increase is <2.5 times.
- Serum albumin may be decreased.

Serum trypsinogen <10 ng/mL in 75–85% of patients with severe chronic pancreatitis with steatorrhea and 15–20% of those with mild to moderate disease; normal (10–75 ng/mL) in nonpancreatic causes of malabsorption.

Bentiromide is used to differentiate pancreatic exocrine insufficiency (abnormal result) from intestinal mucosal disease (normal result).

Secretin-cholecystokinin is the most sensitive and reliable test of chronic pancreatic disease.

Schilling test is useful adjunct to intestinal culture to detect bacterial overgrowth.

Breath tests

Electrolyte absorption indices
- Serum calcium, magnesium, potassium, and vitamin D may be decreased.

$^{51}$Cr albumin test shows increased excretion in 4-day stool collection due to protein-losing enteropathy.

Biopsy of small intestine mucosa is excellent for verification of sprue, celiac disease, and Whipple's disease.

Culture for bacterial overgrowth should be considered in malabsorption associated with abnormal intestinal motility or anatomic abnormalities.

Anemia is due to decreased absorption of iron, folic acid, vitamin $B_{12}$.

Most common laboratory abnormalities are decreased serum carotene, albumin, and iron, increased ESR, increased stool weight ($>300$ gm/24 hrs) and stool fat ($>7$ gm/24 hrs), anemia.

Normal D-xylose test, low serum trypsinogen, pancreatic calcification on x-ray of abdomen, abnormal contents of pancreatic secretion after secretin-cholecystokinin stimulation or abnormal bentiromide tests establish diagnosis of chronic pancreatitis.

## Regional Enteritis (Crohn's Disease)

No pathognomonic findings for this disease
Increased WBC, ESR, CRP, other acute phase reactants
Anemia due to iron deficiency or vitamin $B_{12}$ or folate deficiency
Mild liver function test changes due to pericholangitis

## Ulcerative Colitis, Chronic Nonspecific

Laboratory findings parallel severity of the disease.
* Anemia due to blood loss (frequently Hb = 6 gm/dL)
* WBC and ESR usually normal unless complication occurs (e.g., abscess)
Stools
* Positive for blood (gross and/or occult)
* Negative for usual enteric organisms
Rectal biopsy

## Viral Gastroenteritis

See Fig. 7-2.
Suspected by exclusion by negative tests for other causes of the symptoms (e.g., failure to find *Entamoeba histolytica*, *Shigella*, *Salmonella*)
Antigen detection—Commercial kits for rotavirus permit rapid diagnosis.
Antibody detection (e.g., Norwalk virus) can be diagnosed by presence of serum IgM; 4 times rise in specific IgG antibody titers used to identify cause of an outbreak.
Direct electron microscopy of stool can detect and identify enteric viruses (e.g., rotaviruses, adenoviruses, astroviruses, caliciviruses, Norwalk virus) by characteristic appearance.
Usually only during first 48 hrs of viral diarrhea. Required for conclusive diagnosis of Norwalk virus.
Culture
* Rotavirus, adenoviruses, astrovirus culture available in research centers; not useful for routine diagnosis. Other viruses cannot be cultured.

## Whipple's Disease (Intestinal Lipodystrophy)
### (due to *Tropheryma whippleii*)

Characteristic biopsy of proximal intestine (especially duodenum) and mesenteric lymph nodes establishes the diagnosis showing bacilli.
PCR to amplify bacterial ribosomal RNA in infected tissues and cells

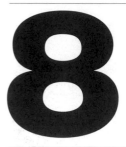

# Hepatobiliary Diseases and Diseases of the Pancreas

---

# Liver Function Tests

## Generalizations on Liver Function Test Interpretation

Patterns rather than single test changes are most useful.

Tests may be abnormal in many conditions that are not primarily hepatic (e.g., heart failure, sepsis, infections) and individual tests may be normal in high proportions of patients with proven specific liver diseases.

## Some Common Patterns (Test Combinations) of Liver Function Change

See Fig. 8-1.

Serum bilirubin (direct:total ratio)

| | |
|---|---|
| <20% direct | Constitutional (e.g., Gilbert syndrome, Crigler-Najjar syndrome) |
| | Hemolytic states |
| 20–40% direct | Favors hepatocellular disease rather than extrahepatic obstruction |
| 40–60% direct | Occurs in either hepatocellular or extrahepatic type |
| >50% direct | Favors extrahepatic obstruction rather than hepatocellular disease |

Total serum bilirubin
- Must exceed 2.5 mg/dL to produce clinical jaundice.
- >5 mg/dL seldom occurs in uncomplicated hemolysis unless hepatobiliary disease is also present.
- Is generally less markedly elevated in hepatocellular jaundice (<10 mg/dL) than in periampullary carcinomas (≤ 20 mg/dL) or intrahepatic cholestasis.
- In extrahepatic biliary obstruction, bilirubin may rise progressively to a plateau of 30–40 mg/dL. Such a plateau tends not to occur in hepatocellular jaundice and bilirubin may exceed 50 mg/dL.
- Concentrations are generally higher in obstruction due to carcinoma than due to stones.
- Increased serum bilirubin with normal ALP suggests constitutional hyperbilirubinemias or hemolytic states.
- Normal serum bilirubin, AST, ALT with increased ALP, and LD suggest obstruction of one hepatic duct or metastatic or infiltrative disease of liver. Metastatic and granulomatous lesions of liver cause 1.5–3.0 times increase of serum ALP and LD.

AST and ALT. See Table 8-1.
- Most marked increase (100–2000 IU/L) occurs in viral hepatitis, drug injury, carbon tetrachloride poisoning.

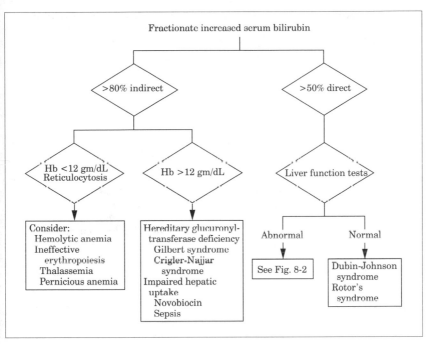

**Fig. 8-1.** Algorithm illustrating work-up for jaundice.

- >4000 indicates toxic injury (e.g., acetaminophen).
- Patient is rarely asymptomatic with level >1000 IU/L.
- AST >10 times normal indicates acute hepatocellular injury but lesser increases are nonspecific and may occur with virtually any other form of liver injury.
- Usually <200 IU/L in posthepatic jaundice and intrahepatic cholestasis.
- <200 IU/L in 20% of patients with acute viral hepatitis.
- Usually <50 IU/L in fatty liver.
- <100 IU/L in alcoholic cirrhosis.
- <150 IU/L in alcoholic hepatitis.
- <200 IU/L in 65% of patients with cirrhosis.
- <200 IU/L in 50% of patients with metastatic liver disease, lymphoma, and leukemia.
- Normal values may not rule out liver disease: ALT is normal in 50%, and AST is normal in 25%, of cases of alcoholic cirrhosis.
- AST soaring to peak of 1000–9000 IU/L, declining by 50% within 3 days and to <100 IU/L within a week suggests shock liver with centrolobular necrosis (e.g., due to congestive heart failure, sepsis, GI hemorrhage); serum bilirubin and ALP reflect underlying disease.
- Rapid rise of AST and ALT to very high levels (e.g., >600 U/L and often >2000 U/L) followed by a sharp fall in 12–72 hrs is said to be typical of acute biliary duct obstruction.
- Abrupt AST rise may also be seen in acute fulminant viral hepatitis (rarely >4000 IU and decline more slowly; positive serologic tests) and acute chemical injury.
- Degree of increase has low prognostic value.
- Serial transaminase determinations reflect clinical activity of liver disease.

**Table 8-1.** Liver Function Test Patterns in Jaundice and Hepatobiliary Disorders

| Disorder | Bilirubin (mg/dL) | AST, ALT (IU/L)* | ALP |
|---|---|---|---|
| Hemolysis | N to 5 mg/dL<br>>85% indirect<br>No bilirubinuria | N | N |
| Gilbert syndrome | N to 5 mg/dL<br>>85% indirect<br>No bilirubinuria | N | N |
| Acute necrosis (e.g., viral, drug, toxic, acute CHF) | Direct and indirect may be I<br>Bilirubinuria | I; often >500; ALT > AST | N to <3 × N |
| Chronic liver disease (e.g., alcoholic hepatitis, cirrhosis) | Direct and indirect may be I<br>Bilirubinuria | I; usually <300; AST:ALT >2 suggests alcoholic etiology | N to <3 × N |
| Intrahepatic cholestasis | Direct and indirect may be I<br>Bilirubinuria | N or I; rarely >500 | I to >3 × N |
| Infiltrative disease (e.g., TB, granuloma, tumor, amyloid) | Usually N | N or sl I | I to >3 × N |
| Partial bile duct obstruction (e.g., biliary stone) | Usually N | N or sl I | I to >3 × N |
| Complete bile duct obstruction (e.g., carcinoma of common bile duct, stone) | I direct; N or sl I indirect<br>≤ 20 due to carcinoma;<br><10 due to stones<br>May increase abruptly due to stones | N or sl I | I to >3 × N |

sl = slightly; CHF = congestive heart failure.
*Increase during preicteric phase of acute viral hepatitis to peak by the time jaundice appears, then rapid decline in several days; usually N 2–5 wks after onset of jaundice.

- Mild increase of AST and ALT (usually <500 IU/L) with ALP increased >3 times normal indicates cholestatic jaundice, but more marked increase of AST and ALT (especially >1000 IU/L) with ALP increased <3 times normal indicates hepatocellular jaundice.

AST:ALT ratio >1 with AST <300 IU/L favors alcoholic hepatitis in cases of liver disease. Increased AST > ALT also occurs in cirrhosis and metastatic liver disease. Increased AST < ALT favors viral hepatitis, posthepatic jaundice, intrahepatic cholestasis. *ALT is more specific for liver disease than AST.*

GGT:ALP ratio >5 favors alcoholic liver disease.

Isolated elevation of GGT is a sensitive screening and monitoring test for alcoholism.

Serum 5'-nucleotidase and LAP parallel the increase in ALP in obstructive type of hepatobiliary disease, but the 5'-nucleotidase is increased only in the latter and is normal in pregnancy and bone disease, whereas the LAP is increased in pregnancy but usually normal in bone disease. GGT is normal in bone disease and pregnancy. Therefore, these enzymes are useful in determining the source of increased serum ALP.

Serum ALP is the best indicator of biliary obstruction.

- But does not differentiate intrahepatic cholestasis from extrahepatic obstruction.
- Increases before jaundice occurs.

- High values (>5 times normal) favor obstruction and normal levels virtually exclude this diagnosis.
- Markedly increased in infants with congenital intrahepatic bile duct atresia but is much lower in extrahepatic atresia.
- Increase (3–10 times normal) with only slightly increased transaminases may be seen in biliary obstruction and converse in liver parenchymal disease (e.g., cirrhosis, hepatitis).
- Increased (2–10 times normal) in early infiltrative (e.g., amyloid) and space-occupying diseases of the liver (e.g., tumor, granuloma, abscess).
- Increased >3 times in 5% of patients with acute hepatitis.

Test for antimitochondrial antibodies to rule out primary biliary cirrhosis in females and radiologic studies to rule out primary sclerosing cholangitis.

Bilirubin (bile) in urine implies increased serum direct bilirubin and excludes hemolysis as the cause. Often precedes or occurs without jaundice.

Complete absence of urine urobilinogen strongly suggests complete bile duct obstruction; normal in incomplete obstruction. Decreased in some phases of hepatic jaundice. Increased in hemolytic jaundice and subsiding hepatitis. Increase may evidence hepatic damage even without clinical jaundice. Presence in viral hepatitis depends on phase of disease. (Normal is <1 mg or 1 Ehrlich unit/2-hr specimen.)

Serum cholesterol
- May be normal or slightly decreased in hepatitis.
- Markedly decreased in severe hepatitis or cirrhosis.
- Increased in posthepatitic jaundice or intrahepatic cholestasis.
- Markedly increased in primary biliary cirrhosis.

PT may be markedly prolonged due to lack of vitamin K absorption in obstruction or lack of synthesis in hepatocellular disease and may herald onset of fulminant hepatic necrosis.
- Corrected by parenteral administration of vitamin K in obstructive but not in hepatocellular disease

Serum gamma globulin tends to increase with most forms of chronic liver disease; marked increases (e.g., >3 gm/dL) are suggestive of chronic active hepatitis.

Serum albumin is slow to reflect liver damage.
- Is usually normal in hepatitis and cholestasis
- Increase toward normal by 2–3 gm/dL in treatment of cirrhosis implies improvement and more favorable prognosis than if no increase with therapy

Some patients do not present the usual pattern.
- Liver function test abnormalities may occur in systemic diseases (e.g., SLE, sarcoidosis, TB, SBE).
- A confusing pattern may occur in mixed forms of jaundice (e.g., sickle-cell disease producing hemolysis and complicated by pigment stones causing duct obstruction).

# Disorders of the Liver, Gallbladder, Biliary Tree, and Pancreas

See Fig. 8-2.

## Hemochromatosis

See Fig. 8-3.

### Due to

Hereditary hemochromatosis (HH) is an autosomal recessive defect in ability of duodenum to regulate iron absorption.

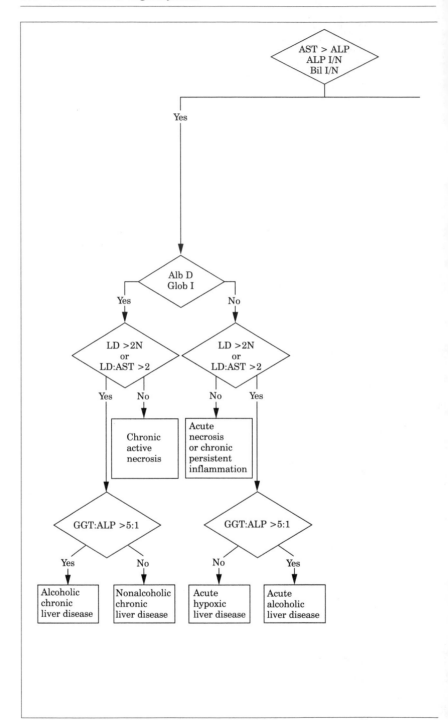

**Fig. 8-2.** Algorithm illustrating sequential abnormal liver function test interpretation. (Bil = bilirubin; Alb = albumin; Glob = globulin; CHF = congestive heart failure. Enzymes all in same U/L.)

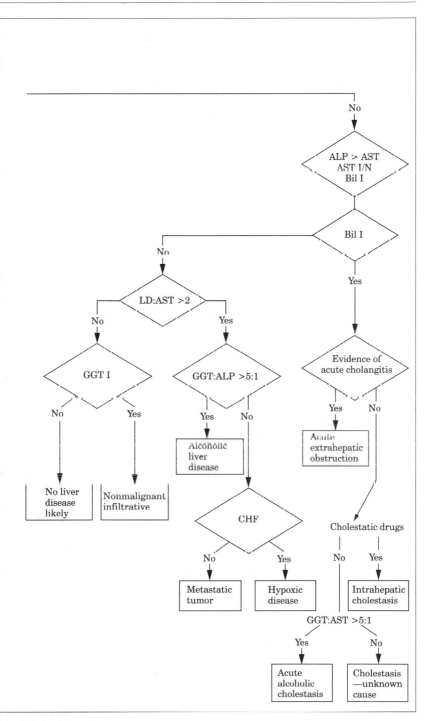

**Fig. 8-2.** (continued)

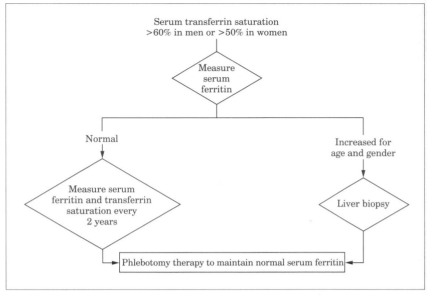

**Fig. 8-3.** Sequence of tests for hemochromatosis screening and treatment.

Secondary
- Increased intake (e.g., excessive medicinal iron ingestion, long-term frequent transfusions)
- Anemias with increased erythropoiesis (especially thalassemias)
- Porphyria cutanea tarda (minor)
- Alcoholic liver disease (minor; deposited in Kupffer's cells, not hepatocytes)
- After portal-systemic shunt
- Congenital atransferrinemia

Best screening method is increased transferrin saturation ([serum iron divided by total iron-binding capacity] × 100); usually >70% and frequently approaches 100%; >62% in fasting men and >50% in women is recommended for screening. 50–62% usually indicates heterozygous state but occasionally found in homozygous persons. Most heterozygous persons have no detectable changes unless there is a secondary cause. An elevated value should be repeated twice at weekly intervals. See Fig. 8-3.

Increased serum ferritin (usually >1000 $\mu$g/L); increased in approximately two-thirds of patients with HH. Is good index of total body iron, but has limited value for screening because it may be increased in acute inflammatory conditions and less sensitive than transferrin saturation in early cases. >5000 $\mu$g/L indicates tissue damage (e.g., liver degeneration) with release of ferritin into circulation.

Serum iron (SI) is increased (usually >200 $\mu$g/dL in women and >300 $\mu$g/dL in men and typically >1000 $\mu$g/dL). *SI may show marked diurnal variation with lowest values in evening and highest between 7 AM and noon.* Confirmed increases of SI, serum ferritin, and transferrin saturation are indication for needle biopsy of liver to confirm or refute diagnosis, grade amount of iron, and assess tissue damage.

TIBC is decreased (~200 $\mu$g/dL; often approaches zero; generally higher in secondary than primary type).

Liver biopsy is needed to confirm the diagnosis. Liver iron is increased (normal 200–2000 $\mu$g/gram in men and 200–1600 in women). >1000 $\mu$g/100 mg of dry liver is consistent with homozygous state but may reach 5000. Some heterozygotes may reach 1000 $\mu g$/100 mg but do not progress beyond this level. Fibrosis or cirrhosis usually does not occur at <2000 $\mu g$/100 mg dry liver unless alcoholism is also present. Liver iron and serum ferritin may also be increased in alcoholic cirrhosis, but levels are not as abnormal (<2 times normal) as in hemochromatosis. Tissue iron must be related to patient age: index in homozygotes $\geq$ 1.9 ([$\mu g$/gm divided by 55.8] × age); in heterozygotes usually $\leq$ 1.5. False negative may be due to phlebotomy treatment; false positive may be due to secondary hemosiderosis.

Presence of excess iron in other tissue biopsy sites (e.g., synovia, GI tract) should arouse suspicion of HH.

Bone marrow biopsy stained for iron is not useful for diagnosis of HH.

Liver function tests depend on presence and degree of liver damage.

Laboratory findings due to involvement of various organs
- Diabetes mellitus in 40–75% of cases.
- Osteoarthritis and chondrocalcinosis (pseudogout) in 50% of cases.
- Cardiomyopathy in 33% of cases.
- Hypogonadism/pituitary dysfunction in ~50% of cases.
- Underlying diseases.
- Increased susceptibility to severe bacterial infection, especially *Yersinia* sepsis.
- Cirrhosis in 69% of cases. Associated alcoholism.
- Hepatocellular carcinoma develops in ~30% of cases and has become the chief cause of death in HH.

When diagnosis of HH established, other family members should be screened.

Adequate treatment with phlebotomy (1–3 U/wk) sufficient to maintain a mild anemia is determined by Hct (37–39%) before each phlebotomy. Serum iron and ferritin are only used to establish whether iron stores are exhausted.

## Hepatitis, Alcoholic

Increased serum GGT and MCV >100 together or separately are useful clues for occult alcoholism.

AST is increased (rarely >300 U/L), but ALT is normal or only slightly increased. AST and ALT are more specific but less sensitive than GGT. AST and ALT do not correlate with severity of liver disease.

AST:ALT ratio >1 associated with AST <300 U/L will identify 90% of patients with alcoholic liver disease; is particularly useful for differentiation from viral hepatitis, in which increase of AST and ALT are about the same.

Cholestasis in $\leq$ 35% of patients.

In acute alcoholic hepatitis, GGT level is usually higher than AST level. GGT is often abnormal in alcoholics, even with normal liver histology. Is more useful as index of occult alcoholism than to follow course of patient for which AST and ALT are most useful.

Serum ALP may be normal or moderately increased in 50% of patients and is not useful as a diagnostic test.

Serum bilirubin may be mildly increased except with cholestasis; is not useful as a diagnostic test.

Decreased serum albumin and increased serum globulin (polyclonal) with disproportionately increased IgA are frequent. Decreased serum albumin means long-standing or relatively severe disease.

Increased PT that is not corrected by parenteral administration of 10 mg/day of vitamin K for 3 days is best indicator of poor prognosis.

Increased WBC (>15,000) in up to one-third of patients with shift to left (WBC is decreased in viral hepatitis); normal WBC may indicate folic acid depletion.

Anemia in >50% of patients may be macrocytic (folic acid or vitamin $B_{12}$ deficiency), microcytic (iron or pyridoxine deficiency), mixed, or hemolytic.

Metabolic alkalosis may occur due to $K^+$ loss with pH normal or increased, but pH <7.2 often indicates disease is becoming terminal.

In terminal stage of chronic alcoholic liver disease, there is often decrease of serum sodium and albumin and increase of PT and serum bilirubin; AST and LD decrease from previously elevated levels.

Liver biopsy should be performed in any alcoholic with enlarged liver; it is the only way to make definite diagnosis of alcoholic hepatitis. Many have normal liver biopsy; others show characteristic alcoholic hyalin.

Compared to nonalcoholics, alcoholics as a group show an increase in some analytes (e.g., AST, phosphorus, ALP, GGT, MCV, MCH, Hb, WBC) and a decrease in others (e.g., TP, BUN); however these variations usually remain within the reference range. These changes may last for >6 wks after abstaining from alcohol.

## Hepatitis, Autoimmune Chronic Active ("Lupoid Hepatitis")

Type I—asymptomatic young woman or girl with icterus or abnormal liver function tests. Hypergammaglobulinemia, positive ANA, and serum smooth muscle antibody tests.

Type II—LD; liver-kidney microsomal (LKM-I) antibodies are present; ANA is absent. ≤ 20% are associated with other autoimmune diseases (e.g., autoimmune thyroid disease, insulin-dependent diabetes mellitus).

Type III—due to various drugs; anti-organelle antibodies that differ from those in types I and II. Generally negative for ANA and LKM antibodies; ≤ 30% have RF, smooth muscle, and other antibodies. Usually resolve in 6–24 months after cessation of drug.

## Hepatitis, Viral, Acute

Only serologic tests can distinguish different types of viral hepatitis.

### Prodromal Period

Serologic markers appear in serum.

Bilirubinuria occurs before serum bilirubin increases.

There is an increase in urinary urobilinogen and total serum bilirubin just before clinical jaundice occurs.

Serum AST and ALT both rise during the preicteric phase and show high peaks (>500 units) by the time jaundice appears.

Leukopenia (lymphopenia and neutropenia) is noted with onset of fever, followed by relative lymphocytosis and monocytosis; may find plasma cells and ≤ 10% atypically lymphocytes.

### Asymptomatic Hepatitis

Biochemical evidence of acute hepatitis is scant and often absent.

### Acute Icteric Period

Serum bilirubin is 50–75% direct in the early stage; later, indirect bilirubin is proportionately more.

Serum AST and ALT fall rapidly in the several days after jaundice appears and become normal 2–5 wks later.

- *In hepatitis associated with infectious mononucleosis*, peak levels are usually <200 units and peak occurs 2–3 wks after onset, becoming normal by week 5.
- *In toxic hepatitis*, levels depend on severity; slight elevations may be associated with therapy with anticoagulants, anovulatory drugs, etc. Poisoning (e.g., carbon tetrachloride) may cause levels ≤ 300 units.
- *In severe toxic hepatitis (especially carbon tetrachloride poisoning)*, serum enzymes may be 10–20 times higher than those in acute hepatitis and show a different pattern (i.e., increase in LD > AST > ALT).

- *In acute hepatitis*, ALT > AST > LD.

Other liver function tests are often abnormal, depending on severity of the disease—bilirubinuria, abnormal serum protein electrophoresis, ALP, etc.

Urine urobilinogen is increased in the early icteric period; at peak of the disease it disappears for days or weeks; urobilinogen simultaneously disappears from stool.

ESR is increased; falls during convalescence.

### Defervescent Period

Diuresis occurs at onset of convalescence.

Bilirubinuria disappears while serum bilirubin is still increased.

Urine urobilinogen increases.

Serum bilirubin becomes normal after 3–6 wks.

ESR decreases.

### Anicteric Hepatitis

Laboratory findings are the same as in the icteric type, but abnormalities are usually less marked and there is slight or no increase of serum bilirubin.

### Acute Fulminant Hepatitis with Hepatic Failure

Findings are the same as in acute hepatitis but more severe (hepatic failure).

Serum bilirubin is very high unless death occurs in the prodromal period. Patient may show anemia, leukocytosis, thrombocytopenia, etc.

Serologic markers are similar in typical cases of acute hepatitis, but seroconversion from HBeAg to HBeAb or from HBsAg to HBsAb is uncommon. As patient deteriorates, titers of HBsAg and HBeAg often fall and disappear.

### Cholangiolitic Hepatitis

Same as acute hepatitis, but evidence of obstruction is more prominent (e.g., increased serum ALP and direct bilirubin), and tests of parenchymal damage are less marked (e.g., AST increase may be 3–6 times normal).

### Chronic Hepatitis

HBV hepatitis is generally divided into three stages:
- Stage of acute hepatitis: usually lasts 1–6 months with mild or no symptoms.
  AST and ALT are increased >10 times.
  Serum bilirubin is usually normal or only slightly increased.
  HBsAg gradually arises to high titers and persists; HBeAg also appears.
- Stage of chronic hepatitis: transaminases increased >50% for >6 months' duration; may last 1 yr or several decades with mild or severe symptoms; most cases resolve, but some develop cirrhosis and liver failure.
  AST and ALT decrease to 2–10 times normal range.
  HBsAg usually remains high, and HBeAg remains present.
- Chronic carrier stage: are usually, but not always, healthy and asymptomatic.
  AST and ALT become normal or <2 times normal.
  HBeAg disappears, and HBeAb appears.
  HBsAg titer falls, although may still be detectable; HBsAb subsequently develops, marking the end of carrier stage.
  HBcAb is usually present in high titer (>1:512).

Laboratory findings due to sequelae
- Glomerulonephritis or nephrotic syndrome due to deposition of HBeAg or HBcAg in glomeruli; often progresses to chronic renal failure.

See Tables 8-2 and 8-3.

## Hepatitis A

See Fig. 8-4.

**Table 8-2.** Comparison of Different Types of Viral Hepatitis

| | A | B | C | D | E |
|---|---|---|---|---|---|
| Genome | RNA | DNA | RNA | RNA | RNA |
| Classification | Picornaviridae | Hepadnaviridae | Flaviviridae | Unclassified | Caliciviridae? |
| Cause of hepatitis (% in United States) | ~30 | ~40 | ~20 | Always associated with HBV; 4% of acute HBV have HDV coinfection | Rare; in travelers to endemic areas |
| Incubation period (days) | 15–60 | 40–160 | 14–180 | 42–180 | 15–64 |
| Transmission | | | | | |
| Enteric | Yes | No | No | No | Yes |
| Sexual | No | Yes | Possible | Possible | Yes |
| Perinatal | No | Yes | Possible | Possible | No |
| Parenteral | Rare | Yes | Yes | Yes | No |
| Post-transfusion incidence (%) | No | 0.002 | 1–4 | Yes | No |
| Viremia | Transient | Prolonged | Prolonged | Prolonged | Transient? |
| Fecal excretion of virus | + | – | – | – | + |

| | | | | | |
|---|---|---|---|---|---|
| Onset | Abrupt | Insidious | Insidious | Abrupt | Abrupt |
| Course | Mild, often subclinical | | | | Mild, self-limited[a] |
| Asymptomatic | Most children | Most children; 50% adults[b] | ~75% | Rare | Often |
| Jaundice | Child: 10% Adult: 70–80% | 15–40%[c] | 10–25% | Varies | 25–50% |
| Fulminant | 1% Causes 5% of fulminant cases | 0.2–2.0% | ~0.5% | High | May cause one-third of fulminant cases with 90% mortality |
| Chronic carrier | No | Adult: 6–10% Child: 25–50% Infant: 70–90% | 50–70% | 10–15% | No |
| Hepatocellular carcinoma | No | Yes | Yes | Yes | No |
| Mortality | 1–2% | 1–2% | 1–2% | ≤ 30% in chronic cases | 1–2%; 20% in pregnancy |

+ = positive; − = negative.

[a]Resembles hepatitis A. Case fatality = 1–2% except ≤ 20% in pregnancy. Usually milder infection and biochemical abnormalities than HBV or HAV infection.

[b]≤ 20% have serum sickness-like prodromata.

[c]Nonicteric patient is more likely to progress to chronic hepatitis. 1% of icteric cases become fulminant ($<8$ wks), and 90% die within 2–4 wks; associated with encephalopathy, renal, electrolyte, acid-base imbalances, hypoglycemia coagulation derangements.

**Table 8-3.** Serologic Markers of Viral Hepatitis

| Stage of Infection | HAV | HBV | HCV | HDV | HEV |
|---|---|---|---|---|---|
| Acute disease | Anti-HAV-IgM | HBcAb-IgM | Anti-HCV | HDAg | Anti-HEV[a] |
| Chronic disease | NA | HBsAg | Anti-HCV | Anti-HDV | NA |
| Infectivity | HAV-RNA[b] | HBeAg, HBsAg, HBV-DNA[c] | Anti-HCV, HCV-RNA | Anti-HDV, HDV-RNA[b] | HEV-RNA[b] |
| Recovery | None | HBeAb, HBsAb | None | None | None |
| Carrier state | NA | HBsAg | None | Anti-HDV, HDAg | NA |
| Immunity screen | Anti-HAV-total (includes anti-HAV-IgG) | HBsAb, HBcAb-total | None | None | Anti-HEV[a] |

Anti-HAV-IgM = antibody to HAV-IgM; HEV = hepatitis E virus; NA = not applicable; HDAg = hepatitis D antigen; anti-HCV = hepatitis C virus antibody; anti-HEV = hepatitis E virus antibody; anti-HDV = hepatitis D antibody.

[a]Not available in United States.
[b]Only available in research laboratories.
[c]Only for investigational use.

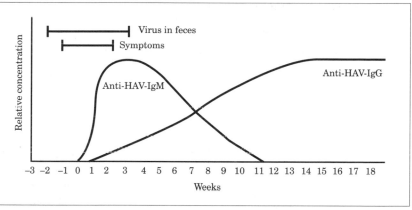

**Fig. 8-4.** Antibody markers in HAV. (anti-HAV-IgM = antibody to hepatitis A virus-IgM; anti-HAV-IgG = antibody to hepatitis A virus-IgG.) (Reproduced with permission of Abbott Laboratories, Pasadena, CA.)

Serum bilirubin usually 5–10 times normal. Jaundice lasts few days to 12 wks. AST and ALT increased to hundreds of units for 1–3 wks.
Relative lymphocytosis is frequent.

### Serologic Tests for Viral Hepatitis A (HAV)

Antibody to HAV-IgM (anti-HAV-IgM) appears at the same time as symptoms and is detectable for 3–24 wks in 80–90% of cases; >6 months in 10–15% of cases. Presence confirms the diagnosis of recent acute infection. Usually order anti-HAV-total and anti-HAV-IgM tests simultaneously; positive anti-HAV-total and negative anti-HAV-IgM indicates anti-HAV-IgG and immunity. Anti-HAV-IgG appears after the acute period and is usually detectable for life; found in 45% of adult population; indicates previous exposure to HAV, recovery, and immunity to type A hepatitis.
Serial testing is usually not indicated.

### Hepatitis B

See Tables 8-2 through 8-8.
Very high serum ALT and bilirubin are not reliable indicators of patient's clinical course, but prolonged PT, especially >20 secs, indicates the likely development of acute hepatic insufficiency; therefore the PT should be performed when patient is first seen. Triad of prolonged PT, increased PMN leukocytes, and nonpalpable liver is omen of massive hepatic necrosis. Acute hepatitis B completely resolves in 90% of patients within 12 wks with disappearance of HBsAg and development of HBsAb. Relapse, usually within 1 yr, recognized in 20% of patients by some elevation of ALT and changes in liver biopsy. ≤ 10% of patients have chronic hepatitis (disease for >6 months and AST and ALT >50% above normal): 70% of these have benign chronic persistent hepatitis and 30% have chronic active hepatitis that can progress to cirrhosis and liver failure. 10% of adult and 90% of perinatal infections become chronic carriers, 25% of whom develop cirrhosis and high risk of hepatoma. HBV carriers should be screened periodically with serum alpha-fetoprotein and ultrasound or CT scan of liver for hepatoma. Effective treatment of chronic HBV hepatitis causes ALT, HBeAg, and HBV-DNA to become normal.

**Table 8-4.** Serologic Test Patterns for HBV

| | | Test | | | | |
|---|---|---|---|---|---|---|
| HBsAg | HBsAb | HBeAg | HBeAb | HBcAb-Total | HBcAb-IgM | Interpretation |
| + | – | – | – | – | – | Late incubation or early acute HBV |
| + | – | + | – | – | – | Early acute HBV; highly infectious |
| + | – | + | – | + | + | Acute HBV |
| + | – | – | + | + | + | "Serologic window/ gap" or acute HBV |
| – | – | – | – | + | + | Serologic gap |
| – | – | – | + | + | + | Convalescence |
| – | + | – | + | + | + | Early recovery |
| – | + | – | + | + | – | Recovery[a] |
| + | – | ± | ± | + | – | Chronic infection (chronic carrier)[a] |
| – | + | – | – | – | – | Old previous HBV with recovery and immunity or HBV vaccination or passive transfer antibody[b] |
| – | – | – | – | – | – | Not HBV infection |

+ = positive; – = negative.
[a]Chronic carriers of HBV may have clinical hepatitis due to non-A, non-B hepatitis rather than HBV.
[b]Various serologic patterns may occur after blood transfusion or injection of immune (gamma) globulin by passive transfer. Anti-HBs can be found for up to 6–8 months after injection of high-titer HB immunoglobulin because of 25-day half-life.

**Table 8-5.** Serologic Test Patterns for HBV Infection Follow-Up

| | Test | | | | |
|---|---|---|---|---|---|
| HBsAg | HBsAb | HBeAg | HBeAb | Interpretation | Follow-Up |
| + | – | – | – | Acute HBV infection | Repeat serology for resolution or chronicity. Serum ALT to monitor disease activity. |
| + | – | + | – | Early acute HBV infection; highly infectious | Repeat serology for resolution or chronicity. Serum ALT to monitor disease activity. |
| + | – | + | + | Decreasing infectivity | Repeat serology for resolution. Serum ALT to monitor disease activity. |
| + | – | – | + | Early seroconversion; HBsAb not yet detected | Repeat for HBsAb and disappearance of HBsAg. |
| – | + | – | + | Recovery; immune | None needed for HBV. |
| – | – | – | – | No evidence of prior HBV infection | Test for other cause of hepatitis. |

+ = positive; – = negative.

**Table 8-6.** Serologic Test Patterns for Prenatal Screening for HBV

| Test | | | Interpretation | Follow-Up |
|---|---|---|---|---|
| HBsAg | HBeAg | HBsAb | | |
| – | – | + | Mother is HBV immune. | Not needed. |
| – | – | – | No evidence of HBV infection. | Not needed unless other evidence of hepatitis. |
| + | + | – | Mother is HBV carrier. Infant at high risk of acquiring HBV infection during delivery and developing chronic hepatitis. | Infant must be vaccinated within 12 hrs of birth. |
| + | – | – | Mother is HBV carrier. Infant at high risk of acquiring HBV infection during delivery and developing chronic hepatitis. | Infant must be vaccinated within 12 hrs of birth. |

+ = positive; – = negative.

**Table 8-7.** Serologic Test Patterns for Candidate for HBV Vaccination

| Test | | | Interpretation | Follow-Up |
|---|---|---|---|---|
| HBsAg | HBsAb | HBcAb | | |
| + | – | – | Acute HBV infection | |
| – | – | + | Acute HBV or carrier | Previous HBV infection; vaccinate |
| – | + | + | Immune; previous HBV infection or vaccination | None |
| + | – | + | Previous HBV infection; may not be immune | Vaccinate |
| – | – | – | Not immune | Vaccinate |

+ = positive; – = negative.

**Table 8-8.** Serologic Tests for HBV Vaccination Follow-Up

| HBsAb | Interpretation | Follow-Up |
|---|---|---|
| + | Effective immunization | Repeat in future years to ensure immunity |
| – | No evidence of immunity | Await appearance of HBsAb or repeat vaccination |

+ = positive; – = negative.

### Serologic Tests for HBV

See Figs. 8-5 and 8-6.

### Use

Differential diagnosis of hepatitis
Screening of blood and organ donors
Determine immune status for possible vaccination

### Hepatitis B Surface Antigen

Earliest indicator of HBV infection. Usually appears in 27–41 days (as early as 14 days). Appears 7–26 days before biochemical abnormalities. Peaks as ALT rises. Persists during the acute illness. Usually disappears 1–13 wks after onset of laboratory abnormalities in 90% of cases. Is the most reliable serologic marker of HBV infection. Persistence >6 months defines carrier state. May also be found in chronic infection. Hepatitis B vaccination does not cause a positive HBsAg. Titers are not of clinical value. Is never detected in some patients in whom diagnosis is based on presence of HBc-IgM.

### Antibody to HBsAg (Anti-HBsAg)

Indicates clinical recovery and immunity to HBV. May also occur after transfusion by passive transfer. Found in 80% of patients after clinical cure. Appearance may take several weeks or months after HBsAg has disappeared and after ALT has returned to normal, causing a "serologic gap" during which (usually 2–6 wks "window") only IgM-anti-HBsAg can identify patients who are recovering but may still be infectious.

In fulminant hepatitis—antibody is produced early and may coexist with low antigen titer.

In chronic carriers—no antibody is present but antigen titers are very high.

Presence of antibody (titer ≥ 10 mIU/mL) (without HBsAg detectable) indicates recovery from HBV infection, absence of infectivity, immunity from future HBV infection and does not need gamma globulin administration if exposed to infection; this blood can be transfused.

Can be used to show efficiency of immunization program. Appears in ~90% of healthy adults after three-dose immunization; 15% of these lose antibodies in 5 yrs and require boosters.

### Hepatitis Be Antigen

Indicates highly infectious state. Appears within 1 wk after HBsAg; in acute cases disappears before disappearance of HBsAg; is found only with HBsAg. Occurs early in disease before biochemical changes. Usually lasts 3–6 wks.

Useful to determine resolution of infection. Persistence >10 wks suggests progression to chronic carrier state and possible chronic hepatitis.

Presence in HBsAg-positive mothers indicates 90% chance of infant acquiring HBV infection.

### Antibody to HBe

Indicates decreasing infectivity, suggesting good prognosis for resolution of acute infection. Association with HBcAb in absence of HBsAg and HBsAb confirms recent acute infection (2–16 wks).

### Antibody to Core Antigen-Total

Occurs early in acute infection, 4–10 wks after appearance of HBsAg, at same time as clinical illness; persists for years or for lifetime.

The earliest specific HBcAb is IgM. This HBcAb-IgM is found in high titer for a short time during the acute disease stage that covers the serologic window and then declines to low levels during recovery. May be the only serologic marker present after HBsAg and HBeAg have subsided but before these antibodies have appeared ("serologic gap" or "window"). Because this is the only test unique to recent infection, it can differentiate acute from chronic HBV.

HBcAb detects persons who have been previously infected with HBV.

### HBV-DNA

Is the most sensitive and specific assay now available for early evaluation of HBV and may be detected when all other markers are negative. For investigational use only at present.

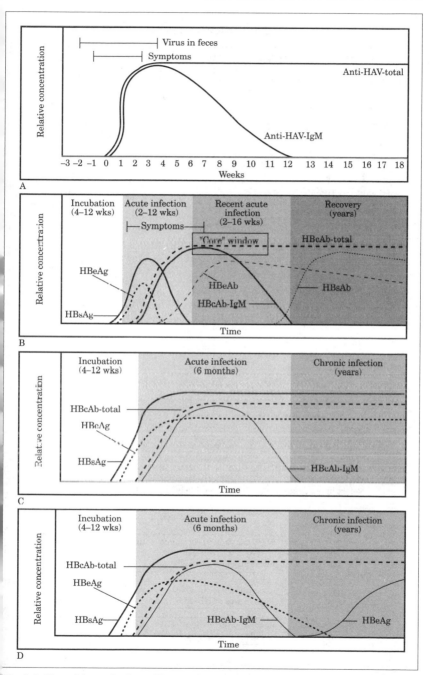

**Fig. 8-5.** Hepatitis serologic profiles. A. Antibody response to hepatitis A. B. Hepatitis B core window identification. C, D. Hepatitis B chronic carrier profiles: no seroconversion (C); late seroconversion (D). (anti-HAV-total = total hepatitis A virus antibody; anti-HAV-IgM = antibody to hepatitis A virus-IgM.) (Reproduced with permission of Hepatitis Information Center, Abbott Laboratories, Abbott Park, IL.)

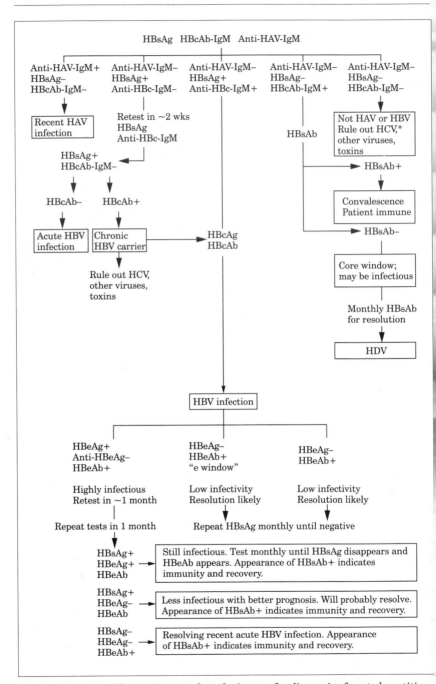

**Fig. 8-6.** Algorithm illustrating use of serologic tests for diagnosis of acute hepatitis. *Do hepatitis C virus antibody. (anti-HAV-IgM = antibody to hepatitis A virus-IgM; + = positive; − = negative.)

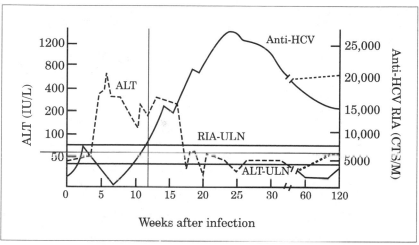

**Fig. 8-7.** Comparison of serum ALT and hepatitis C virus antibody (anti-HCV) findings in acute hepatitis C. Chronic infection is indicated by broken lines.

## Hepatitis C (Formerly Non-A, Non-B Hepatitis [NANB])

See Fig. 8-7.

>50% of acute cases become chronic carriers with or without abnormal ALT values (average time = 10 yrs), 20% of whom develop cirrhosis (average time = 20 yrs). Hepatocellular carcinoma may occur in cirrhosis (average time = 30 yrs). Can remain infectious for years.

Transaminases characteristically show waxing and waning pattern returning to almost normal levels; is highly suggestive but only occurs in 25% of cases. Patients with monophasic transaminase response usually recover completely with no biopsy evidence of residual disease. ALT is usually <800 IU. May have severe liver disease seen on biopsy with normal ALT. Serum ALT is primary marker to monitor therapy. Anicteric patients with ALT >300 IU/L are at high risk for progressing to chronic hepatitis. In chronic disease, >50% remit spontaneously within 3 yrs; death is rare due to chronic disease. Appreciable risk for development of hepatocellular carcinoma; mean time = 20 yrs.

May be associated with essential mixed cryoglobulinemia, membranoproliferative glomerulonephritis, and porphyria cutanea tarda, which should be ruled out in cases of hepatitis C and HCV infection should be ruled out in patients with those disorders.

### Antibody to Hepatitis C Virus (Anti-HCV)

#### Use

Testing persons with clinical or laboratory evidence of hepatitis, especially
- IV drug users
- Transfusion/transplant recipients
- Individuals sustaining needle-stick injuries
- Dialysis patients
- Health care workers and others frequently exposed to blood products
- Individuals who have had intimate or sexual exposure to hepatitis patients
- Individuals with multiple sexual partners
- Infants of infected mothers

#### Interpretation

Anti-HCV reflects active viral replication and infectivity of host rather than immunity (in contrast to HBsAb and HBeAb in HBV infection). Therefore, should consider patient positive for HCVAb infection until proven otherwise. Virus has not been cultured. May be positive in acute or chronic hepatitis C, possible HCV carrier, or past HCV exposure (infection).

Sensitivity is only ~80% in chronic carriers; ~15% for first 6 months following acute HCV infection. Is not seen until 2–6 months after infection or 2–3 months after increase in ALT, so serial specimens (as well as ALT) for up to 1 yr after suspected acute hepatitis may be needed for diagnosis. Does not distinguish between IgG and IgM antibody.

Present in 70–85% of cases of chronic post-transfusion NANB hepatitis but is relatively infrequent in acute cases. Present in 70% of IV drug abusers, 20% of hemodialysis patients, and only 8% of homosexual men positive for HIV.

Surrogate markers fail to detect one-third to one-half of blood units positive for anti-HCV. Is considered chronic only with evidence of activity >12 months.

No tests are presently routinely available for other NANB viruses.

See Fig. 8-5.

## Interferences

False positive
- Autoimmune diseases (≤ 80% of cases of autoimmune chronic active hepatitis).
- RF.
- Hypergammaglobulinemia.
- Paraproteinemia.
- Passive antibody transfer.
- Anti-idiotypes.
- Repeat freezing and thawing or prolonged storage of blood specimens.
- Due to shortcomings in HCV-ELISA, recombinant immunoblot assay (RIBA II) has been used as supplementary test to document HCV infection and help delineate course. Detection of HCV-RNA by PCR is used to confirm RIBA and to monitor clearance of virus after interferon therapy. ELISA and RIBA are also found in polyarteritis nodosa (~10%) and SLE (~2%).

False negative
- Early acute infection
- Immunosuppression
- Immunoincompetence
- Repeat freezing and thawing or prolonged storage of blood specimens

### HCV-RNA Assay

#### Use

Monitors viral replication in liver. Absence after therapy is associated with remission. Patients with low pretreatment level are most likely to respond to interferon alfa therapy.

## Hepatitis D (Delta)

See Tables 8-9 and 8-10.

Due to a transmissible virus (HDV) that depends on HBV for replication. It consists of hepatitis D antigen (HDAg) within external coat of HBsAg. It may be found for 7–14 days in the serum during acute infection. Can be an important cause of acute or chronic hepatitis. Is often severe with relatively high mortality in acute disease and frequent development of cirrhosis in chronic disease. Chronic HDV infection is more severe and has higher mortality than other types of viral hepatitis.

*Coinfection* means simultaneous acute HBV and acute HDV infection. Usually causes acute limited illness with additive liver damage due to each virus followed by recovery. Usually is self-limited; <5% become chronic, ~3% have fulminant course.

### Serologic Tests for HDV

See Tables 8-9 and 8-10.

**Table 8-9.** Comparison of Types of HDV Infections

|  | Coinfection | Superinfection | Chronic HDV |
|---|---|---|---|
| HBV infection | Acute | Chronic | Chronic |
| HDV infection | Acute | Acute to chronic | Chronic |
| Chronicity rate | <5% | >75% | Cirrhosis in >70% |
| Serology |  |  |  |
|   HBsAg | + | Usually persistent | Persistent |
|   HBcAb-IgM | + | Negative | Negative |
|   Anti-HDV-total | Negative or low titer | + | + |
|   Anti-HDV-IgM* | Transient + | Transient | High titer |
|   HDV-RNA (HDAg) | Transient + | Usually persistent | Persistent |
| Liver HDAg | Transient + | Usually persistent | Persistent |

HDAg = hepatitis D antigen; anti-HDV-total = total hepatitis D antibody; anti-HDV-IgM = antibody to hepatitis D-IgM; + = positive.
*Decrease in anti-HDV-IgM usually predicts resolution of acute HDV. Persistent anti-HDV-IgM typically predicts progression to chronic HDV infection. High titer correlates with active liver inflammation.

**Table 8-10.** Serologic Diagnosis of HBV/HDV Hepatitis

|  | Test |  |  |  |
|---|---|---|---|---|
| HB$_s$Ag | HBcAb-IgM | Anti-HDV-IgM | Anti-HDV-IgG | Interpretation |
| Transient + | + High titer | Transient + | Transient low titer | Acute HBV and acute HDV[a] |
| Transient decrease due to inhibitory effect of HDV on HBV synthesis | Negative or low titers | High titer first, low titer later | Increasing titers | Acute HDV and chronic HBV[b] |
| May remain + in chronic HBV | Replaced by HBcAb-IgG in chronic HBV | + correlates with HDAg in hepatocytes | High titers correlate with active infection; may remain + for years after infection resolves | Chronic HDV and chronic HBV[c] |

HDAg = hepatitis D antigen; anti-HDV-IgM = antibody to hepatitis D-IgM; anti-HDV-IgG = antibody to hepatitis D-IgG; + = positive.
[a]Clinically resembles acute viral hepatitis; fulminant hepatitis is rare, and progression to chronic hepatitis is unlikely. If HBV does not resolve, HDV can continue to replicate indefinitely.
[b]Clinically resembles exacerbation of chronic liver disease or of fulminant hepatitis with liver failure.
[c]Clinically resembles chronic liver disease progressing to cirrhosis.

Serum HDAg and HDV-RNA appear during incubation period after HBsAg and before rise in AST, which often shows a biphasic elevation. HBsAg and HDAg are transient; HDAg resolves with clearance of HBsAg. Anti-HDV appears soon after clinical symptoms but titer is often low and short-lived.

*Superinfection* means acute HDV infection in a chronic HBV carrier. Mortality = 2–20%; >80% develop chronic hepatitis. Serum anti-HDV appears and rises to high sustained titers, indicating continuing replication of HDV; intrahepatic HDAg is present. HDV-RNA persists in low titers.

Diagnosis of HDV hepatitis is made by presence of anti-HDV in patient with HBsAg-positive hepatitis.

Acute coinfection is distinguished from superinfection by presence of serum HBsAg and HBcAb-IgM, which indicate acute HBV.

Chronic HDV infection occurs in ≤ 80% of acute cases; shows presence of HBsAg and high titer of anti-HDV (>1:100 suggests chronic HDV hepatitis) and absence of HBcAb-IgM in serum.

Confirm by liver biopsy showing HDAg by immunofluorescence or immunoperoxidase.

Serum anti-HDV-IgM documents acute HDV infection; low levels will remain in persistent infection. Western blot can demonstrate serum HDVAg when radioimmunoassay is negative. Persistence correlates with development of chronic HDV hepatitis and viral antigen in liver biopsy.

DNA probe for HDV-RNA in serum to monitor HDV replication.

Serum anti-HDV may be sought in patients with HBsAg-positive hepatitis in high-risk group or with severe disease, or with biphasic acute hepatitis or acute onset in chronic hepatitis.

## Hepatitis E

Serologic markers for hepatitis A, B, and C and other causes of acute hepatitis are absent.

Antibody to hepatitis E can be detected.

## Hepatitis G

Flavivirus similar to HCV. Can cause acute or chronic hepatitis. Active infection can persist for years.

Compared to HCV infection, is milder, less frequently chronic.

Serum ALT is often persistently normal.

Hepatitis G virus and HCV can be transmitted simultaneously in blood transfusion and cause persistent coinfection.

Prevalence in blood donors is higher than that of HCV and unrelated to ALT status of donor.

Serologic assays under development.

## Gallbladder and Bile Ducts, Cancer of

Laboratory findings reflect varying location and extent of tumor infiltration that may cause partial intrahepatic duct obstruction or obstruction of hepatic or common bile duct, metastases in liver, or associated cholangitis; 50% of patients have jaundice at the time of hospitalization.

Laboratory findings of duct obstruction are of progressively increasing severity in contrast to the intermittent or fluctuating changes due to duct obstruction caused by stones.

Stool is frequently positive for occult blood.

Cytologic examination of aspirated duodenal fluid may demonstrate malignant cells.

## Cholangitis, Acute

Marked increase in WBC (≤ 30,000/cu mm) with increase in granulocytes

Blood culture positive in ~30% of cases; 25% of these are polymicrobial.

Laboratory findings of incomplete duct obstruction due to inflammation or of preceding complete duct obstruction (e.g., stone, tumor, scar).

Laboratory findings of parenchymal cell necrosis and malfunction
- Increased serum AST, ALT, etc.
- Increased urine urobilinogen.

## Cholangitis, Primary Sclerosing

Chronic fibrosing inflammation of intrahepatic and extrahepatic bile ducts; slow, relentless, progressive chronic cholestasis to liver failure. 25% of patients are asymptomatic at time of diagnosis. Diagnosis should not be made if previous bile duct surgery, gallstones, suppurative cholangitis, bile duct tumor or damage due to floxuridine, AIDS, congenital duct anomalies. Characteristic cholangiogram is required for diagnosis to distinguish from primary biliary cirrhosis.
Cholestatic biochemical profile for >6 months
- Serum ALP may fluctuate but is always increased >1.5 times ULN (usually ≥ 3 times ULN).
- Serum GGT is increased.
- AST is mildly increased in >90%. ALT > AST in three-fourths of cases.
- Bilirubin is increased in one-half of patients; occasionally is very high; may fluctuate markedly; gradually increases as disease progresses. Persistent value >1.5 mg/dL is poor prognostic sign that may indicate irreversible, medically untreatable disease.

Increased gamma globulin in 30% and increased IgM in 40–50% of cases
Anti-neutrophil cytoplasmic in ~65% and ANA in <35% of cases are present at higher levels than in other liver diseases but diagnostic significance is not yet known.
In contrast to primary biliary cirrhosis, antimitochondrial antibody, smooth-muscle antibody, RF, ANA are negative in >90% of patients. HBsAg is negative.
Liver biopsy provides only confirmatory evidence in patients with compatible history, laboratory and x-ray findings.
Liver copper is usually increased, but serum ceruloplasmin is also increased.
Laboratory findings due to sequelae
- Cholangiocarcinoma in 10–15% of patients
- Portal hypertension, biliary cirrhosis, secondary bacterial cholangitis, steatorrhea and malabsorption, cholelithiasis, liver failure
- Associated with syndrome of retroperitoneal and mediastinal fibrosis

## Cholecystitis, Acute

Increased ESR, WBC (average 12,000/cu mm; if >15,000, suspect empyema or perforation)
Increased serum bilirubin in 20% of patients (if >4 mg/dL, suspect associated choledocholithiasis)
Increased serum ALP even if serum bilirubin is normal
Increased serum amylase and lipase
*Serum AST is increased in 75% of patients.*

## Cholestasis

Increased serum ALP, GGT, and serum cholesterol but not triglycerides
*Cholestasis may occur without hyperbilirubinemia.*

## Cirrhosis of Liver

Criteria for diagnosis by liver biopsy or ≥ 3 of the following:
- Hyperglobulinemia, especially with hypoalbuminemia.
- Low-protein (<2.5 g/dL) ascites.
- Evidence of hypersplenism.
- Evidence of portal hypertension.
- Characteristic "corkscrew" hepatic arterioles on celiac arteriography.

- Shunting of blood to bone marrow on radioisotope scan.
- *Abnormality of serum bilirubin, transaminases, or ALP is often not present and therefore not required for diagnosis.*

Serum bilirubin is often increased; may be present for years. Fluctuations may reflect liver status due to insults to the liver (e.g., alcoholic debauches). Most bilirubin is of the indirect type unless cirrhosis is of the cholangiolitic type. Higher and more stable levels occur in postnecrotic cirrhosis; lower and more fluctuating levels occur in Laënnec's cirrhosis. Terminal icterus may be constant and severe.

Serum AST is increased (<300 units) in 65–75% of patients. Serum ALT is increased (<200 units) in 50% of patients. Transaminases vary widely and reflect activity of the process.

Serum ALP is increased in 40–50% of patients.

Total serum protein is usually normal or decreased. Serum albumin parallels functional status of parenchymal cells and may be useful for following progress of liver disease; may be normal in the presence of considerable liver cell damage. Serum globulin level is usually increased; it reflects inflammation and parallels the severity of the inflammation. Increased serum globulin (usually gamma) may cause increased total protein, especially in chronic (viral) hepatitis and posthepatitic cirrhosis.

Total serum cholesterol is normal or decreased.

Urine bilirubin is increased; urobilinogen is normal or increased.

BUN is often decreased (<10 mg/dL).

Serum uric acid is often increased.

Electrolytes and acid-base balance are often abnormal and reflect various combinations of circumstances at the time.

Blood ammonia level is increased in liver coma and cirrhosis and with portacaval shunting of blood.

Anemia reflects increased plasma volume and some increased destruction of RBCs. If more severe, rule out hemorrhage in GI tract, folic acid deficiency, excessive hemolysis, etc.

WBC is usually normal with active cirrhosis; increased (<50,000/cu mm) with massive necrosis, hemorrhage, etc.; decreased with hypersplenism.

Abnormalities of coagulation
- Prolonged PT
- Prolonged BT in 40% of cases

Hepatorenal syndrome

## Cirrhosis, Primary Biliary (PBC) (Cholangiolitic Cirrhosis, Hanot's Hypertrophic Cirrhosis, Chronic Nonsuppurative Destructive Cholangitis)

(**multisystem autoimmune disease; chronic inflammation and destruction of small intrahepatic bile ducts producing chronic cholestasis and cirrhosis**)

### Diagnostic Criteria

Laboratory findings of cholestatic pattern of long duration (may last for years) not due to known cause (e.g., drugs)
- Antimitochondrial antibodies present.
- Confirmed patency of bile ducts (e.g., with ultrasound or CT scan).
- Compatible liver biopsy is highly desirable.

Serum bilirubin is normal in early phase but increases in 60% of patients with progression of disease and is a reliable prognostic indicator. Direct serum bilirubin is increased in 80% of patients; levels >5 mg/dL in only 20% of patients; levels >10 mg/dL in only 6% of patients. Indirect bilirubin is normal or slightly increased.

Serum ALP is markedly increased. Reaches a plateau early in the course and then fluctuates within 20% thereafter; changes have no prognostic value. GGT parallels the ALP. *This is one of the few conditions that will elevate both serum ALP and GGT to striking levels.*

Serum IgM is increased in ~75% of patients; may be very high (4–5 times normal). Other serum immunoglobulins are also increased.

Serum mitochondrial antibody titer is strongly positive in 90–95% of patients (1:40–1:80) and is hallmark of disease; titer >1:40 strongly suggests PBC even in absence of symptoms or laboratory abnormalities. Similar titers occur in 5% of patients with chronic hepatitis; low titers occur in 10% of patients with other liver disease. Many other circulating antibodies are present (e.g., ANA, antithyroid) although not useful diagnostically.

Biopsy of liver categorizes the four stages and helps assess prognosis but needle biopsy is subject to sampling error; findings consistent with all four stages may be found in one specimen.

Marked increase in total cholesterol and phospholipids with normal triglycerides; serum triglycerides become elevated in late stages.

Laboratory findings show relatively little evidence of parenchymal damage.
- AST and ALT may be normal or slightly increased (up to 1–5 times normal) and fluctuate within a narrow range and have no prognostic significance.
- Serum albumin, globulin, and PT normal early.

Serum ceruloplasmin is characteristically elevated (in contrast to Wilson's disease) and liver copper may be increased 10–100 times normal.

ESR is increased 1–5 times normal in 80% of patients.

Laboratory findings due to associated diseases
- >80% have one and >40% have at least two other autoimmune diseases (e.g., RA, thyroiditis, Sjögren's syndrome, scleroderma).

*Should be ruled out in an asymptomatic female with elevated serum ALP without obesity, diabetes mellitus, alcohol abuse, some drugs.*

## Biliary Atresia, Congenital Extrahepatic

Direct serum bilirubin increased in early days of life in some infants but not until week 2 in others. Is often <12 mg/dL during first months, with subsequent rise later in life.

Laboratory findings as in complete biliary obstruction

Liver biopsy to differentiate from neonatal hepatitis. Most important to differentiate this condition from neonatal hepatitis for which surgery may be harmful.

Laboratory findings due to sequelae (e.g., biliary cirrhosis, portal hypertension, frequent infections, rickets, hepatic failure)

>90% of cases of extrahepatic biliary obstruction in newborns are due to biliary atresia; occasional cases may be due to choledochal cyst, bile plug syndrome, or bile ascites.

## Liver Function Abnormalities in Congestive Heart Failure

Pattern of abnormal liver function tests is variable depending on severity of heart failure; the mildest show only slightly increased ALP and slightly decreased serum albumin; moderately severe also show slightly increased serum bilirubin and GGT; one-fourth to three-fourths of the most severe will also show increased AST and ALT (up to ≤ 200 U/L) and LD (up to ≤ 400 U/L). All will return to normal when heart failure responds to treatment. Serum ALP is usually the last to become normal, and this may be weeks to months later.

Serum bilirubin is frequently increased (indirect more than direct); usually 1–5 mg/dL.

AST and ALT are disproportionately increased compared with other liver function tests.

Increased LD (mild to moderate)

*These findings may occur with marked liver congestion due to other conditions (e.g., Chiari's syndrome [occlusion of hepatic veins] and constrictive pericarditis).*

## Dubin-Johnson Syndrome (Sprinz-Nelson Disease)
**(Autosomal recessive disease due to inability to transport bilirubin-glucuronide through hepatocytes into canaliculi, but conjugation of bilirubin-glucuronide is normal.)**

Serum direct bilirubin is increased (3–10 mg/dL); rarely ≤ 30 mg/dL; mild, chronic, recurrent.

Urine contains bile and urobilinogen.

Bromsulphalein excretion is impaired with late (1½- to 2-hr) increase.

Other liver function tests are normal.

Liver biopsy shows large amounts of yellow-brown or slate-black pigment in centrolobular hepatic cells (lysosomes) and small amounts in Kupffer's cells.

## Fatty Liver

Biopsy of liver establishes the diagnosis.

Liver function tests are normal in >50% of patients; may show abnormalities of one or several tests, especially serum ALP.

Cirrhosis occurs in ≤ 25% of chronically obese females.

A biochemically different form occurs in acute fatty liver of pregnancy, Reye's syndrome, and tetracycline administration.

## Fatty Liver of Pregnancy, Acute

Often associated with toxemia

Increased AST and ALT to ~300 units (rarely >500 units) is used for early screening in suspicious cases; ratio is not helpful in differential diagnosis.

Increased WBC in >80% of cases (often >15,000/cu mm)

Evidence of DIC

Serum uric acid is increased disproportionately to BUN and creatinine, which may also be increased.

Serum bilirubin may be normal early but will rise unless pregnancy terminates.

Blood glucose is often decreased, sometimes markedly.

## Gilbert Syndrome (Unconjugated Hyperbilirubinemia without Overt Hemolysis)
**(Chronic, benign, familial [autosomal dominant with incomplete penetrance], nonhemolytic unconjugated hyperbilirubinemia with an evanescent increase of indirect serum bilirubin due to defective uptake, transportation, and conjugation of unconjugated bilirubin.)**

Indirect serum bilirubin is increased but had been previously normal at least once in ≤ 33% of patients. It may rise to 18 mg/dL but usually is <4 mg/dL. Fasting (<400 calories/day) for 72 hrs causes elevated indirect bilirubin to increase >100% in Gilbert syndrome but not in healthy persons (increase <0.5 mg/dL) or those with liver disease or hemolytic anemia. Combination of basal total bilirubin >1.2 mg/dL, and fasting increase of unconjugated bilirubin >1 mg/dL has good sensitivity and specificity.

Liver function tests are usually normal.

## Liver Abscess

Gram's stain and culture
- Gram-negative bacilli (e.g., *Escherichia coli*, *Klebsiella* spp.).
- Anaerobes (e.g., *Bacteroides fragilis*).
- *Staphylococcus aureus* or streptococci are found in children with bacteremia.

Abnormalities of liver function tests (e.g., space-occupying lesions)
- Decreased serum albumin in 50% of cases; increased serum globulin.

- Increased serum ALP in 75% of cases.
- Increased serum bilirubin in 20–25% of cases; >10 mg/dL usually indicates pyogenic rather than amebic and suggests poorer prognosis because of more tissue destruction.

Increase in WBC due to increase in granulocytes

Anemia

Ascites is unusual compared to other causes of space-occupying lesions.

Patients with amebic abscess of liver due to *Entamoeba histolytica* also show positive serologic tests for ameba.

- Stools may be negative for cysts and trophozoites.
- Needle aspiration of abscess may show *E. histolytica* in 50% of patients.
  *Characteristic brown or anchovy-sauce color may be absent; secondary bacterial infection may be superimposed.*

## Neonatal Hyperbilirubinemia, Differential Diagnosis

Unconjugated hyperbilirubinemia is serum level >1.5 mg/dL. Conjugated hyperbilirubinemia (direct-reacting) serum level >1.5 mg/dL when this fraction is >10% of total serum bilirubin (because newborn with marked increase of unconjugated bilirubin level, up to 10% of the unconjugated bilirubin will act as direct reacting).

Mixed hyperbilirubinemia shows conjugated bilirubin as 20–70% of total and usually represents disorder of hepatic cell excretion or bile transport.

Visible icterus before 36 hrs old indicates hemolytic disorder.

Diagnostic studies should be performed whenever serum bilirubin >12 mg/dL.

After hemolytic disease and hepatitis, the most frequent cause of hyperbilirubinemia is enterohepatic circulation of bilirubin.

Visible icterus persisting after day 7 is usually due to impaired hepatic excretion, most commonly due to breast milk feeding or congenital hypothyroidism.

Increase in direct bilirubin usually indicates infection or inflammation of liver, but can also be seen in galactosemia and tyrosinosis.

## Neonatal Physiologic Hyperbilirubinemia
(Transient unconjugated hyperbilirubinemia ["physiologic jaundice"] that occurs in almost all newborns.)

In normal full-term neonate, average maximum serum bilirubin is 6 mg/dL (up to 12 mg/dL is in physiologic range) occurs during days 2–4 and then rapidly falls to about 2.0 mg/dL by day 5 (phase I physiologic jaundice). Declines slowly to <1.0 mg/dL during days 5–10, but may take 1 month to fall to <2 mg/dL (phase II physiologic jaundice). Phase I due to deficiency of hepatic bilirubin glucuronyl transferase activity and 6 times increase in bilirubin load presented to liver. Serum bilirubin >5 mg/dL during first 24 hrs of life is indication for further work-up because of risk of kernicterus.

*In newborns, clinical icterus is not apparent until serum bilirubin is >5–7 mg/dL; therefore only half of the full-term newborns show clinical jaundice during first 3 days of life.*

In premature infants—average maximum serum bilirubin is 10–12 mg/dL and occurs during days 5–7. Serum bilirubin may not fall to normal until day 30. Further work-up is indicated in all premature infants with clinical jaundice because of risk of kernicterus in some low-birth-weight infants with serum levels of 10–12 mg/dL.

In postmature infants and half of small-for-dates infants, serum bilirubin is <2.5 mg/dL and physiologic jaundice is not seen.

*When a pregnant woman has unconjugated hyperbilirubinemia, similar levels occur in cord blood, but when the mother has conjugated hyperbilirubinemia (e.g., hepatitis), similar levels are not present in cord blood.*

Cause should be sought for underlying pathologic jaundice if

- Total serum bilirubin >7 mg/dL during first 24 hrs or increases >5 mg/dL/day or visible jaundice

- Peak total serum bilirubin >12.5 mg/dL in white or black full-term or >15 mg/dL in Hispanic or premature infants
- Direct serum bilirubin >1.5 mg/dL
- Clinical jaundice longer than 7 days in full-term or 14 days in premature infants or before age 36 hrs or with dark urine (containing bile)

## Obstruction, Complete Biliary (Intrahepatic or Extrahepatic)

Typical pattern of extrahepatic obstruction includes increased serum ALP (>2–3 times normal), AST <300 U/L, increased direct serum bilirubin.

In extrahepatic type, the increase in ALT is related to the completeness of obstruction. Normal ALP is extremely rare in extrahepatic obstruction. Very high levels may also occur in cases of intrahepatic cholestasis.

AST is increased (≤ 300 units), and ALT is increased (≤ 200 units); they usually become normal 1 wk after relief of obstruction. In *acute* biliary duct obstruction (e.g., due to common bile duct stones), AST and ALT are increased >300 IU (and often >2000 IU) and decline 58–76% in 72 hrs without treatment; simultaneous serum total bilirubin shows less marked increase and decline; ALP changes are inconsistent and unpredictable.

Direct serum bilirubin is increased; indirect serum bilirubin is normal or slightly increased.

Serum cholesterol is increased (acute, 300–400 mg/dL; chronic, ≤ 1000 mg/dL).

PT is prolonged.

Urine bilirubin is increased; urine urobilinogen decreased.

There is decreased stool bilirubin and urobilinogen (clay-colored stools).

## Obstruction of One Hepatic Bile Duct

Characteristic pattern is serum bilirubin that remains normal in the presence of markedly increased serum ALT.

## Rotor's Syndrome
### (autosomal recessive benign defective uptake and storage of conjugated bilirubin and possibly in transfer of bilirubin)

Mild chronic conjugated hyperbilirubinemia (usually <10 mg/dL)

Other liver function tests are normal.

Liver biopsy is normal; no pigment is present.

Urine coproporphyrin is increased and coproporphyrin I may be greater than coproporphyrin III.

## Space-Occupying Lesions of Liver

Increased serum ALP is the most useful index of partial obstruction of the biliary tree in which serum bilirubin is usually normal and urine bilirubin is increased.

- Increased in 80% of patients with metastatic carcinoma
- Increased in 50% of patients with TB
- Increased in 40% of patients with sarcoidosis
- Increased frequently in patients with amyloidosis

AST is increased in 50% of patients.

ALT is increased less frequently.

Detection of metastases by panel of blood tests (ALP, LD, transaminase, bilirubin) has sensitivity of 85%.

Blind needle biopsy of the liver is positive in 65–75% of patients.

### Hepatoma

Serum AFP is found in 50% of white and 75–90% of nonwhite patients; may be present for up to 18 months before symptoms; is sensitive indicator of recur-

rence in treated patients. >500 ng/dL in adults strongly suggest primary carcinoma of liver.

Laboratory findings associated with underlying disease

- Hemochromatosis (≤ 20% of patients die of hepatoma).
- More frequent in postnecrotic than in alcoholic cirrhosis.
- Cirrhosis associated with alpha$_1$-antitrypsin deficiency and other inborn
  errors of metabolism (e.g., tyrosinemia).
- *Clonorchis sinensis* infection is associated with cholangiosarcoma.

Sudden progressive worsening of laboratory findings of underlying disease (e.g.,
increased serum ALT, LD, AST, bilirubin)

Hemoperitoneum—ascites in ~50% of patients but tumor cells found irregularly.

Laboratory findings due to obstruction of hepatic (Budd-Chiari syndrome) or portal veins or inferior vena cava may occur.

Anemia is common; polycythemia occurs occasionally.

## Wilson's Disease
**(Autosomal recessive defect impairs copper excretion by liver, causing
copper accumulation in liver.)**

Serum ceruloplasmin

### *Decreased (<20 mg/dL) in*

Wilson's disease *(It is normal in 2–5% of patients with overt Wilson's disease.)*
May not be decreased in Wilson's disease with acute or fulminant liver involvement (ceruloplasmin is an acute phase reactant).

Normal infants (therefore, cannot use test for Wilson's disease before 1 yr of age).

10–20% of persons heterozygous for Wilson's disease

Renal protein loss (e.g., nephrosis)

Malabsorption (e.g., sprue)

Malnutrition

*Decreased serum ceruloplasmin (<20 mg/dL) with increased hepatic copper (>250
μg/gm) occurs only in Wilson's disease or normal infants aged <6 months.*

### *Increased in*

Pregnancy
Use of estrogen or birth control pills
Thyrotoxicosis
Cirrhosis
Cancer
Acute inflammatory reactions (e.g., infection)

*Heterozygous gene for Wilson's disease* occurs in 1 of 200 in the general population; 10% of these have decreased serum ceruloplasmin; liver copper is not
increased (<250 μg/gm of dry liver). Serum copper and ceruloplasmin and
urine copper are inadequate to detect heterozygous state.

*Homozygous gene (clinical Wilson's disease)* occurs in 1 of 200,000 in the general
population.

Total serum copper is decreased and generally parallels serum ceruloplasmin.

Free (nonceruloplasmin) copper in serum is increased and causes excess copper deposition in tissues and excretion in urine. Free copper (μg/dL) = (total serum copper
[μg/dL] – ceruloplasmin [mg/dL]) × 3. Is virtually 100% sensitive and specific.

Urinary copper is increased (>100 μg/24 hrs); may be normal in presymptomatic
patients and increased in other types of cirrhosis.

Liver biopsy shows high copper concentration (>250 μg/gm of dry liver; normal =
20–45) and should be used to confirm the diagnosis. May also be increased in
cholestatic syndromes (e.g., primary biliary cirrhosis), which are easily differentiated from Wilson's disease by increased serum ceruloplasmin.

Liver biopsy may show no abnormalities, moderate to marked fatty changes with
or without fibrosis, or active or inactive cirrhosis.

Findings of liver function tests may not be abnormal, depending on the type and severity of disease. *In patients presenting as acute fulminant hepatitis, Wilson's disease is suggested if there is a disproportionately low serum ALP and relatively mild increase in AST and ALT. Should also be ruled out in any patient <30 yrs with hepatitis (with negative serology for viral hepatitis), Coomb-negative hemolysis, or neurologic symptoms to allow early diagnosis and treatment of Wilson's disease.*

Radiocopper loading test: Serum $^{64}Cu$ disappears within 4–6 hrs and then reappears in persons without Wilson's disease; secondary reappearance is absent in Wilson's disease; useful in patients with normal ceruloplasmin levels or increased hepatic copper due to other forms of liver disease, heterozygous carriers of Wilson's disease gene, or when liver biopsy is contraindicated.

Laboratory findings due to complications
- Cirrhosis.
- Hypersplenism.
- Acute liver failure characterized by very high serum bilirubin (often >30 mg/dL) and decreased ALP; ALP:bilirubin ratio <2.0 is said to distinguish this from other causes of liver failure.

# Tests for Differential Diagnosis of Pancreatic Diseases

## Amylase, Serum
**(composed of pancreatic and salivary types; nonpancreatic etiologies are almost always salivary; both types may be increased in renal insufficiency)**

### Increased in

Acute pancreatitis. Urine levels reflect serum changes 6–10 hrs later.

Acute exacerbation of chronic pancreatitis

Obstruction of pancreatic duct by
- Stone or carcinoma
- Drug-induced spasm of sphincter (e.g., opiates, codeine, methyl choline, chlorothiazide) to levels 2–15 times normal
- Partial obstruction
- Drug stimulation

Biliary tract disease
- Common bile duct obstruction
- Acute cholecystitis

Complications of pancreatitis (pseudocyst, ascites, abscess)

Pancreatic trauma (abdominal injury; after ERCP)

Altered GI permeability
- Ischemic bowel disease or frank perforation
- Esophageal rupture
- Perforated or penetrating peptic ulcer
- Postoperative upper abdominal surgery, especially partial gastrectomy

Acute alcohol ingestion or poisoning

Salivary gland disease (mumps, suppurative inflammation, duct obstruction due to calculus, radiation)

Malignant tumors (especially of pancreas, lung, ovary, esophagus; also breast, colon); usually >25 times ULN, which is rarely seen in pancreatitis

Advanced renal insufficiency

Macroamylasemia

Others—burns, pregnancy (including ruptured tubal pregnancy), ovarian cyst, diabetic ketoacidosis, recent thoracic surgery, myoglobinuria, presence of myeloma proteins, some cases of intracranial bleeding (unknown mechanism), splenic rupture, dissecting aneurysm

*Increased serum amylase with low urine amylase* may be seen in renal insufficiency and macroamylasemia. Serum amylase ≤4 times normal in renal disease only when creatinine clearance is <50 mL/min due to pancreatic or salivary isoamylase but rarely >4 times normal in absence of acute pancreatitis.

### Decreased in

Extensive marked destruction of pancreas (e.g., acute fulminant pancreatitis)
Decreased levels are clinically significant only in occasional cases of fulminant pancreatitis.
Severe liver damage (e.g., hepatitis, poisoning, toxemia of pregnancy, severe thyrotoxicosis, severe burns)

### Amylase:Creatinine Clearance Ratio

- Normal: 1–5%
- Macroamylasemia: <1%; very useful for this diagnosis
- Acute pancreatitis: >5%; use is presently discouraged for this diagnosis

### May Be Normal in

Relapsing chronic pancreatitis
Hypertriglyceridemia (technical interference with test)
Acute alcoholic pancreatitis

## Lipase, Serum

### Increased in

Acute pancreatitis
Penetrating peptic ulcer, especially with involvement of pancreas
Obstruction of pancreatic duct by
- Stone
- Drug-induced spasm of sphincter
- Partial obstruction
- Drug stimulation
Chronic pancreatitis
Acute cholecystitis
Small-bowel obstruction
Intestinal infarction
Acute and chronic renal failure
Organ transplant (kidney, liver, heart) especially with complications (e.g., organ rejection, CMV infection, cyclosporin toxicity)
Alcoholism
Diabetic ketoacidosis
After ERCP
Some cases of intracranial bleeding (unknown mechanism)
Macro forms in lymphoma, cirrhosis

### Usually Normal in

Mumps
Values are lower in neonates.

# Diseases of the Pancreas

See Fig. 8-8.

## Carcinoma of Pancreas

### Body or Tail

Laboratory tests are often normal.

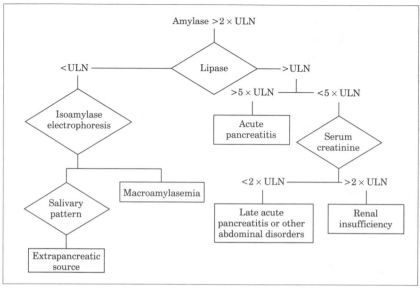

**Fig. 8-8.** Algorithm for increased serum amylase and lipase.

Serum markers for tumor CA 19-9, CEA, etc.
- In carcinoma of pancreas, CA 19-9 is sensitive and specific for local and metastatic disease. High levels may also occur in other GI cancers, especially colon and bile duct. Often normal in early stages, and therefore not useful for screening. Increased level may help differentiate benign disease from cancer. Falls if cancer is completely removed so may be useful for prognosis and follow-up.
- Testosterone:dihydrotestosterone ratio <5 (normal ~10) in >70% of men with pancreatic cancer (due to increased conversion by tumor). Less sensitive but more specific than CA 19-9; present in higher proportion of stage I tumors.

Serum amylase and lipase may be slightly increased in early stages (<10% of cases); with later destruction of pancreas, they are normal or decreased. They may increase following secretin-pancreozymin stimulation.

Glucose tolerance curve is of the diabetic type with overt diabetes in 20% of patients with pancreatic cancer.

Flat blood sugar curve with IV tolbutamide tolerance test indicates destruction of islet cell tissue. *Unstable, insulin-sensitive diabetes that develops in an older man should arouse suspicion of carcinoma of the pancreas.*

Secretin-cholecystokinin stimulation evidences duct obstruction when duodenal intubation shows decreased volume of duodenal contents (<10 mL/10-min collection period) with usually normal bicarbonate and enzyme levels in duodenal contents. Acinar destruction (as in pancreatitis) shows normal volume (20–30 mL/10-min collection period), but bicarbonate and enzyme levels may be decreased. Abnormal volume, bicarbonate, or both is found in 60–80% of patients with pancreatitis or cancer.

In carcinoma, the test result depends on the relative extent and combination of acinar destruction and of duct obstruction. Cytologic examination of duodenal contents shows malignant cells in 40% of patients. Malignant cells may be found in up to 80% of patients with periampullary cancer.

Needle biopsy has reported sensitivity of 57–96%; false positives are rare.

### Head

The abnormal pancreatic function tests that occur with carcinoma of the body of the pancreas may be evident.

Laboratory findings due to complete obstruction of common bile duct
- Serum bilirubin increased (12–25 mg/dL), mostly direct (increase persistent and nonfluctuating).
- Serum ALP increased.
- Urine and stool urobilinogen absent.
- Increased PT; normal after IV vitamin K administration.
- Increased serum cholesterol (usually >300 mg/dL) with esters not decreased.
- Other liver function tests are usually normal.

## Cystic Fibrosis of Pancreas (Mucoviscidosis)

### Quantitative Pilocarpine Iontophoresis Sweat Test

Striking increase in sweat sodium (>60 mEq/L) and chloride (>60 mEq/L) and, to a lesser extent, potassium is present in virtually all homozygous patients; is 3–5 times higher than in healthy persons or other diseases. It is consistently present throughout life from time of birth and degree of abnormality is not related to severity of disease or organ involvement. There is a broad range of values in this disease and in normal but minimal overlap. *Sweat chloride is somewhat more reliable than sodium for diagnostic purposes.* Increased sweat sodium and chloride are not useful for detection of heterozygotes (who have normal values) or for genetic counseling.
- In children, chloride >60 mEq/L is considered positive for cystic fibrosis.
- 40–60 mEq/L is considered borderline and requires further investigation.
- <40 mEq/L is considered normal.
- ≤ 80 mEq/L may be normal for adults.

Sweat Values (mEq/L)

|  | Chloride | | Sodium | | Potassium | |
|---|---|---|---|---|---|---|
|  | Mean | Range | Mean | Range | Mean | Range |
| Cystic fibrosis | 115 | 79–148 | 111 | 75–145 | 23 | 14–30 |
| Normal | 28 | 8–43 | 28 | 16–46 | 10 | 6–17 |

*Sweat testing is fraught with problems and technical and laboratory errors are very frequent; should be performed in duplicate and repeated at least once on separate days on samples >100 mg of sweat.*

On occasion, 1–2% of cystic fibrosis patients have normal, borderline, or variable values.

### Interferences

Values may be increased to cystic fibrosis range in healthy persons when sweat rate is rapid (e.g., exercise, high temperature), but pilocarpine test does not increase sweating rate.

Sweat electrolytes may also be increased in untreated adrenal insufficiency, hypothyroidism, malnutrition, ectodermal hyperplasia, and some unusual syndromes (e.g., G6PD deficiency, glycogen storage disease, vasopressin-resistant diabetes insipidus).

Serum and urine electrolytes are normal.

Serum protein electrophoresis shows increasing gamma globulin with progressive pulmonary disease, mainly due to IgG and IgA. Serum albumin is often decreased.

Glucose intolerance in ~40% of patients.

Findings of chronic lung disease.

Bacteriology: Special culture techniques should be used in these patients.
- Hemolytic *S. aureus* is the most frequent and important organism in the respiratory tract.

- *Pseudomonas aeruginosa* is found increasingly often after treatment of staphylococcus and special identification and susceptibility tests should be performed on *P. aeruginosa.*
- *Pseudomonas cepacia* is becoming more important in older children.

Laboratory changes secondary to complications

- Excessive loss of electrolytes in sweat and stool may cause hypochloremic metabolic alkalosis and hypokalemia.
- Pancreatic deficiency with decrease or absence of all pancreatic enzyme activity.
- Cirrhosis.
- Chronic lung disease (especially upper lobes); sinusitis, nasal polyps.
- Meconium ileus during early infancy.
- Aspermia in 98% of patients with cystic fibrosis.

Stool and duodenal fluid show lack of trypsin digestion of x-ray film gelatin; this is a useful screening test up to age 4 yrs; decreased chymotrypsin production gauged by bentiromide test.

## Macroamylasemia

Serum amylase persistently increased (often 1–4 times normal) without apparent cause. Serum lipase is normal.

Urine amylase normal or low

Amylase:creatinine clearance ratio <1% with normal renal function is very useful for this diagnosis.

Macroamylase is identified in serum by special methods.

## Pancreatitis, Acute

Serum lipase increases within 3–6 hrs with peak at 24 hrs and usually returns to normal in 8–14 days. Is superior to amylase. Pancreatitis is highly likely when lipase ≥ 5 times ULN. *Lipase should always be determined whenever amylase is determined.* Urinary lipase is not useful. It has been suggested that a lipase:amylase ratio >3 (and especially >5) indicates alcoholic rather than nonalcoholic pancreatitis). If lipase ≥ 5 times ULN, acute pancreatitis or organ rejection is highly likely but unlikely if <3 times ULN.

Serum amylase increase begins in 3–6 hrs, rises rapidly within 8 hrs in 75% of patients, reaches maximum in 20–30 hrs, and may persist for 48–72 hrs. The increase may be ≤ 40 times normal. An increase >7–10 days suggests an associated cancer of pancreas or pseudocyst, pancreatic ascites, nonpancreatic etiology. *Similar high values may occur in obstruction of pancreatic duct; they tend to fall after several days. >10% of patients with acute pancreatitis (especially when seen more than 2 days after onset of symptoms) may have normal values, even when dying of acute pancreatitis.* May also be normal in relapsing chronic pancreatitis and patients with hypertriglyceridemia, acute alcoholic pancreatitis. Acute abdomen due to GI infarction or perforation rather than acute pancreatitis is suggested by only moderate increase in serum amylase and lipase (<3 times ULN), evidence of bacteremia. 10–40% of patients with acute alcoholic intoxication have elevated serum amylase (usually <3 times ULN; about half are salivary type). Levels >25 times ULN indicates metastatic tumor rather than pancreatitis.

Serum pancreatic isoamylase can distinguish increases due to salivary amylase that may account for 25% of all elevated values. (In healthy persons, 40% of total serum amylase is pancreatic type and 60% is salivary type.)

Only slight increase in serum amylase and lipase values suggest a different diagnosis than acute pancreatitis. *Many drugs increase both amylase and lipase in serum.* In patients with signs of acute pancreatitis, acute pancreatitis is highly likely if serum lipase >5–10 times ULN, values change significantly with time, and if amylase and lipase changes are concordant.

Serum calcium is decreased in severe cases 1–9 days after onset. The decrease usually occurs after amylase and lipase levels have become normal. *(Rule out hyperparathyroidism if serum calcium is high or fails to fall in hyperamylasemia of acute pancreatitis.)*

Increased urinary amylase tends to reflect serum changes by a time lag of 6–10 hrs. The 24-hr level may be normal even when some of the 1-hr specimens are increased. Ratio of amylase clearance to creatinine clearance is increased (>5%) and avoids the problem of timed urine specimens; also increased in any condition that decreases tubular reabsorption of amylase (e.g., severe burns, diabetic ketoacidosis, chronic renal insufficiency, multiple myeloma, acute duodenal perforation).

Serum bilirubin may be increased when pancreatitis is of biliary tract origin but is usually normal in alcoholic pancreatitis. Serum ALP, ALT, and AST may increase and parallel serum bilirubin rather than amylase, lipase, or calcium levels.

Serum trypsin is increased. A normal value is useful for excluding acute pancreatitis. Poor specificity limits use.

WBC is slightly to moderately increased (10,000–20,000/cu mm). Hemoconcentration occurs (increased Hct).

Methemalbumin may be increased in serum and ascitic fluid in hemorrhagic (severe) but not edematous (mild) pancreatitis; may distinguish these two conditions but not useful in diagnosis of acute pancreatitis.

## Pancreatitis, Chronic

Cholecystokinin-secretin test measures the effect of IV administration of cholecystokinin and secretin on volume, bicarbonate concentration, and amylase output of duodenal contents and increase in serum lipase and amylase. This is the gold standard test for chronic pancreatitis, especially in the early stages. Amylase output is the most frequent abnormality. When all three are abnormal, there is a greater frequency of abnormality in the following tests.

Normal duodenal contents

Serum amylase and lipase increase after administration of cholecystokinin and secretin in ~20% of patients with chronic pancreatitis.

Normally serum lipase and amylase do not rise above normal limits.

Fasting serum amylase and lipase are increased in 10% of patients with chronic pancreatitis.

Diabetic oral GTT in 65% of patients with chronic pancreatitis and frank diabetes in >10% of patients with chronic relapsing pancreatitis. When GTT is normal in the presence of steatorrhea, the cause should be sought elsewhere than in the pancreas.

Laboratory findings due to malabsorption and steatorrhea
  • Bentiromide test is usually abnormal with moderate to severe pancreatic insufficiency.

Starch tolerance test is abnormal in 25% of patients with chronic pancreatitis.

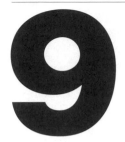

# Central and Peripheral Nervous System Disorders

# Laboratory Tests for Disorders of the Nervous System

## Normal CSF Values

*These analytes should always be measured on simultaneously drawn blood samples.*

| | |
|---|---|
| Appearance | Clear, colorless: no clot |
| Cell count | |
|     Adults, children | 0–6/cu mm (all mononuclear cells) |
|     Infants | <19/cu mm |
|     Neonates | <30/cu mm |
| Glucose | 45–80 mg/dL (20 mg/dL less than blood) |
| Ventricular fluid | 5–10 mg/dL > lumbar |
| TP | |
|     Cisternal | 15–25 mg/dL |
|     Ventricular | 5–15 mg/dL |
|     Lumbar | |
|         3 months–60 yrs | 15–45 mg/dL |
|         Neonates | 15–100 mg/dL |
|         >60 yrs | 15–60 mg/dL |
| Albumin | 10–35 mg/dL |
| Protein electrophoresis | |
|     Transthyretin (Prealbumin) | 2–7% |
|     Albumin | 56–76% |
|     Alpha$_1$ globulin | 2–7% |
|     Alpha$_2$ globulin | 4–12% |
|     Beta globulin | 8–18% |
|     Gamma globulin | 3–12% |
| IgG | <4.0 mg/dL; <10% of total CSF protein |
| Albumin index (ratio) | <9.0 |
| IgG synthesis rate | 0.0–8.0 mg/day |
| IgG index (ratio) | 0.28–0.66 |
| CSF IgG:albumin ratio | 0.09–0.25 |
| Oligoclonal bands | Negative |
| Myelin basic protein | 0.0–4.0 ng/mL |
| Chloride | 120–130 mEq/L (20 mEq/L > serum values) |
| Sodium | 142–150 mEq/L |
| Potassium | 2.2–3.3 mEq/L |
| Carbon dioxide | 25 mEq/L |
| pH | 7.35–7.40 |
| Transaminase (AST) | 7–49 units |

| | |
|---|---|
| LD | ~10% of serum level |
|    LD-1 | 38–58% (LD-1 > LD-2) |
|    LD-2 | 26–36% |
|    LD-3 | 12–24% |
|    LD-4 | 1–7% |
|    LD-5 | 0–5% |
| CK | 0–5 IU/L |
| Bilirubin | 0 |
| Urea nitrogen | 5–25 mg/dL |
| Amino acids | 30% of blood level |
| Xanthochromia | 0 |
| Volume (adults) | ~140 mL |
| Generation rate | 0.35 mL/min = 500 mL/day |

Enzymes in CSF (AST, LD, CK) are generally not useful in CNS diseases.

## Abnormal CSF

### Gross Appearance

Viscous CSF may occur with metastatic mucinous adenocarcinoma, large numbers of cryptococci, severe meningeal infection, or, rarely, injury to annulus fibrosus.

Turbidity may be due to increased WBC (>200/cu mm), RBC (>400/cu mm), bacteria (>$10^5$/mL), fungi, amebae, contrast media, epidural fat.

For clots or pellicles to occur: protein >150 mg/dL.

Protein >100 mg/dL usually causes CSF to look faintly yellow.

CSF with RBC >6000/cu mm appears grossly bloody; with RBC = 500–6000/cu mm, it appears cloudy, xanthochromic, or pink-tinged. Test for occult blood may be positive before xanthochromia develops. In intracerebral hemorrhage, bloody CSF clears by day 10 in 40% of patients. CSF is persistently abnormal after 21 days in 15% of patients. ~5% of cerebrovascular episodes due to hemorrhage are wholly within the parenchyma and CSF findings are normal. See Table 9-1.

Xanthochromia may be due to prior (within 2–36 hrs) bleeding, including traumatic tap, markedly elevated protein (>150 mg/dL), or serum bilirubin >6 mg/dL.

Yellow color may be due to serum bilirubin >10 mg/dL or prior hemorrhage (10 hrs–4 wks).

**Table 9-1.** Differentiation Between Bloody CSF Due to Subarachnoid Hemorrhage and Traumatic Lumbar Puncture

| CSF Finding | Subarachnoid Hemorrhage | Traumatic Lumbar Puncture |
|---|---|---|
| CSF pressure | Often increased | Low |
| Blood in tubes for collecting CSF | Mixture with blood is uniform in all tubes | Earlier tubes more bloody than later tubes; RBC count decreases in later tubes |
| CSF clotting | No clots | Often clots |
| Xanthochromia | Present if >8–12 hrs since subarachnoid hemorrhage | Absent unless patient is icteric; may appear if CSF examination delayed ≥ 2 hrs |
| Immediate repeat of lumbar puncture at higher level | CSF same as initial puncture | CSF clear |

## Blood Cells

CSF WBC may be corrected for presence of blood (e.g., traumatic tap, subarachnoid hemorrhage).
In normal CSF, minimal blood contamination may cause ≤ 2 PMNs/25 RBCs, or ≤ 10 PMNs/25–100 RBCs.
CSF WBC count (>3000/cu mm) predominantly PMNs strongly suggests bacterial cause. *WBCs are usually PMNs in early stages of all types of meningitis; mononuclear cells only appear in a second specimen 18–24 hrs later.* Low WBC counts do not rule out acute bacterial meningitis (ABM).
Neutrophilic leukocytes are found in meningitis due to bacteria, fungi, chemicals, other conditions (e.g., SLE).
Lymphocytes are found in
  • Bacterial, fungal, viral infections
  • Parasitic diseases
  • Parameningeal disorders (e.g., brain abscess)
  • Noninfectious disorders (e.g., neoplasms, sarcoidosis, multiple sclerosis)
Eosinophils may be found in
  • Lymphoma
  • Helminthic infection

## Microbiology/Serology

Smears for Gram's and acid-fast stains must be routinely *centrifuged* on all CSF specimens because other findings may be normal in meningitis. Gram's stain of CSF sediment is negative in 20% of cases of bacterial meningitis because at least $10^5$ bacteria/mL CSF must be present to demonstrate 1–2 bacteria/100× microscopic field. Gram's stain is positive in 90% of cases due to pneumococci, 85% of cases due to *Haemophilus influenzae*, 75% of cases due to meningococci, 50% of cases due to *Listeria monocytogenes*, 30–50% of cases due to gram-negative enteric bacilli. Stains are positive in <60% of cases of treated bacterial meningitis, <5% of cases of TB meningitis, 20–70% of cases of fungal meningitis, and <2% of cases of brain abscess.
Positive CSF culture has high sensitivity and specificity.
Limulus amebocyte lysate is a rapid specific indicator of endotoxin produced by gram-negative bacteria (e.g., *Neisseria meningitidis, H. influenzae* type B, *Escherichia coli, Pseudomonas*).
Latex agglutination for antigen detection of *H. influenzae* type B, *Cryptococcus neoformans, N. meningitidis, Streptococcus pneumoniae, Streptococcus agalactiae* in CSF is more sensitive than urine and serum. Negative results are not conclusive; positive results should be confirmed by culture.
Serologic methods are often preferred in cases of coccidiosis, syphilis, brucellosis, Lyme disease. PCR to detect herpes simplex virus and human enteroviruses.

## CSF Chemistries

Glucose is decreased by use by organisms, WBCs, or occasionally cancer cells in CSF. CSF glucose lags behind blood glucose by about 1 hr. May rapidly become normal after onset of antibiotic therapy. Is decreased in only ~50% of cases of bacterial meningitis. CSF glucose <45 mg/dL is almost always abnormal. Normally is ~50–65% of blood glucose, which should *always* be drawn simultaneously. In ABM, CSF:serum ratio of glucose is usually <0.5; a ratio of <8.0 is significant in infants. May also be decreased in acute infection due to syphilis or Lyme disease but is generally rare in viral infections or parameningeal processes. May also be decreased in rheumatoid meningitis, lupus myelopathy, and other causes of chronic meningitis (e.g., bacteria, syphilis, fungi, and parasites; granulomatous, chemical, and carcinomatous meningitis; hypoglycemia; and subarachnoid hemorrhage).

*CSF protein, glucose, and WBC levels may not return to normal in ~50% of patients with clinically cured bacterial meningitis and are not recommended as a test of cure.*

CSF total protein may be corrected for presence of blood (e.g., due to traumatic tap or intracerebral hemorrhage) by subtracting 1 mg/dL of protein for each 1000 RBCs/cu mm if serum protein and CBC are normal and are determined on same tube of CSF. *Serum protein levels must be normal to interpret any CSF protein values and should always be measured concurrently.*

CSF protein
- May not be increased in treated or early stages of many types of meningitis
- Normal in >10% of patients with bacterial meningitis
- Usually >150 mg/dL in bacterial meningitis
- Rarely >200 mg/dL in viral meningitis
- May show mild to moderate elevation in myxedema (25% of cases), uremia, connective tissue disorders, and Cushing's syndrome

Increased tumor markers CSF (e.g., CEA) are occasionally helpful in diagnosis of suspected metastatic carcinoma with negative cytology and leukemia.

# Diseases of the Nervous System

See Table 9-2.

## Bacterial Meningitis

Bacteria can be identified in CSF in only 90% of patients; when Gram's stain is positive, CSF is more likely to show decreased glucose, increased protein, and increased RBCs. 75% of cases are due to *N. meningitidis, S. pneumoniae, H. influenzae.*

In listeria meningitis, the Gram's stain is usually negative and the cellular response is usually monocytic.

Gram's stain of scrapings from petechial skin lesions, buffy coat of peripheral blood, and less often, peripheral blood smear demonstrate the pathogen in meningococcemia.

Latex agglutination for bacterial antigen in CSF for *S. pneumoniae, S. agalactiae, H. influenzae,* some strains of *N. meningitidis.* Not affected by previous antimicrobial therapy. Not likely to be useful if CSF chemistry and cell count are normal unless patient is immunocompromised. False positive for group B *Streptococcus* and *H. influenzae* antigen in urine is common.

Blood culture is usually positive if patient has not received antibiotics.

Most frequent and important differential diagnosis is between ABM and acute viral meningitis (AVM). The most useful test results that favor the diagnosis of ABM rather than AVM are
- CSF positive by bacterial stain, culture, or antigen detection.
- Decreased CSF glucose.
- Decreased CSF:serum ratio of glucose (<0.25 in <1% of AVM cases and 44% of ABM cases) even if CSF glucose is normal.
- Increased CSF protein >1.72 gm/L (1% of AVM and 50% of ABM cases).
- CSF WBC >2000/cu mm in 38% of ABM cases and PMN >1180/cu mm but low counts do not rule out ABM.
- Peripheral WBC is only useful if very high WBC (>27,200/cu mm) and total PMN (>21,000/cu mm) counts, which occur in relatively few patients; leukopenia is common in infants and elderly.
- Combination of findings can exclude AVM and rule in ABM, but none of them can establish the diagnosis of AVM, and absence of these findings cannot exclude ABM.

**Table 9-2.** CSF Findings in Various Conditions

| | Appearance | Protein (mg/dL) | Glucose (mg/dL) | WBC/cu mm | Page Nos. in 6th ed. |
|---|---|---|---|---|---|
| Normal | C, colorless no clot | | | 0–10 | |
| Ventricular | | 5–15 | 45–80 | | |
| Cisternal | | 10–25 | | | |
| Lumbar | | 10–45 | | | |
| TB meningitis | O, sl yellow, delicate clot | 45–500 | 10–45 | 10–1000, chiefly L | 748–750 |
| Tuberculoma | | I | | Small number of cells | 258 |
| Acute pyogenic meningitis | O to Pu, sl yellow, delicate clot | 50–1500 | 0–45 | 25–10,000, chiefly P | 253 |
| Aseptic meningitis[a] | C, T, or X | 20 to >200 | N | ≤ 500, occ 2000; first PMNs, later mononuclear cells | 255–256 |
| AIDS | | 50–100 | N | ≤ 300 | 256, 763–771 |
| Acute anterior polio | C or sl O, may be sl yellow, may be delicate clot | 20–350 | N | 10 to >500, L > P | 756–757 |
| Mumps | N or O | 20–125 | N | 0 to >2000 | 760 |
| Measles | N or O | sl I | N | ≤ 500 | 760–761 |
| Herpes zoster | N | 20–110 | N | ≤ 300 in 40% of patients | 761–762 |
| Equine, St. Louis encephalitis, choriomeningitis | N or sl T | 20 to > 200 | N | 10–200; occ to 3000 | 758 |
| Herpes simplex | | I | N | 10–1000, chiefly L | 257 |

| | N or sl I | | N or ≤ 100 mononuclear cells | |
|---|---|---|---|---|
| Rabies | | | | 257, 759 |
| Postinfectious | N | 15–75 | N | 5–200, rarely ≤ 1000 | 257, 759 |
| Coccidioidomycosis | | I | N early, then D | ≤ 200 early; may be higher later | 784 |
| Cryptococcal meningitis | N | ≤ 500 in 90% | Moderate D in 55% | ≤ 800 (L > P) | 782 |
| Toxoplasmosis | X | ≤ 200 | N | 50–500; chiefly monocytes | 788–789 |
| Syphilis | | | | | 742 |
| Tabes dorsalis | N | 25–100 I gamma globulin less marked than in general paresis | N | 10–80 | |
| General paresis[b] | N | ≤ 100 marked in gamma globulin | N | ≤ 175, mononuclear | |
| Meningovascular syphilis | N | ≤ 60 in 66%; I gamma globulin in 75% of cases | N | 10–100, N in 60% | |
| Syphilitic meningitis | N | | | ≤ 2000 L | |
| Asymptomatic CNS lues | N | I protein and cell count are index of activity | | | |
| Leptospirosis | | I ≤ 80 | N | ≤ 500 M | 738 |

**Table 9-2.** (continued)

| | Appearance | Protein (mg/dL) | Glucose (mg/dL) | WBC/cu mm | Page Nos. in 6th ed. |
|---|---|---|---|---|---|
| Lyme disease | | I IgG and oligoclonal bands | | ≤ 450 L | 738–740 |
| Primary amebic (*Naegleria*) meningitis | Sanguino-Pu, may be T or Pu | I | Usually D | 400–21,000, mostly P; also RBC | 259 |
| Chronic meningitis[c] | Symptoms for 1–4 wks | Moderate to marked I | D | 100–400, mostly L | 256 |
| Cavernous sinus thrombophlebitis | Usually N; may be B | | Usually N | | 257 |
| Brain abscess[d] | | May be ≤ 75–300 | N | 25–300; PMN, L, RBCs | 258 |
| Extradural abscess | | 100–400 | N | Relatively few PNMs and L | 258 |
| Subdural empyema | | I | N | ≤ Few hundred, mostly PMNs | 258 |
| Cord tumor | C, occ X | ≤3500 in 85%; N in 15% | N | ≤ 100, chiefly L; N in 60% | 263 |
| Brain tumor[e] | C, occ X; B if hemorrhage into tumor | ≤ 500 | May be D if cells are present | ≤ 150; N in 75% | 253 |
| Leukemia | | I | D to 50% of blood | | 253 |
| Pseudotumor cerebri | N | N | N | N | 252 |
| Cerebral thrombosis | N | ≤ 100, N in 60% | N | ≤ 50, N in 75%, rarely ≤ 2000 | 251 |

Cerebral embolism¹

| | | | | | |
|---|---|---|---|---|---|
| Bland | Sl X in one-third of cases in few days; may be B | | | May be 10,000 RBC | 252 |
| Septic | Sl X | I | N | ≤ 200 with varying L and PMNs; ≤ 1000 RBCs | 252 |
| Cerebral hemorrhage^g | N in 15%, X in 10%, B in 75% | Usually ≤ 2000 | N | Same as in blood; N in 10% | 253 |
| Subarachnoid hemorrhage | B; X in 24 hrs; no clot | Usually ≤ 1000 | N | Same as in blood | 251 |
| Hypertensive encephalopathy | | ≤ 100 | | | 253 |
| Postoperative neurosurgery (especially posterior fossa) | | I | <40 | 1000–2000, mostly P | |
| Traumatic tap | B | I by blood | N | Same as in blood | 251 |
| Head trauma | N, B, or X | I if bloody | N | Same as in blood | 245 |
| Acute epidural hemorrhage | C unless associated injuries | | | | 245 |
| Subdural hematoma | C, B, or X, depending on associated injuries | N or sl I | | | 251 |
| Chronic subdural hematoma | Usually X | 300–2000 | | | 251 |
| Multiple sclerosis | N | N | | | 261–262 |
| Polyarteritis; porphyria; beriberi; alcohol effect; arsenic poisoning | N, X if protein very I | Usually N | N | N but albuminocytologic dissociation in Guillain-Barré syndrome that may occur in heavy metal poisoning, infection, etc. | |

**Table 9-2.** (continued)

| | Appearance | Protein (mg/dL) | Glucose (mg/dL) | WBC/cu mm | Page Nos. in 6th ed. |
|---|---|---|---|---|---|
| Diabetes mellitus | Same as polyarteritis, etc. | Often ≤ 300 | N | Same as polyarteritis, etc. | |
| Acute infection | Same as polyarteritis, etc. | ≤ 1500 | N | Same as polyarteritis, etc. | |
| Lead encephalopathy | N or sl yellow | ≤ 100 | N | 0–100 | 851, 853–855 |
| Sarcoidosis (findings in ≤ 50%) | | | D in 10% | I in 40% | 825–827 |
| Behçet's disease (25% have meningoencephalitis) | | I | N | I | 256 |
| Alcoholism | N | N | N | Usually N | 845–847 |
| Diabetic coma | N | N | N | Usually N | 569–571 |
| Uremia | N | N or I | N or I | Usually N | 676–678 |
| Epilepsy | N | N | N | N | |
| Eclampsia | May be B | Usually ≤ 200 | N | May be RBCs | 708 |
| Guillain-Barré syndrome | | 50–100 average albumino-cytologic dissociation | | N | 259 |

C = clear; O = opalescent; T = turbid; X = xanthochromic; B = bloody; Pu = purulent; IL = lymphocytes; sl = slightly; occ = occasionally.
[a]Possible underlying disorders:

- Infections (e.g., viral, bacterial [e.g., incompletely treated or very early bacterial meningitis], spirochetes [e.g., leptospirosis, syphilis, Lyme disease], TB, fungal, amebic, mycoplasma, rickettsia, helminths).
- Chemical meningitis.
- Drug-induced meningitis.
- Systemic disorders.
    - Vasculitis
        - Collagen vascular disease
        - Sarcoid
    - Neoplasm (e.g., leukemia, metastatic carcinoma).
    - SLE.

*If glucose levels are decreased, rule out TB, cryptococcosis, leukemia, lymphoma, metastatic carcinoma, sarcoidosis, drug-induced meningitis.*

[b]CSF always abnormal in untreated general paresis.

[c]Possible underlying disorder:

- Various infections: TB (most common cause), bacteria, spirochetes, fungi, protozoa, amebae, mycoplasma, rickettsia, helminths
- Systemic disorders (e.g., vasculitis, collagen vascular disease, sarcoid, neoplasm)

[d]Findings depend on stage and duration of abscess.

[e]*Protein is particularly increased with meningioma of the olfactory groove and with acoustic neuroma.* Usually normal in brain stem gliomas and "diencephalic syndrome" of infants due to glioma of hypothalamus.

[f]Usually same as in cerebral thrombosis.

[g]*Especially if blood pressure is normal, always rule out ruptured berry aneurysm, hemorrhage into tumor, and angioma.*

## Multiple Sclerosis (MS)

No diagnostic changes in peripheral blood or routine CSF tests.

Diagnosis should not be made on the basis of CSF findings unless there are *multiple clinical lesions in time and anatomic location*.

CSF WBC is usually <20 mononuclear cells/cu mm in ~25% of patients. >50 cells/cu mm should cast doubt on diagnosis. Albumin, glucose, and pressure are normal.

CSF total protein may be mildly elevated in ~25% of patients. Levels >100 mg/dL should cast doubt on diagnosis. CSF gamma globulin is increased in 60–75% of patients regardless of whether the total CSF protein is increased. Gamma globulin ≥ 12% of CSF TP is abnormal if there is not a corresponding increase in serum gamma globulin; but may also be increased in other CNS disorders (e.g., syphilis, subacute panencephalitis, meningeal carcinomatosis) or when serum electrophoresis is abnormal due to non-CNS diseases (e.g., RA, sarcoidosis, cirrhosis, myxedema, multiple myeloma).

CSF IgG concentration is increased (reference range <4.0 mg/dL) in ~70% of cases, often when TP is normal. Increase in *production* of IgG is expressed as ratio of CSF to serum albumin to rule out increased IgG due to disruption of blood-brain barrier. CSF IgG does not correlate with duration, activity, or course of MS. Increase may also be found in other inflammatory demyelinating diseases (e.g., two-thirds of cases of neurosyphilis, acute Guillain-Barré syndrome), 5–15% of patients with miscellaneous neurologic diseases, and a few normal persons; recent myelography is said to invalidate the test. See Table 9-3.

CSF IgG:albumin ratio indicates in-situ production of IgG. Abnormal in 90% of MS patients and 18% of non-MS neurologic patients.

CSF IgG synthesis rate is increased in 90% of MS patients and 4% of non-MS patients.

IgG index indicates IgG synthesis in CNS. Occurs in 90% of MS patients; may also occur in other neurologic diseases (e.g., meningitis).

Increased albumin index used to prevent misinterpreting falsely increased CSF IgG concentrations. Indicates CSF contaminated with blood or increased permeability of blood-brain barrier (e.g., aged persons, obstruction of CSF circulation, diabetes mellitus, SLE of CNS, Guillain-Barré syndrome, polyneuropathy, cervical spondylosis).

Discrete bands of oligoclonal proteins (abnormal gamma globulins) in 85–95% of patients with definite MS and 30–40% with possible MS can be demonstrated by high-voltage electrophoresis or isoelectric focusing of concentrated CSF; *is the most sensitive marker of MS*. Positive results also occur in ≤ 10% of patients with noninflammatory neurologic disease (e.g., meningeal carcinomatosis, cerebral infarction), and ≤ 40% of patients with inflammatory CNS disorders (e.g., neurosyphilis, viral encephalitis, progressive rubella encephalitis, subacute sclerosing panencephalitis, bacterial meningitis, toxoplasmosis, cryptococcal meningitis, inflammatory neuropathies, trypanosomiasis). Not known to correlate with severity, duration, or course of MS. Persists during remission. During steroid treatment, prevalence of oligoclonal bands and other gamma globulin abnormalities may be reduced by 30–50%.

CSF IgM and IgA are not useful for diagnosis.

A few patients with definite MS may have normal CSF immunoglobulins and lack oligoclonal bands.

Myelin basic protein indicates recent myelin destruction; it is increased in 70–90% of MS patients during an acute exacerbation and usually returns to normal within 2 wks. Useful for following course of MS but not for screening. It is frequently increased in other causes of demyelination and tissue destruction (e.g., meningoencephalitis, leukodystrophies, metabolic encephalopathies, SLE of CNS, cranial irradiation and intrathecal chemotherapy, 45% of patients with recent stroke) and other disorders (e.g., diabetes mellitus, chronic renal failure, vasculitis, carcinoma of pancreas). Falsely increased by contamination with blood.

**Table 9-3.** Formulas for CNS IgG Synthesis*

$$\text{Albumin index} = \frac{\text{CSF albumin}}{\text{Serum albumin}} \times 1000 \ (\text{reference range} = 0.09\text{--}0.25)$$

$$\text{IgG:albumin ratio} = \frac{\text{CSF IgG}}{\text{CSF albumin}} \ (\text{reference range} < 9)$$

$$\text{IgG synthesis rate} = \left(\text{CSF IgG} - \frac{\text{Serum IgG}}{369}\right) - \left(\text{CSF albumin} - \frac{\text{Serum albumin}}{230}\right) \times$$
$$\left(\frac{0.43 \text{ Serum IgG}}{\text{Serum albumin}}\right) \ (\text{reference range} = 0\text{--}8.0 \text{ mg/day})$$

$$\text{IgG index} = \frac{\text{CSF IgG/Serum IgG}}{\text{CSF albumin/Serum albumin}} \ (\text{reference range} = 0.28\text{--}0.66)$$

*All serum and CSF analytes drawn simultaneously, reported in mg/dL.

## Skull Fractures

If 100 $\mu$L of CSF can be obtained to perform immunofixation, CSF transferrin shows a double band but only a single transferrin band is seen in other fluids (serum, nasal secretions, saliva, tears, lymph). In CSF, IgM is 5 times higher, prealbumin is 12 times higher, and transferrin is 2 times higher than levels in serum. To differentiate nasal secretions from CSF by absence of glucose (using test tapes or tablets) in nasal secretions is not reliable because nasal secretions may normally contain glucose.

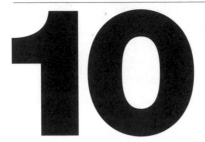

# Musculoskeletal and Joint Diseases

# Laboratory Tests for Skeletal Muscle Diseases

## Enzymes, Serum, in Some Diseases of Muscle

CK is the measurement of choice. It is more specific and sensitive than AST and LD, but AST is more significantly associated with inflammatory myopathy and more useful in these cases.

## Myoglobinemia and Myoglobinuria

See Chapter 4.

# Diseases of Skeletal Muscles

## Metabolic Diseases of Muscle

Endocrine
- Hypothyroidism
- Hyperthyroidism
- Acromegaly
- Cushing's syndrome and adrenal corticosteroid therapy
- Other endocrinopathies (e.g., hypoadrenalism, hyperparathyroidism)

Inherited metabolic myopathies
- Glycogen storage diseases (types II, III, V, and VII)
- Disordered lipid metabolism (muscle carnitine deficiency)

Alcoholism

## Muscular Dystrophy
### (genetic primary myopathies)

See Table 10-1 and Fig. 10-1.

Serum enzymes (CK is most useful) are increased.

Serum CK is useful for
- Preclinical diagnosis of Duchenne's and Becker's dystrophies in families with history of disease or for screening
- Clinical diagnosis
- Identifying female carriers

Antibodies to muscle protein (dystrophin) establishes diagnosis by showing dystrophin to be absent in Duchenne's dystrophy and decreased or qualitatively abnormal in Becker's dystrophy.

**Table 10-1.** Laboratory Findings in Differential Diagnosis of Some Muscle Diseases

| Disease | Complete Blood Count | ESR | Thyroid Function Tests | Percentage of Patients with Increase in Various Serum Enzyme Levels | Muscle Biopsy | Comment |
|---|---|---|---|---|---|---|
| Myasthenia gravis | N | N | N | N | Lymphorrhages | Cancer of lung should always be ruled out; high frequency of associated diabetes mellitus, especially in older patients<br>Serum electrolytes N |
| Polymyositis | Total eosinophil count frequently I | Moderately to markedly I; occasionally N | N | CK in 65%; levels may vary greatly and become N with steroid therapy; marked increase may occur in children LD in 25%, AST in 25% | Necrosis of muscle with phagocytosis of muscle fibers; infiltration of inflammatory cells | Associated cancer in ≤ 17% of cases (especially lung; also breast)<br>Serum alpha$_2$ and gamma globulins may be I |
| Muscular dystrophy | N | N | N | In active phase, CK in 50%, LD in 10%, AST in 15% | Various degenerative changes in muscle; late muscle atrophy; no cellular infiltration | |

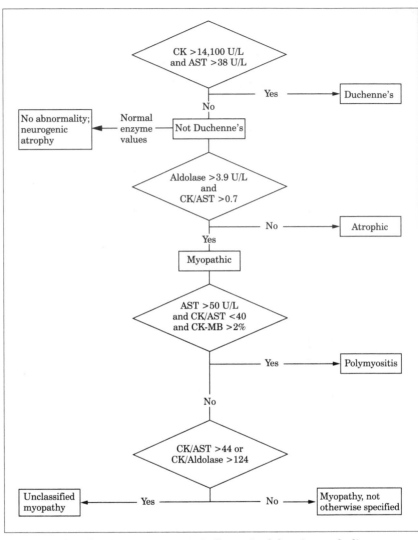

**Fig. 10-1.** Algorithm for serum enzymatic diagnosis of chronic muscle disease. Serum enzymes are not useful diagnostically in patients receiving immunosuppressive therapy in which the cause of muscle weakness is uncertain and muscle biopsy is required.

Dystrophin protein determined on biopsy of muscle is absent in Duchenne's dystrophy and decreased or abnormally formed in Becker's dystrophy.
Recombinant DNA technology allows
- Prenatal diagnosis by chorionic villous sampling at week 12 of gestation
- Diagnosis of carriers
- Diagnosis and differential diagnosis (e.g., from limb-girdle dystrophy)
Muscle biopsy specimen shows muscle atrophy but no cellular infiltration.

### Limb-Girdle Dystrophy
*(autosomal recessive disorder)*

Serum CK is increased. Not useful to detect carriers or to distinguish it from other disorders.

### Facioscapulohumeral Dystrophy

Serum CK is increased.

## Myasthenia Gravis (MG)

See Fig. 10-1 and Table 10-1.
Acetylcholine receptor (AChR) binding antibodies
AChR blocking antibodies
AChR modulating antibodies
Striational antibodies to skeletal muscle cross-striations
>90% of seropositive patients have more than one type of autoantibody.
Other immunologic abnormalities are frequent (e.g., anti-DNA antibodies).
*Thymic tumor develops in up to 15–20% of generalized MG patients.*
*Always rule out lung cancer.*

## Myotonic Dystrophy
**(autosomal dominant disorder)**

Serum CK is increased.
Findings due to atrophy of testicle and androgenic deficiency are noted.

## Polymyositis
**(nongenetic primary inflammatory myopathy; may be idiopathic or due to infection or may be associated with dermatomyositis, or collagen or malignant disease)**

See Fig. 10-1 and Table 10-1.
Serum enzymes
  • Serum CK is the most useful. Serum LD and AST are increased in 25% of patients.
Muscle biopsy findings are definitive.
Total eosinophil count is frequently increased. WBC may be increased in fulminant disease.
Increased ANA titers and positive RF may be found.
*Associated carcinoma may occur (especially cancer of lung or breast).*

# Laboratory Tests for Bone Diseases

## Alkaline Phosphatase (ALP), Bone-Specific, Serum

### Use

Marker for bone formation

### Increased in

Paget's disease; may be more sensitive than total ALP
Primary hyperparathyroidism
Osteomalacia
Osteoporosis
Pregnancy

### Calcium, Serum

See Chapters 3 and 13.

### Osteocalcin

*Use*

Marker of bone turnover rather than just of resorption or formation. Assesses
patients at risk for osteoporosis.
Classifies patients with established osteoporosis.
Determine efficacy of therapy in osteoporosis or bone metastases.

*Increased in*

Increased bone formation (e.g., Paget's disease, primary hyperparathyroidism,
osteogenic sarcoma)

*Decreased in*

Hypoparathyroidism
Cushing's syndrome

### Pyridinium Cross-Links and Deoxypyridinoline, Urine
**(stabilizing factors to type I bone collagen within organic matrix of
mineralized bone; released into circulation)**

*Use*

Increase is marker of increased osteoclastic activity and bone demineralization.

### Telopeptide, N-Terminal and C-Terminal, Urine
**(antibodies to intermolecular cross-links of bone type I collagen)**

*Use*

Serial changes decide course of therapy and monitor response to therapy of osteoporosis. Failure to change >30% after 4–8 wks of therapy may suggest need to
change therapy. Not for diagnosis.
More specific to bone than pyridinoline, hydroxyproline, or calcium.

*Increased in*
*(indicates bone resorption)*

Paget's disease
Osteoporosis
Primary hyperparathyroidism
Metastatic bone cancer

---

# Diseases of Skeletal System

---

### Fat Embolism
**(occurs after trauma [e.g., fractures, insertion of femoral head prosthesis])**

Unexplained decrease in Hb
Decreased platelet count
Free fat in urine
Fat globules in sputum, bronchoalveolar washings, and blood
Arterial blood gas values are always abnormal in clinically significant fat
embolism syndrome; are the most useful and important laboratory data.
*Laboratory findings alone are inadequate for diagnosis.*

## Osteomyelitis

Organism is identified by bone biopsy material culture and blood culture.
Microbiology
- *Staphylococcus aureus* causes almost all infections of hip and two-thirds of infections of skull, vertebrae, and long bones. Other bacteria may be present simultaneously.
- *S. aureus* causes 90% of cases of hematogenous osteomyelitis.
- Group B streptococci, *S. aureus*, and *Escherichia coli* are chief organisms in neonates. *Haemophilus influenzae* type b; *S. aureus*, group A; *Streptococcus* and *Salmonella* are chief organisms in older children. *S. aureus*, coagulase-negative staphylococci, and gram-negative bacilli are frequent organisms.
- *Staphylococcus epidermidis* is the most common organism involved in total hip arthroplasty infection.
- Gram-negative bacteria cause most infections of mandible, pelvis, and small bones.
- *Salmonella* is found in patients with hemoglobinopathies.
- Diabetic patients with foot ulcers and surgical infections that extend to bone usually have polymicrobial infection.
- Most infections due to *Candida, Aspergillus*, and other fungi occur in diabetic and immunocompromised patients. *Candida* infection also occurs in patients with central and hyperalimentation lines. Patients are often on steroid and antibiotic therapy.
- *Mucor* infection occurs in poorly controlled diabetics.
- IV drug abusers frequently have osteomyelitis of sternoclavicular joints.
- Puncture wounds of calcaneus usually involve pseudomonal organisms.
- Cranial involvement in neonates after scalp fetal monitoring during labor is mainly associated with group B streptococci, *E. coli*, and staphylococci.
- *Coccidioides immitis* may occur in endemic areas.
Vertebral osteomyelitis
- May be due to unusual organisms (e.g., *Mycobacterium tuberculosis*, fungi, *Brucella*).
- Blood culture may be positive.
- Aspiration of involved site with stains, cultures, and histologic exam.

## Osteopenia
(generic term for decreased mineralized bone on x-ray study, but x-ray study cannot distinguish osteomalacia from osteoporosis in most patients)

Diagnosis is established by bone biopsy that may be combined with tetracycline labeling.
All serum chemistry values may be normal in any form of osteopenia; are commonly normal in osteomalacia, especially that coexisting with osteoporosis. Serum 25-hydroxyvitamin D <15 ng/mL suggests osteomalacia.

## Paget's Disease of Bone (Osteitis Deformans)

Marked increase in serum ALP (in 90% of cases) is directly related to severity and extent of disease.
Serum calcium increased during immobilization (e.g., due to intercurrent illness or fracture).
Normal or slightly increased serum phosphorus
Frequently increased urine calcium; renal calculi common
Increase in hydroxyproline in urine may be marked.

## Osteogenic Sarcoma

Marked increase in serum ALP ($\leq$ 40 times normal); reflects new bone formation and parallels clinical course (e.g., metastasis, response to therapy).

## Rickets

Serum ALP is increased. This is the earliest and most reliable biochemical abnormality.
Serum calcium is usually normal or slightly decreased.
Serum phosphorus is usually decreased.
Serum calcium and phosphorus rapidly become normal after institution of vitamin D therapy.
Serum 25-hydroxyvitamin D is low (usually <5 ng/mL; normal = 10–20 ng/mL).

# Diseases of Joints

See Table 10-2.

## Synovial Fluid, Normal Values

| | |
|---|---|
| Volume | 1.0–3.5 mL |
| pH | Parallels serum |
| Appearance | Clear, pale yellow, or straw-colored; viscous; does not clot |
| Fibrin clot | 0 |
| Mucin clot | Good |
| WBC (per cu mm) | <200 (even in presence of leukocytosis in blood) |
| Neutrophils | <25% |
| Crystals | |
|     Free | 0 |
|     Intracellular | 0 |
| Fasting uric acid, bilirubin | Approximately the same as serum |
| TP | ~25–30% of serum protein |
| Mean = 1.8 gm/dL | |
|     Abnormal if >2.5 gm/dL; inflammation is moderately severe if >4.5 gm/dL | |
| Glucose | <10 mg/dL lower than serum level of simultaneously drawn blood |
| Culture | No growth |

## Chondrocalcinosis ("Pseudogout")

Joint fluid contains crystals identified as calcium pyrophosphate dihydrate.
Blood and urine findings are normal.

## Gout

Presence of crystals of monosodium urate from tophi or joint fluid viewed microscopically under polarized light establish the diagnosis and differentiate it from calcium pyrophosphate crystals of pseudogout and calcium oxalate crystals.
Histologic examination of gouty nodule is characteristic.
Increased serum uric acid does *not* establish the diagnosis of gout. Is normal in 30% of acute attacks. Many gout patients never have an elevated level.
Serum uric acid levels are increased in ~25% of asymptomatic relatives.
Only 1–3% of patients with hyperuricemia have gout.
With primary gout, ≤ 25% of patients develop uric acid stones.

**Table 10-2.** Synovial Fluid Findings in Various Diseases of Joints

| Property | Normal | Noninflammatory[a] | Hemorrhagic[b] | Acute Inflammatory[c] | | | Septic | | |
|---|---|---|---|---|---|---|---|---|---|
| | | | | Acute Gouty Arthritis | RF | RA | TB Arthritis | Gonorrheal Arthritis | Septic Arthritis[d,e] |
| Volume | 3.5 mL | I | I | I | | | I | | |
| Appearance | Clear, colorless | Clear, straw | Bloody or xanthochromic | Turbid yellow | | | Turbid yellow | | |
| Viscosity | High | High | V | D | | | D | | |
| Fibrin clot | 0 | Usually 0 | Usually 0 | + | | | + | | |
| Mucin clot | Good | Good | V | Fair to poor | | | Poor | | |
| WBC (no./cu mm)[f] | <200 | <5000 | <10,000 | Range 750–45,000 / Average 13,500 | 300–98,000 / 17,800 | 300–75,000 / 15,500 | 2500–105,000 / 23,500 | 1500–108,000 / 14,000 | 15,600–213,000 / 65,400 |
| Neutrophils (%) | <25 | <25 | <50 | Range 48–94 / Average 83 | 8–98 / 46 | 5–96 / 65 | 29–96 / 67 | 2–96 / 64 | 75–100 / 95 |
| Blood-synovia glucose difference (mg/dL)[g] | <10 | <10 | <25 | Range 0–41 / Average 12 | 6 | 0–88 / 31 | 0–108 / 57 | 0–97 / 26 | 40–122 / 71 |

**Table 10-2.** (continued)

| Property | Normal | Noninflam-matory[a] | Hemor-rhagic[b] | Acute Gouty Arthritis | RF | RA | TB Arthritis | Gonorrheal Arthritis | Septic Arthritis[d,e] |
|---|---|---|---|---|---|---|---|---|---|
| Culture[h] | Neg | Neg | Neg | Neg | Neg | Neg | See Infective Arthritis. | | |

Neg = negative; + = positive.

[a]For example, degenerative joint disease, traumatic arthritis, some cases of pigmented villonodular synovitis.

[b]For example, tumor, hemophilia, neuroarthropathy, trauma, some cases of pigmented villonodular synovitis.

[c]For example, RA, Reiter's syndrome, acute gouty arthritis, acute pseudogout, SLE.

[d]For example, pneumococcal.

[e]In purulent arthropathy of undetermined cause, very high synovial fluid lactate (>2000 mg/dL) indicates a nongonococcal septic arthritis (gram-negative bacilli, gram-positive cocci, fungi). Lactate is <100 mg/dL in gonococcal infection, gout, RA, osteoarthritis, trauma.

[f]Use saline instead of acetic acid, which clumps the joint fluid.

[g]Joint tap should be performed, preferably after the patient has been fasting for >4 hrs, and a blood glucose determination should be performed simultaneously. Culture for tubercle bacilli should be performed.

[h]Material should be cultured aerobically and anaerobically. Culture to rule out infectious arthritis, gout, or pseudogout.

*Synovial fluid analysis is primarily useful to diagnose or to rule out infectious arthritis, gout, or pseudogout.*

*To distinguish inflammatory from noninflammatory conditions, synovial fluid WBC >2000/cu mm and >75% PMNs have sensitivities of 84% and 75% and specificities of 84% and 92%, respectively.*

Drug-induced gout may cause ≤ 50% of all new cases of gouty arthritis.
Moderate leukocytosis and increased ESR occur during acute attacks; normal at
other times. Low-grade proteinuria may occur for many years before further
evidence of renal disease appears.

## Gout, Secondary

### Occurs in

Lead intoxication
Neoplastic and hemolytic conditions (e.g., leukemia, polycythemia vera, sec-
ondary polycythemia, malignant lymphomas). Blood dyscrasias are found in
~10% of patients with clinical gout.
Cytotoxic drug therapy
Psoriasis

## Infective Arthritis

Joint fluid
- Bacterial
    In purulent arthritis, organism is recovered from joint and blood. Most
    often due to *S. aureus* and *Streptococcus* spp. Positive Gram's stain is
    useful for prompt diagnosis and when cultures are negative.
    In tuberculous arthritis, acid-fast stain, culture for tubercle bacilli, and
    biopsy of synovia confirm diagnosis.
    In children, most common organisms are *H. influenzae* type b, *S. aureus*,
    various streptococci, and gram-negative bacilli.
    In young adults, >50% of cases are due to *Neisseria gonorrhoeae*; the rest
    are due to *S. aureus*, streptococci, or gram-negative bacilli.
- Viral
- Fungal
Infection of prosthetic joints
- Early onset (within first 3 months).
- Delayed onset (within first 2 yrs—two-thirds of patients).
    Due to organisms introduced during surgery or to those of nosocomial
    infection, which multiply slowly; most common are skin flora.
- Late onset (after 2 yrs—one third of cases).
    Due to hematogenous seeding from infected focus (e.g., GU tract, dental).
- If five biopsies are cultured, bacterial growth in fewer than two biopsies or
    only in broth media indicates contamination, but growth in all five biopsies
    in solid and broth media suggests infection.

## Osteoarthritis

Laboratory tests are all normal and not helpful.

## Polymyalgia Rheumatica

ESR is markedly increased; this is a criterion for diagnosis.
Mild hypochromic or normochromic anemia is common.
Abnormalities of serum proteins are frequent, although there is no consistent or
    diagnostic pattern.
Serum enzymes (e.g., AST, ALP) may be increased in one-third of patients.
Temporal artery biopsy findings are often positive because one-third of patients
    with giant cell arteritis present with polymyalgia rheumatica, which ultimately
    develops in 50–90% of them.

## Reiter's Syndrome
**(This triad of arthritis, urethritis, and conjunctivitis is present in only one-third of patients.)**

Increased acute phase reactants
- Increased ESR parallels the clinical course.
- Increased CRP and WBC.

## Rheumatoid Arthritis (RA)

American Rheumatism Association has 11 criteria for diagnosis of RA; seven are required for diagnosis of classic RA, five for definite RA, and three for probable RA. Four lab findings included in these criteria are (1) positive serum test for RF, (2) poor mucin clotting of synovial fluid, (3) characteristic histologic changes in synovium, and (4) characteristic histologic changes in rheumatoid nodules.

Serologic tests for RF (autoantibodies to immunoglobulins)
- Significant titer is ≥ 1:80; in conditions other than RA, it is usually <1:80.
- Negative in one-third of patients with definite RA. Becomes positive after disease is active for 3–6 months. Titer may decrease during remission but rarely becomes negative.
- Positive in normal population; increasingly more common with age; ≤ 30% of persons older than 70 yrs.
- May be positive in other conditions. See Chapter 16.

Increased ESR, positive CRP, and other acute phase reactants may be present.

Moderate normocytic hypochromic anemia of chronic disease with decreased serum iron, normal TIBC, and normal iron stores. If Hct <26%, search for other cause of anemia.

Synovial biopsy is especially useful in monoarticular form to rule out TB, gout, etc.

Synovial fluid glucose may be greatly decreased (<10 mg/dL). See Amyloidosis in Chapter 16.

## Rheumatoid Arthritis, Juvenile

Usual serologic tests for RF are negative, but RF and circulating immune complexes can be demonstrated by special techniques.

## Sjögren's Syndrome (SS)
**(may be secondary to RA, SLE, scleroderma, or vasculitis in one-half to two-thirds of patients, or may be primary; immunologic abnormality associated with decreased salivary and lacrimal gland secretion)**

Diagnosis is established by biopsy of salivary gland (lower lip is easiest).
ANAs may be present. See Chapter 16.
RF is present in ≤ 90% of primary and secondary types.
Mild normochromic, normocytic anemia occurs in 50% of patients.
Leukopenia occurs in more than one-third of patients.
ESR is usually increased.
Serum protein electrophoresis shows increased gamma globulins (usually polyclonal) largely due to IgG.
Primary biliary cirrhosis is found in 3% of patients with SS; SS is found in 50–100% of patients with primary biliary cirrhosis.
Other associated diseases include generalized scleroderma, mixed connective tissue disease, and chronic active hepatitis.

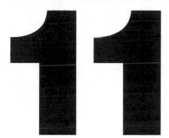

# Hematologic Diseases

# Hematologic Laboratory Tests

## Coombs' (Antiglobulin) Test

### Positive Direct Coombs' (Antiglobulin) Test

#### Use
Detects immunoglobulin antibodies and/or complement on patient's RBC membrane (e.g., autoimmune hemolysis, hemolytic disease of newborn, drug-induced hemolysis, transfusion reactions)

#### Positive In
Erythroblastosis fetalis

Most cases of autoimmune hemolytic anemia, including ≤ 15% of certain systemic diseases, especially acute and chronic leukemias, malignant lymphomas, collagen diseases

Delayed hemolytic transfusion reaction

Drug induced
- Alpha methyldopa (in 30% of patients but <1% show hemolysis)
- L-Dopa
- Others

Healthy blood donors (1:4000–1:8000 persons)

### Positive Indirect Coombs' Test
(using patient's serum that contains antibody)

#### Use
Cross matching for blood transfusion

Detect and identify antibodies
- Specific antibody—usually isoimmunization from previous transfusion
- "Nonspecific" autoantibody in acquired hemolytic anemia

RBC phenotyping
- In genetic and forensic medicine
- To identify syngeneic twins for bone marrow transplantation

## Erythropoietin (Ep), Plasma
(Normal = 3.7–16.0 IU/L by radioimmunoassay)

#### Use

Differential diagnosis of polycythemia vera

Indicator of need for Ep therapy in patients with renal failure

#### Interferences

Decreased by high plasma viscosity, estrogens, beta-adrenergic blockers, agents that increase renal blood flow (e.g., enalapril, an inhibitor of angiotensin-converting enzyme)

Circadian rhythm in hospitalized adults with lowest values at 0800–1200 and 40% higher values in late evening

### Increased Appropriately*

Extremely high: usually transfusion dependent anemia with Hct = 10–25 and Hb = 3–7 gm/dL; e.g., aplastic anemia, severe hemolytic anemia, hematologic cancers

Very high: Patients have mild to moderate anemia with Hct = 25–40 or Hb = 7–12 gm/dL.

High: Patients are more anemic, e.g., hemolytic anemia, myelodysplasia, exposure to chemotherapeutic or immunosuppressive drugs, AIDS.

### Increased Inappropriately*

Some renal disorders (cysts, postrenal transplant)
Some neoplasms
  Malignant
  • Renal tumors
  • Hepatocellular carcinoma, or hemangiosarcoma
  • Testicular carcinoma
  • Malignant pheochromocytoma
  • Breast carcinoma
  Nonmalignant
  • Meningioma
  • Capillary hemangioblastoma of brain (20% of cases), liver, or adrenal
  • Leiomyoma

### Decreased Inappropriately*

Renal failure
Autonomic neuropathy
AIDS before zidovudine therapy
Weeks 3 and 4 after bone marrow transplant
Polycythemia vera

### Decreased Appropriately*

Renal failure, RA, multiple myeloma, cancer

## Ferritin, Serum
### (chief iron-storage protein in the body)

### Use

Diagnosis of iron deficiency or excess; correlates with total body iron stores
  • Predict and monitor iron deficiency
  • Determine response to iron therapy or compliance with treatment
  • Differentiate iron deficiency from chronic disease as cause of anemia
  • Monitor iron status in patients with chronic renal disease with or without dialysis
  • Detect iron overload states and monitor rate of iron accumulation and response to iron-depletion therapy

### Decreased in

Iron deficiency. Is most sensitive and specific test for iron deficiency if is not increased (e.g., pregnancy, infancy, polycythemia) or there is no vitamin C deficiency. *Decreases before anemia and other changes occur. No other condition causes a low level. Returns to normal range within few days after onset of oral*

*Ep is inversely related to RBC volume, Hb, or Hct.

*iron therapy; failure to produce serum ferritin level >50 ng/mL suggests non-compliance or continued iron loss.*

<18 ng/mL is associated with absent stainable iron in marrow.

<12 ng/mL always indicates iron deficiency.

>80 ng/mL essentially excludes iron deficiency.

### Increased in

Ferritin is an acute phase reactant and thus is increased in many patients with various acute and chronic liver diseases, alcoholism, malignancies, infection and inflammation, hyperthyroidism, Gaucher's disease, AMI, etc. *Serum ferritin may not be decreased when iron deficiency coexists with these conditions, and then bone marrow stain for iron may be the only way to detect the iron deficiency.*

Iron overload (e.g., hemosiderosis, idiopathic hemochromatosis). Can be used to monitor therapeutic removal of excess storage iron. Transferrin saturation is more sensitive to detect early iron overload in hemochromatosis; serum ferritin is used to confirm diagnosis and as indication to proceed with liver biopsy. Ratio of serum ferritin (in ng/mL) to ALT (in IU/L) >10 in iron overloaded thalassemic patients but average $\leq 2$ in viral hepatitis; ratio decreases with successful iron chelation therapy.

Anemias other than iron deficiency (e.g., megaloblastic, hemolytic, sideroblastic, thalassemia major and minor, spherocytosis, porphyria cutanea tarda)

Renal cell carcinoma due to hemorrhage within tumor

RBC transfusion $\geq 6$ units within last 6 months

## Flow Cytometry

### Use

Diagnosis of leukemias and lymphomas

Diagnose DNA content and DNA synthetic activity of tumors

Enumeration of lymphocyte subsets (e.g., CD4+ T cells as surrogate marker for disease progression in AIDS)

## Haptoglobins, Serum

### Use

Indicator of chronic hemolysis. Such patients should not have splenectomy if serum haptoglobin is >40 mg/dL if infection and inflammation have been ruled out.

Following splenectomy, increased haptoglobin level indicates success of surgery for these conditions (e.g., haptoglobin reappears at 24 hrs and becomes normal in 4–6 days in hereditary spherocytosis treated with splenectomy).

In diagnosis of transfusion reaction by comparison of concentrations in pre-transfusion and post-transfusion samples

In paternity studies by determination of haptoglobin phenotypes

### Increased in

Conditions associated with increased ESR and alpha$_2$ globulin (haptoglobin is also an acute phase reactant)

One-third of patients with obstructive biliary disease

Therapy with steroids or androgens

Aplastic anemia (normal to very high)

Diabetes mellitus

### Decreased or Absent in

Hemoglobinemia (related to the duration and severity of hemolysis) due to

- Intravascular hemolysis (e.g., hereditary spherocytosis with marked hemolysis, pyruvate kinase deficiency, autoimmune hemolytic anemia, some transfusion reactions)
- Extravascular hemolysis
- Intramedullary hemolysis (e.g., thalassemia, megaloblastic anemias)

Genetically absent in 1% of general population
Parenchymatous liver disease (especially cirrhosis)
Protein loss via kidney, GI tract, skin
Infancy

## Hemoglobin, Fetal (Hb F)
**(alkali denaturation method; confirmed by examination of Hb bands on electrophoresis)**

### Normal

>50% at birth; gradual decrease to ~5% by age 5 months
<2% older than age 2 yrs

### Use

Diagnosis of various hemoglobinopathies

### Increased in

Various hemoglobinopathies. See Table 11-1. ~50% of patients with beta-thalassemia minor have high levels of Hb F; even higher levels are found in virtually all patients with beta-thalassemia major.
Hereditary persistence of Hb F
Nonhereditary refractory normoblastic anemia (one-third of patients)
Some patients with leukemia, especially juvenile myeloid leukemia
Multiple myeloma
Molar pregnancy
Patients with an extra D chromosome (trisomy 13–15, D1 trisomy) or an extra G chromosome (trisomy 21, Down syndrome, mongolism)
Acquired aplastic anemia (due to drugs, toxic chemicals, or infections, or idiopathic)

## Hemoglobin, Serum
**(normal <10 mg/dL; <30 mg/dL is not accurate technically; >150 mg/dL causes hemoglobinuria; >200 mg/dL adds clear cherry red color to serum)**

### Use

Increase indicates intravascular hemolysis

## Iron, Serum

### Use

Differential diagnosis of anemias
Diagnosis of hemochromatosis and hemosiderosis

### Increased in

Idiopathic hemochromatosis
Hemosiderosis of excessive iron intake (e.g., repeated blood transfusions, iron therapy) (may be >300 μg/dL)
Decreased formation of RBCs (e.g., thalassemia, pyridoxine-deficiency anemia, pernicious anemia in relapse)
Increased destruction of RBCs (e.g., hemolytic anemias)

**Table 11-1.** Representative Laboratory Values of Some Common Hemoglobinopathies

| Laboratory Test | Hemoglobinopathy | | | | |
|---|---|---|---|---|---|
| | AS | SS | SC* | S-beta+ | S-beta0 |
| Hb (gm/dL) | N | 7.5 | 11 | 11 | 8 |
| Range | | (6–9) | (9–14) | (8–13) | (7–10) |
| Hct (%) | N | 22 | 30 | 32 | 25 |
| Range | | (18–30) | (26–40) | (25–40) | (20–36) |
| MCV (fL) | N | 93 | 80 | 76 | 69 |
| Reticulocyte count (%) | N | 11 | 3 | 3 | 8 |
| Range | | (4–30) | (1.5–6.0) | (1.5–6.0) | (3–18) |
| RBC morphology | N | | | | |
| Sickle cells | | Many | Rare | Rare | Varies |
| Target cells | | Many | Many | | Many |
| Microcytosis | | | | Mild | Marked |
| Hypochromia | | | | Mild | Marked |
| Nucleated RBC | | Many | | | |
| Hb electrophoresis (%) | N | | | | |
| S | 38–45 | 80–95 | 45–55 | 55–75 | 50–85 |
| F | N | 2–20 | <8 | 1–20 | 2–30 |
| $A_2$ | 1–3 | <3.6 | | >3.6 | >3.6 |
| A | 55–60 | 0 | 0 | 15–30 | 0 |
| C | 0 | 0 | 45–55 | 0 | 0 |
| Clinical severity | No symptoms | Moderate/severe | Mild/moderate | Mild/moderate | Mild/severe |
| Presence in U.S. blacks | 10% | 1:625 | 1:833 | 1:1667 | 1:1667 |

*Blood smear shows tetragonal crystals within RBC in 70% of patients; RBCs tend to be microcytic with low or low/normal MCV but high MCHC; typical distorted RBCs in which Hb is concentrated more in one area of cell than another.

Acute liver damage (degree of increase parallels the amount of hepatic necrosis) (may be >1000 $\mu g$/dL); some cases of chronic liver disease
Progesteronal birth control pills (may be >200 $\mu g$/dL) and pregnancy
Premenstrual elevation 10–30%

### Decreased in

Iron deficiency anemia
Normochromic (normocytic or microcytic) anemias of infection and chronic diseases (e.g., neoplasms, active collagen diseases)
Nephrosis (due to loss of iron-binding protein in urine)
Pernicious anemia at onset of remission
Menstruation (decreased 10–30%)
*Diurnal variation—normal values in mid-morning, low values in mid-afternoon, very low values (~10 $\mu g$/dL) near midnight. Diurnal variation disappears at levels <45 $\mu g$/dL.*

## Iron-Binding Capacity (TIBC), Total, Serum

TIBC ($\mu mol$/L) = transferrin (mg/L) × 0.025

### Use

Differential diagnosis of anemias

### Increased in

Iron deficiency
Acute and chronic blood loss
Acute liver damage
Late pregnancy
Progesteronal birth control pills

### Decreased in

Hemochromatosis
Cirrhosis of the liver
Thalassemia
Anemias of infection and chronic diseases (e.g., uremia, RA)
Nephrosis
Hyperthyroidism

## Iron (Hemosiderin), Stainable, in Bone Marrow

### Use

*Is a most reliable index of iron deficiency; its presence almost invariably rules out
iron deficiency anemia.*
Diagnosis of iron overload

### Increased in

Idiopathic hemochromatosis
Hemochromatosis secondary to
  • Increased intake (e.g., Bantu siderosis, excessive medicine ingestion).
  • Anemias with increased erythropoiesis (especially thalassemia major; also
    thalassemia minor, some other hemoglobinopathies, paroxysmal nocturnal
    hemoglobinuria, "sideroachrestic" anemias, refractory anemias with hyper-
    cellular bone marrow, etc.). In hemolytic anemias, decrease or absence may
    signify acute hemolytic crisis.
  • Liver injury (e.g., after portal shunt surgery).
  • Atransferrinemia.
Megaloblastic anemias in relapse
Uremia
Chronic infection
Chronic pancreatic insufficiency

### Decreased in

Iron deficiency (e.g., inadequate dietary intake, chronic bleeding, malignancy,
  acute blood loss). *Rapidly disappears after hemorrhage.*
Polycythemia vera (usually absent in polycythemia vera but usually normal or
  increased in secondary polycythemia). See Table 11-2.
Pernicious anemia in early phase of therapy
Collagen diseases (especially RA, SLE)
Infiltration of marrow (e.g., malignant lymphomas, metastatic carcinoma,
  myelofibrosis, miliary granulomas)
Uremia
Chronic infection (e.g., pulmonary TB, bronchiectasis, chronic pyeloneph-
  ritis)
Myeloproliferative diseases
*One may have a normal serum iron and TIBC in iron deficiency anemia, espe-
  cially if Hb is <9 gm/dL.*

**Table 11-2.** Comparison of Polycythemia Vera, Secondary Polycythemia, and Relative Polycythemia

| Test | Polycythemia Vera | Secondary Polycythemia[a] | Relative Polycythemia[b] |
|---|---|---|---|
| Hct | I | I | I |
| Blood volume | I | I | D or N |
| Red cell mass | I | I | D or N |
| Plasma volume | I or N | N or I | D |
| Platelet count | I | N | N |
| WBC with shift to left | I | N | N |
| Nucleated RBC, abnormal RBC | I | N | N |
| Serum uric acid | I | I | N |
| Serum vitamin $B_{12}$ | I | N | N |
| Leukocyte alkaline phosphatase | I | N | N |
| Oxygen saturation of arterial blood | N | D | N |
| Bone marrow | Hyperplasia of all elements | Erythroid hyperplasia | N |
| Erythropoietin level | D | I | N |

[a]Diagnosis of secondary polycythemia is suggested by erythrocytosis without increased WBC, platelets, or splenomegaly; causes should be sought.
[b]Relative polycythemia is not secondary to hypoxia but results from decreased plasma volume due to unknown mechanism or to decreased fluid intake and/or excess loss of body fluids (e.g., diuretics, dehydration, burns) with high normal RBC mass.

## Mean Corpuscular Hemoglobin (MCH)
**(Hb divided by RBC count)**

### Use

Limited value in differential diagnosis of anemias
Instrument calibration

### Decreased in

Microcytic and normocytic anemias

### Increased in

Macrocytic anemias
Infants and newborns

## Mean Corpuscular Hemoglobin Concentration (MCHC)
**(Hb divided by Hct)**

### Use

For laboratory quality control
Instrument calibration

### Decreased in
**( <30.1 gm/dL)**

Hypochromic anemias. *Normal value does not rule out any of these anemias.*

**Table 11-3.** RBC Indices in Various Anemias[a]

| Type of Anemia | MCV[b] (fL) | MCH[c] (pg) | MCHC[d] (gm/dL) |
|---|---|---|---|
| Normal | 82–92 | 27–31 | 32–36 |
| Normocytic | 82–92 | 25–30 | 32–36 |
| Macrocytic | 95–150 | 30–50 | 32–36 |
| Microcytic (usually hypochromic) | 50–80 | 12–25 | 25–30 |

[a]Use: Classification and differential diagnosis of anemias.
[b]MCV (fL) = Hct/RBC.
[c]MCH (pg) = Hb/RBC; represents weight of Hb in average RBC. Not as useful as MCHC.
[d]MCHC (gm/dL) = Hb/Hct; represents concentration of Hb in average RBC.
*Formula for estimating Hct from Hb*:
Hct = Hb (gm/dL) × 2.8 + 0.8 or Hct = 3 × Hb

*Low MCHC may not occur in iron deficiency anemia when performed with auto-mated instruments* or occurs very late in iron deficiency when anemia is severe.

### Increased in

Only in hereditary spherocytosis; should be suspected whenever MCHC >36 gm/dL
Infants and newborns

## Mean Corpuscular Volume (MCV)

See Table 11-3.

### Use

Classification and differential diagnosis of anemias
Useful screening test for occult alcoholism

### Increased in

Macrocytic anemias (MCV >95 fL and often >110 fL; MCHC >30 gm/dL)
  • Megaloblastic anemia
      Pernicious anemia (Vitamin $B_{12}$ or folate deficiency)
      Sprue (e.g., steatorrhea, celiac disease, intestinal resection or fistula)
      Macrocytic anemia of pregnancy
      Megaloblastic anemia of infancy
      Fish tapeworm infestation
      Carcinoma of stomach, following total gastrectomy
      Drugs
      Oral contraceptives
      Anticonvulsants (e.g., phenytoin, primidone, phenobarbital)
      Antitumor agents (e.g., methotrexate, hydroxyurea, cyclophosphamide)
      Antimicrobials (e.g., sulfamethoxazole, sulfasalazine, trimethoprim, zido-vudine, pyrimethamine)
      Orotic aciduria
      Di Guglielmo's disease
  • Nonmegaloblastic macrocytic anemias; are usually normocytic (MCV usually <110 fL)
      Alcoholism
      Liver disease
      Anemia of hypothyroidism
      Accelerated erythropoiesis (some hemolytic anemias, posthemorrhage)
      Myelodysplastic syndromes (aplastic anemia, acquired sideroblastic anemia)
      Myelophthisic anemia

Postsplenectomy
* Infants and newborns

## Normal in

Normocytic anemias (MCV = 80–94 fL; MCHC >30 gm/dL)
* After acute hemorrhage
* Some hemolytic anemias
* Some hemoglobinopathies
* Anemias due to inadequate blood formation (myelophthisic, hypoplastic, aplastic)
* Endocrinopathies (e.g., hypopituitarism, hypothyroidism, hypoadrenalism)
* Anemia of chronic disease

## Decreased in

Microcytic anemias (MCV <80 fL; MCHC <30 gm/dL)
* Usually hypochromic
    Iron deficiency anemia
        Inadequate intake
        Poor absorption
        Excessive iron requirements
        Chronic blood loss
    Pyridoxine-responsive anemia
    Thalassemia (major or combined with hemoglobinopathy)
    Sideroblastic anemia (hereditary)
    Lead poisoning
    Anemia of chronic diseases (usually normocytic)
* Usually normocytic
    Anemia of chronic diseases
    Hemoglobinopathies

# Osmotic Fragility

## Use

Diagnosis of hereditary spherocytic anemia

## Increased in

Hereditary spherocytic anemia
Hereditary nonspherocytic hemolytic anemia
Acquired hemolytic anemia
Hemolytic disease of newborn due to ABO incompatibility

# Protoporphyrin, Free Erythrocyte (FEP)
(normal <100 μg/dL/packed RBCs)

## Use

Screening for lead poisoning and iron deficiency

## Increased in

Iron deficiency (even before anemia; early sensitive sign, useful for screening)
Range 100–1000 μg/dL; average ~200 μg/dL
Chronic lead poisoning
Most sideroblastic anemias (e.g., acquired idiopathic)
Anemia of chronic diseases

## Normal or Decreased in

Primary disorders of globin synthesis

- Thalassemia minor (useful to differentiate from iron deficiency)

Pyridoxine-responsive anemia

One form of sideroblastic anemia due to block proximal to protoporphyrin synthesis

## Red Cell Distribution Width (RDW)

Normal = 11.5–14.5. No subnormal values have been reported.

Is quantitative measure of anisocytosis

$$CV = \frac{\text{Standard deviation of RBC size}}{\text{MCV}}$$

### Use

Classification of anemias based on MCV and RDW is most useful to distinguish iron deficiency anemia from that of chronic disease or heterozygous thalassemia and to improve detection of early iron or folate deficiency.

The RDW is more sensitive in microcytic than macrocytic RBC conditions. Not helpful for patients without anemia.

### Classification of RBC Disorders by MCV and RDW

| | |
|---|---|
| RDW low, MCV low | Thalassemia minor |
| RDW normal, MCV low | Thalassemia minor |
| | Anemia of chronic disease |
| RDW high, MCV low | Iron deficiency |
| | Hb H disease |
| | S-beta-thalassemia |
| | Fragmentation of RBCs |
| | Hemoglobinopathy traits (AC) |
| | Some patients with anemia of chronic disease |
| RDW normal, MCV normal | Normal |
| | Anemia of chronic disease |
| | Hereditary spherocytosis |
| | Some hemoglobinopathy traits (e.g., AS) |
| RDW high, MCV normal | Early deficiency of iron or vitamin $B_{12}$ or folate |
| | Sickle cell (SC) anemia |
| | Hb SC disease |
| RDW normal, MCV high | Aplastic anemia |
| | Myelodysplastic syndrome |
| RDW high, MCV high | Deficiency of vitamin $B_{12}$ or folate |
| | Immune hemolytic anemia |
| | Cold agglutinins |
| | Alcoholism |

## Reticulocytes

### Use

Diagnosis of ineffective erythropoiesis or decreased RBC formation.

Increase indicates effective RBC production. Is a useful index of therapeutic response to iron, folate or vitamin $B_{12}$ therapy and to blood loss.

### Increased in

After iron therapy for iron deficiency anemia. After blood loss or increased RBC destruction: Normal increase is 3–6 times.

After specific therapy for megaloblastic anemias

Possibly other hematologic conditions (e.g., polycythemia, metastatic carcinoma in bone marrow, Di Guglielmo's disease)

## Decreased in

Ineffective erythropoiesis or decreased RBC formation
- Severe autoimmune type of hemolytic disease
- Aregenerative crises
- Megaloblastic disorders

Alcoholism

Myxedema

Reticulocyte index (RI) corrects count for degree of anemia.

$$RI = \text{Reticulocyte count} \times \frac{\text{Patient's Hct}}{45} \times \frac{1}{1.85}$$

(45 is assumed normal Hct; 1.85 is number of days for reticulocyte to mature into an RBC.)

RI <2% indicates hypoproliferative component to anemia.

RI >2–3% indicates increased RBC production.

## Transferrin, Serum

### Use

Differential diagnosis of anemias

### Increased in

Iron deficiency anemia

Pregnancy, estrogen therapy, hyperestrogenism

### Decreased in

Hypochromic microcytic anemia of chronic disease

Acute inflammation

Protein deficiency or loss (e.g., burns, chronic diseases, nephrosis, malnutrition)

Genetic deficiency

## Transferrin Saturation, Serum

Normal ≥ 16%

$$\text{Transferrin saturation (\%)} = \frac{\text{Serum iron (}\mu\text{g/dL)}}{\text{TIBC (}\mu\text{g/dL)}} \times 100$$

Unsaturated iron-binding capacity = TIBC minus serum iron ($\mu$g/dL)

### Use

Screening for hemochromatosis

Differential diagnosis of anemias

### Increased in

Hemochromatosis

Hemosiderosis

Thalassemia

Progesteronal birth control pills (up to 75%)

Ingestion of iron (up to 100%)

Iron dextran administration causes increase for several weeks (may be >100%).

### Decreased in

Iron deficiency anemia (usually <10% in established deficiency)

Anemias of infection and chronic diseases (e.g., uremia, RA, some neoplasms)

## WBC Differential Count

### Use

Diagnosis of myeloproliferative disorders, myelodysplasias, various other hematologic disorders
Support diagnosis of various infections and inflammation
Often ordered inappropriately and has almost no value as a *screening* test

### Causes of Neutropenia/Leukopenia
*(absolute neutrophil count [total WBC × % segmented neutrophils and bands] <1800/cu mm; <1000 in black persons)*

Decreased/ineffective production of WBCs
  • Infections
  • Drugs and chemicals
  • Ionizing radiation
  • Hematopoietic diseases
      Folic acid and vitamin $B_{12}$ deficiency
      Aleukemic leukemia
      Aplastic anemia
      Myelophthisis
Decreased survival of WBCs
  • Felty's syndrome
  • SLE
  • Autoimmune and isoimmune neotropenias
  • Splenic sequestration
  • Drugs
Abnormal distribution of WBCs
  • Hypersplenism
Miscellaneous
  • Severe renal injury
Certain inborn errors of metabolism (e.g., maple syrup urine disease)
Immune defects
  • X-linked agammaglobulinemia
  • Dysgammaglobulinemia
  • Cyclic neutropenia
Disorders of myeloid stem cell proliferation
  • Kostmann's agranulocytosis.
  • Pregnancy—progressive decrease in granulocyte count during pregnancy. *Serum $B_{12}$ is normal in megaloblastic anemia of pregnancy.*

### Causes of Neutrophilia
*(absolute neutrophil count >8000/cu mm)*

See Tables 11-4 and 11-5.
Acute infections
Inflammation (e.g., vasculitis)
Intoxications
  • Metabolic (uremia, acidosis, eclampsia, acute gout)
  • Poisoning by chemicals, drugs, venoms, etc.
  • Parenteral (foreign protein and vaccines)
Acute hemorrhage
Acute hemolysis of RBCs
Myeloproliferative diseases
Tissue necrosis
Physiologic conditions (e.g., exercise, emotional stress, menstruation, obstetric labor)
Steroid administration

**Table 11-4.** Some Common Causes of Leukemoid Reaction

| Cause | Myelocytic | Lymphocytic | Monocytic |
|---|---|---|---|
| Infections | Endocarditis<br>Pneumonia<br>Septicemia<br>Leptospirosis<br>Other | Infectious mononucleosis<br>Infectious lymphocytosis<br>Pertussis<br>Chickenpox<br>TB | TB |
| Toxic conditions | Burns<br>Eclampsia<br>Poisoning<br>  (e.g., mercury) | | |
| Neoplasms | Carcinoma of colon<br>Embryonal carci-<br>  noma of kidney | Carcinoma of stomach<br>Carcinoma of breast | |
| Miscellaneous | Treatment of megalo-<br>  blastic anemia (of<br>  pregnancy, perni-<br>  cious anemia)<br>Acute hemorrhage<br>Acute hemolysis<br>Recovery from<br>  agranulocytosis | Dermatitis herpetiformis | |
| Myeloproliferative<br>  diseases | | | |

**Table 11-5.** Comparison of Leukemia and Leukemoid Reaction

| | Leukemia | Leukemoid Reaction |
|---|---|---|
| WBC | May be >100,000 | Usually <50,000 |
| Neutrophils | May have myeloid cells earlier<br>  than bands | Mature; <10% bands |
| Leukocyte alkaline<br>  phosphatase | Decreased in CML; variable<br>  in others | Increased |
| Basophilia, eosinophilia,<br>  monocytosis | Frequently present | Absent |
| Platelets | Frequently abnormal morphology<br>Frequently >1 million<br>  Thrombocytopenia may occur | Usually small<br>Normal aggregation<br>Rarely >600,000<br>No thrombocytopenia |
| Peripheral smear RBC | Nucleated RBCs, abnormal forms<br>  (tear drop, polychromatophilia)<br>  may occur | RBCs appear normal<br>No nucleated RBCs |
| Bone marrow | Abnormal | Hyperplastic |
| Karyotype | May be abnormal<br>$Ph^1$ may be present in CML | Normal<br>$Ph^1$ absent |
| Clone demonstrated | By X-linked inactivation | No clone demonstrated |
| *bcr-abl* demonstrated | By Southern blot or PCR | Not demonstrated |

$Ph^1$ = Philadelphia chromosome; CML = chronic myelogenous leukemia.

### Causes of Lymphocytosis
*(>4000/cu mm in adults, >7200/cu mm in adolescents, >9000/cu mm in young children and infants)*

Viral infections
Thyrotoxicosis (relative)
Addison's disease
Neutropenia with relative lymphocytosis
Lymphatic leukemia
Crohn's disease
Ulcerative colitis
Serum sickness
Drug hypersensitivity
Vasculitis

### Causes of Lymphocytopenia
*(<1500/cu mm in adults, <3000/cu mm in children)*

Increased destruction of lymphocytes
  • Chemotherapy or radiation treatment
  • Corticosteroids
Increased loss via GI tract
  • Intestinal lymphectasia
  • Thoracic duct drainage
  • Obstruction to intestinal lymphatic drainage (e.g., tumor, Whipple's disease)
  • Congestive heart failure
Decreased production
  • Aplastic anemia
  • Malignancy, especially Hodgkin's disease
  • Inherited immunoglobulin disorders (e.g., Wiskott-Aldrich, combined immunodeficiency, ataxia-telangiectasia)
  • Infection (e.g., AIDS)
Others (e.g., SLE, renal failure, miliary TB, myasthenia gravis, aplastic anemia)

### CD4 Lymphocytes
*(by flow cytometry)*
#### Use
Diagnosis of immune dysfunction, especially AIDS
#### Decreased in
Acute minor viral infections

### Causes of Atypical Lymphocytes

Lymphatic leukemia
Viral infections
Pertussis
Brucellosis
Syphilis (in some phases)
Toxoplasmosis
Drug reactions and serum sickness
Normal persons may show up to 12% atypical lymphocytes.
"Heterophile negative" infectious mononucleosis syndrome is seen in
  • Early stage of infectious mononucleosis
  • Toxoplasmosis
  • Cytomegalovirus
  • Infectious hepatitis

### Basophilic Leukocytes
#### Use
May be first sign of blast crisis or accelerated phase of chronic myelogenous leukemia

*Persistent basophilia may indicate unsuspected myeloproliferative disease.*
Diagnosis of basophilic leukemia
**Increased in (>50/cu mm or >1%)**
Chronic myelogenous leukemia
Basophilic leukemia
Polycythemia
Myeloid metaplasia
Hodgkin's disease
Postsplenectomy
Chronic hemolytic anemia
Chickenpox
Smallpox
Myxedema
Nephrosis
Foreign protein injection
Ionizing radiation
**Decreased in**
Hyperthyroidism
Pregnancy
Period after irradiation, chemotherapy, and glucocorticoids
Acute phase of infection

## Causes of Monocytosis
**(>10% of differential count; absolute count >500/cu mm)**

Monocytic leukemia, other leukemias
Myeloproliferative disorders
Malignant lymphomas
Lipid storage diseases (e.g., Gaucher's disease)
Postsplenectomy
Recovery from agranulocytosis and subsidence of acute infection
Many protozoan infections (e.g., malaria, kala-azar, trypanosomiasis)
Some rickettsial infections (e.g., Rocky Mountain spotted fever, typhus)
Certain bacterial infections (e.g., subacute bacterial endocarditis, TB, brucellosis)
Chronic ulcerative colitis, regional enteritis, and spruc
Sarcoidosis
Collagen diseases (e.g., RA, SLE)
Most common causes are indolent infections (e.g., mycobacteria, subacute bacterial endocarditis) and recovery phase of neutropenia.
*Monocyte phagocytosis of RBCs in peripheral smears from earlobe is said to occur often in subacute bacterial endocarditis.*

### Plasma Cells
**Increased in**
Plasma cell leukemia
Multiple myeloma
Hodgkin's disease
Chronic lymphocytic leukemia
Other neoplasias (cancer of liver, kidney, breast, prostate)
Cirrhosis
RA
SLE
Serum reaction
Bacterial infections (e.g., syphilis, TB)
Parasitic infections (e.g., malaria, trichinosis)
Viral infections (e.g., infectious mononucleosis, rubella, measles, chickenpox, benign lymphocytic meningitis)
**Decreased in**
Not clinically significant

### Causes of Eosinophilia
*(>250/cu mm; diurnal variation, with highest levels in morning)*

Allergic diseases (e.g., bronchial asthma, hay fever, urticaria, drug therapy, allergic rhinitis)

Parasitic infestation, especially with tissue invasion (e.g., trichinosis, echinococcus disease, schistosomiasis, filariasis, fascioliasis)

Mycoses (e.g., coccidioidomycosis)

Some infectious diseases (e.g., scarlet fever, erythema multiforme, *Chlamydia*)

Collagen-vascular diseases (e.g., periarteritis nodosa, SLE, RA, scleroderma, dermatomyositis, Churg-Strauss syndrome)

Some diffuse skin diseases (e.g., eczema, pemphigus, dermatitis herpetiformis)

Some hematopoietic diseases (e.g., pernicious anemia, chronic myelogenous leukemia, acute myelomonocytic leukemia, polycythemia, Hodgkin's disease, T-cell lymphomas, eosinophilic leukemia); postsplenectomy

Some immunodeficiency disorders (e.g., Wiskott-Aldrich syndrome, graft-versus-host disease [GVHD], cyclic neutropenia, IgA deficiency)

Some GI diseases (e.g., eosinophilic gastroenteritis, ulcerative colitis, regional enteritis)

Some endocrine diseases (e.g., hypopituitarism, Addison's disease)

Postirradiation

Drugs (e.g., aspirin sensitivity)

Hypereosinophilic syndrome

Highest levels occur in trichinosis, *Clonorchis sinensis* infection, and dermatitis herpetiformis.

# Hematologic Diseases

## Agranulocytosis

In acute fulminant form, WBC is decreased to ≤ 2000/cu mm, sometimes as low as 50/cu mm. Granulocytes are 0–2%.

In chronic or recurrent form, WBC is down to 2000/cu mm with less marked granulocytopenia.

There is relative lymphocytosis and sometimes monocytosis.

Bone marrow shows absence of cells in granulocytic series but normal erythroid and megakaryocytic series.

ESR is increased.

Hb and RBC count and morphology, platelet count, and coagulation tests are normal.

## Anemia, Classification

Anemias may be classified according to pathogenesis or RBC indices and peripheral blood smear and reticulocyte count. See Fig. 11-1.

Marrow hypofunction with decreased RBC production

- Marrow replacement (myelophthisic anemias due to tumor or granulomas)
    Marrow injury (hypoplastic and aplastic anemias)
        Nutritional deficiency (e.g., megaloblastic anemias due to lack of vitamin $B_{12}$ or folic acid)
        Endocrine hypofunction (e.g., pituitary, adrenal, thyroid; anemia of chronic renal failure)
- Marrow hypofunction due to decreased Hb production (hypochromic microcytic anemias)
        Deficient heme synthesis (iron deficiency, pyridoxine-responsive anemias)
        Deficient globin synthesis (thalassemias, hemoglobinopathies)
- Excessive loss of RBCs (hemolytic anemias due to genetically defective RBCs)

Abnormal shape (hereditary spherocytosis, hereditary elliptocytosis)
Abnormal Hb (sickle cell anemia, thalassemias, Hb C disease)
Abnormal RBC enzymes (G6PD deficiency, congenital nonspherocytic
  hemolytic anemias)
- Excessive loss of RBCs
  Hemolytic anemias with acquired defects of RBC and positive Coombs'
    test (autoantibodies, as in SLE, malignant lymphoma; or exogenous
    allergens, as in penicillin allergy) See Anemia, Hemolytic, Classification.
- Excessive loss of normal RBCs
  Hemorrhage
  Hypersplenism
  Chemical agents (e.g., lead)
  Infectious agents (e.g., *Clostridium welchii, Bartonella,* malaria)
  Miscellaneous diseases (e.g., uremia, liver disease, cancers)
  Physical agents (e.g., burns)
  Mechanical trauma (e.g., artificial heart valves, tumor microemboli)
*Anemias are often multifactorial. The diagnosis must be re-evaluated after the
apparent causes have been treated*

## Anemia, Acute Blood Loss

RBC, Hb, and Hct level are not reliable initially because of compensatory vaso-
  constriction and hemodilution. They decrease for several days after hemorrhage ceases.
Anemia is normochromic, normocytic. *(If hypochromic or microcytic, rule out iron
  deficiency due to prior hemorrhages.)*
Reticulocyte count is increased after 1–2 days, reaches peak in 4–7 days ($\leq$ 15%).
  Persistent increase suggests continuing hemorrhage.
Polychromasia and increased number of nucleated RBCs (up to 5:100 WBCs) may
  be found.
Increased WBC (usually $\leq$ 20,000/cu mm) reaches peak in 2–5 hrs, becomes nor-
  mal in 3–4 days. Persistent increase suggests continuing hemorrhage, bleed-
  ing into a body cavity, or infection.
Platelets are increased ($\leq$ 1 million/cu mm) within a few hours.
BUN is increased if hemorrhage into lumen of GI tract occurs.
Serum indirect bilirubin is increased if hemorrhage into a body cavity or cystic
  structure occurs.

## Anemia, Aplastic

Peripheral blood pancytopenia with variable bone marrow hypocellularity in the
  absence of underlying myeloproliferative or malignant disease
- Neutropenia (absolute neutrophil count <1500/cu mm) is always present;
  often monocytopenia is present.
- Lymphocyte count is normal; reduced helper/inducer:cytotoxic/suppressor
  ratio.
- Platelet count <150,000/cu mm; severity varies.
- Anemia is usually normochromic, normocytic but may be slightly macrocytic. RDW is normal. Poikilocytes are not seen on peripheral blood
  smear.
- Bone marrow is hypocellular; aspiration and biopsy should both be performed to rule out leukemia, myelodysplastic syndrome, granulomas, tumor.
Reticulocyte count corrected for Hct is decreased.
Serum iron is increased.
Laboratory findings represent the whole spectrum, from the most severe condition of the classic type with marked leukopenia, thrombocytopenia, anemia,
  and acellular bone marrow, to cases with involvement only of erythroid elements. In some cases, the marrow may be cellular or hyperplastic.

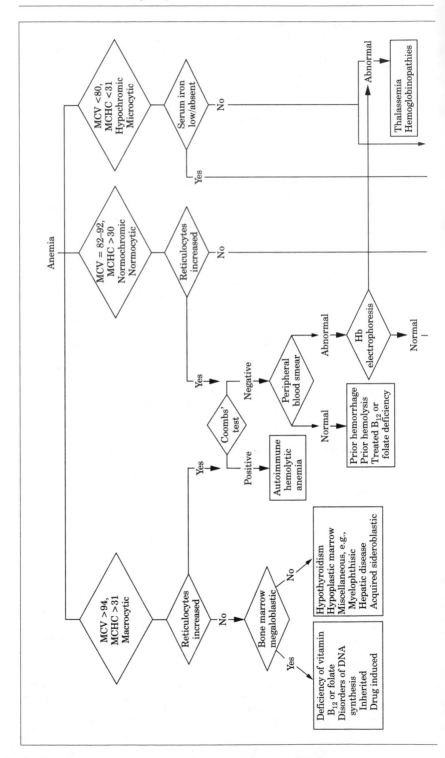

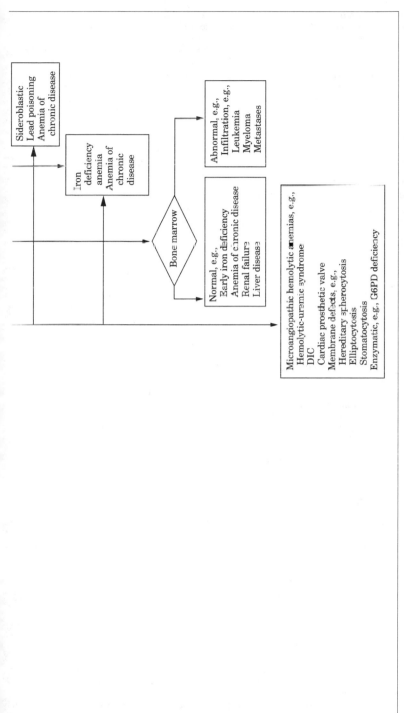

**Fig. 11-1.** Sequence of laboratory tests in work-up of anemia. This algorithm is meant only to illustrate the use of indices for preliminary classification of anemias; many of the subsequent steps in the diagnostic work-up are not included. Note also that some conditions may appear in more than one category.

**Table 11-6.** Comparison of Iron Deficiency Anemia Alone and Combined with Thalassemia Minor or Anemia of Chronic Disease

|  | Iron Deficiency Anemia Alone | Anemia of Chronic Disease | Combined Anemias: Iron Deficiency and Chronic Disease | Thalassemia Minor | Combined Anemias: Iron Deficiency and Thalassemia Minor |
|---|---|---|---|---|---|
| MCV | D | N or D | D | Very D | Very D |
| RDW | I | I or N | I | I or N | I |
| RBC count | D | D | D | N or I | N or D |
| Serum iron | D | D | D | N | D |
| Serum ferritin | D | I or N | N | N | D |
| Marrow iron stain | D to O | N or I | D to O | N | D to O |
| TIBC | I | D | D | N | I |
| Hb electrophoresis | N | N | N | Ab* | Ab* |

O = absent; Ab = abnormal.
*Hb electrophoresis abnormal in beta-thalassemia but not alpha-thalassemia.

Criteria for *severe* aplastic anemia (International Aplastic Anemia Study Group)
- ≥ 2 peripheral blood criteria plus either marrow criteria
  Peripheral blood criteria
    Neutrophils <500/cu mm
    Platelets <20,000/cu mm
    Reticulocyte count <1% (corrected for Hct)
  Marrow criteria
    Severe hypocellularity
    Moderate hypocellularity with <30% of residual cells being hematopoietic

## Anemias of Chronic Diseases

See Table 11-6.

### *Due to*

Subacute or chronic infections (especially TB, bronchiectasis, lung abscess, empyema, bacterial endocarditis)
Neoplasms
RA (anemia parallels activity of arthritis)
Rheumatic fever, SLE
Uremia (BUN >70 mg/dL)
Chronic liver disease
Hypothyroidism
Hypogonadism
Hypoadrenalism

### *Laboratory Findings*

Anemia is usually mild (Hb >9 gm/dL) but may be as low as 5 gm/dL in uremia when other factors are present. Is insidious, *not progressive*. May be due to multiple mechanisms.

Usually normocytic, normochromic. In 25%–33% of these patients, is hypochromic and/or microcytic, in which case it is always less marked than in iron deficiency anemia.

Serum iron and TIBC are decreased. If TIBC is elevated, presence of iron deficiency must be ruled out but TIBC is not sufficiently sensitive or specific to
distinguish this from iron deficiency anemia. Transferrin saturation is usually
normal; >10% if decreased; <10% implies iron deficiency.
Serum ferritin is increased or normal in contrast to iron deficiency. *In RA, liver
disease, or neoplasms, normal serum ferritin does not exclude concomitant iron
deficiency.*
FEP is increased.
Bone marrow cellular elements are normal.
*Increased WBC, increased ESR and other acute phase reactants (e.g., CRP) are
disproportionate to anemia, and may be a useful clue to distinguish this from
iron deficiency anemia.*

## Anemia, Hemolytic, Classification

See Figs. 11-2 and 11-3.
A useful approach to the diagnosis of hemolytic anemias may be based on:
  • Site of RBC destruction (intravascular or extravascular)
  • Site of etiologic defect (intracellular RBC or extracellular)
  • Nature of defect (acquired or hereditary)
Hb disorders
  • Intrinsic
    Autosomal
      SC disease                    Common
      Thalassemias                  Common
      Hb C, D, E disease            Common
      Unstable hemoglobins          Very rare
Membrane disorders
  • Intrinsic
    Congenital or familial (usually autosomal dominant)
      Hereditary spherocytosis                          Common (~.02%
                                                        Northern
                                                        European pop-
                                                        ulation)
      Hereditary elliptocytosis                         Rare
      Hereditary stomatocytosis                         Very rare
      Acanthocytosis (abetalipoproteinemia)             Very rare
      Hereditary pyropoikilocytosis                     Very rare
      Acquired—paroxysmal nocturnal hemoglobinuria      Rare
  • Extrinsic
    Acquired
      Isoimmune (blood transfusion reaction, hemolytic
          disease of newborn)
      Autoimmune (AIHA) (Coombs' test usually positive;
          spherocytes may be present)                   Rare
        Warm antibody
          Idiopathic
          Secondary to disease (e.g., lymphomas/leuke-
              mia, infectious mononucleosis, SLE)
        Cold agglutinin syndrome
          Idiopathic
          Secondary (e.g., *Mycoplasma pneumoniae*
              infection, infectious mononucleosis, viral
              infection, lymphoreticular neoplasms)
        Paroxysmal cold hemoglobinuria                  Rare
          Idiopathic
          Secondary (viral illnesses, syphilis)
        Atypical AIHA
          Coombs' test negative
          Combined cold and warm AIHA

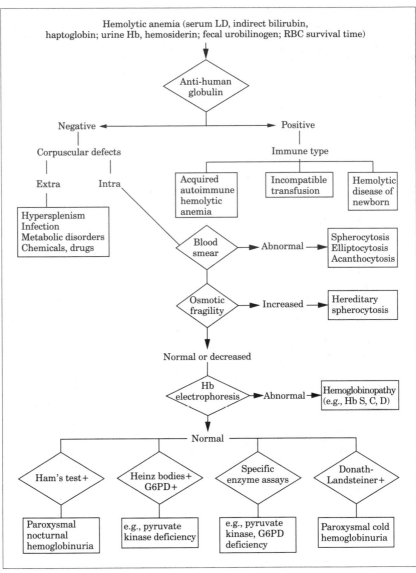

**Fig. 11-2.** Algorithm for work-up of hemolytic anemia. (+ = positive.)

Drug induced (e.g., penicillin, methyldopa)                    Common
Nonimmune (Coombs' test usually negative; mor-
  phologic changes usually found in blood smear)
Physical or mechanical
  Prosthetic heart valves
  Microangiopathic hemolytic disease, includ-
    ing DIC, thrombotic thrombocytopenic
    purpura, hemolytic uremic syndrome, etc.
  March hemoglobinuria
  Severe burns

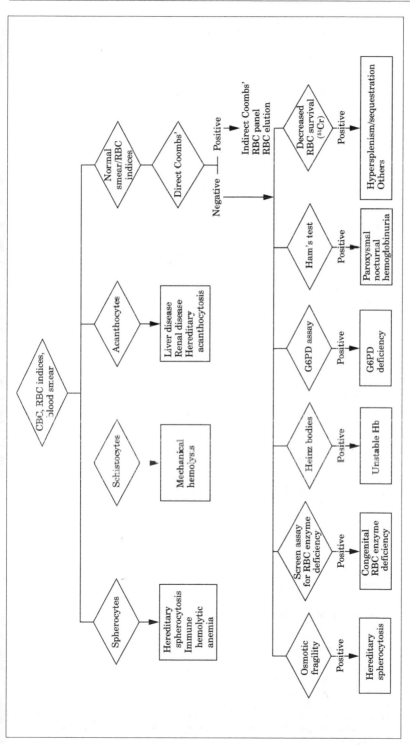

**Fig. 11-3.** Sequence of laboratory tests for hemolytic anemia with normal Hb electrophoresis.

Snakebite
Osmotic—distilled water used
in prostate resection
Infectious
Protozoan
Bacterial
Viral
Metabolic disorders
- Intrinsic
  G6PD deficiency                  Common
  Pyruvate kinase deficiency       Rare
  Hexokinase
  Phosphofructokinase
  Aldolase
  Defects in nucleotide metabolism
  Pyrimidine 5'-nucleotidase
  Erythropoietic porphyria
- Extrinsic
  Drugs in normal RBCs or in G6PD deficiency
  Marked hypophosphatemia (<1 mg/dL) may predispose to hemolysis
  Others (e.g., lead poisoning, Wilson's disease)
15–20% of acquired immune hemolytic anemias are related to drug therapy (e.g., penicillins, cephalosporins, methyldopa). Serologic findings cannot be distinguished from idiopathic warm antibody AIHA.

## Anemia, Hemolytic, Acquired

Laboratory findings due to increased destruction of RBCs
- RBC survival time differentiates intrinsic defect from factor outside RBC.
- Blood smear often shows marked changes.
- Increased indirect serum bilirubin (<6 mg/dL) because of compensatory excretory capacity of liver.
- Hemoglobinemia and hemoglobinuria are present when hemolysis is very rapid.
- Haptoglobins are decreased or absent in chronic hemolytic diseases (removed following combination with free Hb in serum).
- WBC is usually elevated.

## Anemia, Hemolytic, Microangiopathic
**(traumatic intravascular hemolysis due to fibrin strands in vessel lumens)**

Peripheral blood smear establishes the diagnosis by characteristic burr cells, schistocytes, helmet cells, microspherocytes.
Nonimmune hemolytic anemia varies in severity depending on underlying condition.
Laboratory findings of hemolysis
Direct Coombs' test is usually negative.

## Anemia, Iron Deficiency

### Due to
*(usually a combination of these factors)*

Chronic blood loss
Decreased dietary intake
Decreased absorption
Increased requirements (e.g., pregnancy)
*The cause of iron deficiency should always be ascertained to avoid overlooking occult carcinoma. In adults, iron deficiency usually means blood loss.*

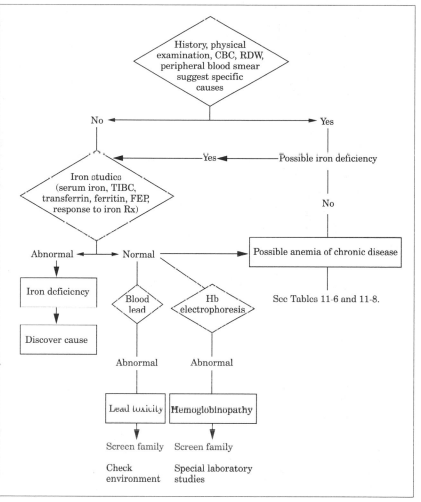

**Fig. 11-4.** Algorithm for work-up for microcytic hypochromic anemia. (CBC = complete blood count; FEP = free erythrocyte protoporphyrin; Rx = therapy.)

### Laboratory Findings

See Fig. 11-4 and Tables 11-7 and 11-8.

Decreased serum ferritin is the most sensitive and specific test and is first test to reflect iron deficiency; *decreased before anemia* but may be increased when there is coexisting liver disease, inflammation, or other conditions that increase acute phase reactants.

Hb is usually 6–10 gm/dL; out of proportion to decrease in RBC (3.5–5.0 million/cu mm); decreased MCV (<80 fL) is a sensitive indicator; MCH is decreased (<30 pg); decreased MCHC (25–30 gm/dL) is poor indicator as is usually normal until anemia is severe.

Increased RDW may be the first indication of iron deficiency.

Hypochromia and microcytosis parallel severity of anemia. Diagnosis from peripheral blood smear is unreliable.

**Table 11-7.** Comparison of Sample Values in Iron Deficiency States

| | Normal | Early Deficiency | Early Anemia | Moderate Anemia | Moderate to Severe Anemia | Severe Anemia |
|---|---|---|---|---|---|---|
| MCV | 82–92 fL | N | N | D | D — Gradually decreases (95→80 fL) — | D |
| MCH | 27–31 pg | N | N | D | D | D |
| Hb (gm/dL) | 12–14 M / 14–16 F | N | Gradually decreases to ~10 | D | D — Usually 7–10 — | D |
| RDW | 11.5–14.5 | N | N | — Gradually increases — | — Gradually increases — | |
| Blood smear | N | N | Only mild microcytosis | Moderate microcytosis; ovalocytes, target cells, leptocytes | Poikilocytes, severe microcytosis, ovalocytes, elliptocytes | Schistocytes |
| % Cells hypochromic | N | N | — Gradually increases — | — Gradually increases — | | |
| Serum iron (μg/dL) | 65–165 | N (115) | D (<60) | D (<40) | D (<40) | D (<40) |
| TIBC (μg/dL) | 250–450 | — Increases to ~480 — | | | | |
| Transferrin saturation | 20–50% | N (30%) | D (<15%) | D (<10%) | D (<10%) | D (<10%) |
| Serum ferritin (μg/L) | 40–160 | 40–160; decreases to 20 | D | <10 | <10 | <10 |
| RE marrow iron | 2–3+ | 0–1+ | 0–1+ | 0 | 0 | 0 |
| Free RBC | <100 μg/dL | N | I | I | I | I |
| Protoporphyrin | Packed RBCs | N | 100 μg/dL | — Gradually increasing to ~200 μg/dL — | | |
| RBC life span | N | N | N | — Gradually decreases — | | |

M = males; F = females; RE = reticuloendothelial.

**Table 11-8.** Laboratory Tests in Differential Diagnosis of Microcytic (MCV <80 fL) and Hypochromic (MCHC <30 gm/dL) Anemias

| Type of Anemia | Serum Iron | TIBC | Transferrin Saturation | Serum Ferritin | FEP* | Marrow Hemo-siderin | Sidero-blasts | Type of Hb | Anemia | RBC Count | RDW |
|---|---|---|---|---|---|---|---|---|---|---|---|
| Normal values | 80–160 μg/dL in men 50–150 μg/dL in women | 250–410 μg/dL | 20–55% | 20–150 ng/dL | | | 30–50% | AA | | | 11.5–14.5 |
| Iron deficiency | D | I | D | D | I | O | D | AA | Hypochromic, normocytic, or microcytic | D | I |
| Normochromic, normocytic or microcytic, of chronic disease | D | D or N | D or N | N or slightly I | I | N or I | D | AA | Normochromic, normocytic, or microcytic | D | N |
| Thalassemia | | | | | | | | | | | |
| Major | I | D | I | I | N | I | I | 20–90% F | Hypochromic | I | N |
| Minor | N or I | N | N or I | I | N | N or I | I | 2–8% F; A₂ is I | Microcytic | I | N |
| Sideroblastic | N or I | D or N | I | I | D | I | I | AA | Hypochromic and/or microcytic with normocytic or macrocytic changes, dimorphic RBC population | D | I |

Notes: (1) Determine serum iron and TIBC (and also perhaps do iron stain on bone marrow smear—the most reliable index of iron deficiency). (2) If serum iron and TIBC are both normal, Hb electrophoresis will establish the diagnosis of thalassemia. If serum iron is abnormal, the cause may be iron deficiency (e.g., blood loss, dietary deficiency) or normochromic microcytic anemia of chronic disease.

O = absent; FEP = free erythrocyte protoporphyrin.

*FEP is useful to distinguish between iron deficiency and beta thalassemia.

*Iron depletion: Early—serum iron is normal; TIBC may be increased. Later—serum iron decreases; anemic is normocytic when mild or of rapid onset; anemia first becomes microcytic, then hypochromic.*

*Iron deficiency may occur without anemia (transferrin saturation <15%; decreased marrow iron and sideroblasts).*

Serum iron is decreased (usually 40 μg/dL), TIBC increased (usually 350–460 μg/dL), and transferrin saturation decreased (<15%). TIBC may be normal or moderately increased in many patients with uncomplicated iron deficiency. Serum transferrin may be normal or increased (calculated transferrin = TIBC × 0.7). These have limited value in differential diagnosis because they are often normal in iron deficiency and abnormal in anemia of chronic disease.

As iron deficiency progresses, decreased serum ferritin is followed in order by anisocytosis, microcytosis, elliptocytosis, hypochromia, decrease in Hb, serum iron, and transferrin saturation.

Bone marrow shows normoblastic hyperplasia. Decreased to absent iron is the gold standard for diagnosis of iron deficiency.

Free erythrocyte protoporphyrin is increased and is useful screening test because it is *increased before anemia* and is also increased in lead poisoning, anemia of chronic disease and most sideroblastic anemias but is normal in thalassemias and can be done on fingerstick sample.

Reticulocytes are normal or decreased, unless there is recent hemorrhage or administration of iron.

WBC is normal or may be slightly decreased in 10% of cases; may be increased with fresh hemorrhage.

Response to oral iron therapy is the final proof of diagnosis

- Increased reticulocytes within 3–7 days with peak of 8–10% on day 5–10.
- Followed by rising Hb (average 0.25–0.4 gm/dL/day) and Hct (average = 1%/day) during first 7–10 days; thereafter Hb increases ≥ 11 gm/dL in 3–4 wks. Should be fully corrected by 8 wks.
- Failure to respond suggests incorrect diagnosis, coexistent deficiencies, or associated conditions.

## Anemias, Megaloblastic

### Pernicious Anemia (PA) (Vitamin B₁₂ Deficiency) and Folate Deficiency

See Fig. 11-5 and Table 11-9.

| Most Commonly Due to | Vitamin B₁₂ Deficiency | Folate Deficiency |
|---|---|---|
| Inadequate intake | Strict vegetarian diet (rare) | Malnutrition, alcoholism |
| Increased need | Pregnancy, lactation | Pregnancy, lactation, infancy |
| Defective absorption | Decreased intrinsic factor (e.g., PA, congenital deficiency of intrinsic factor, 4 yrs after gastrectomy) Z-E syndrome Pancreatitis Ileal mucosal disease (e.g., sprue, regional enteritis, surgery) Tapeworm infestation, bacterial overgrowth in blind loop Drugs (e.g., colchicine, PAS, alcoholism) | Malabsorption due to drugs (e.g., anticonvulsants, antituberculosis, oral contraceptives), jejunal-mucosal disease (e.g., amyloidosis, sprue, lymphoma, surgery) |

Hematologic picture is identical in folate or vitamin B₁₂ deficiency, but neurologic findings are absent in folate deficiency.

Normochromic macrocytic anemia is a relatively late event; RBC may be as low as 500,000/cu mm. Degree of anemia does not correlate with severity of neurologic signs and symptoms, which may precede hematologic abnormalities.

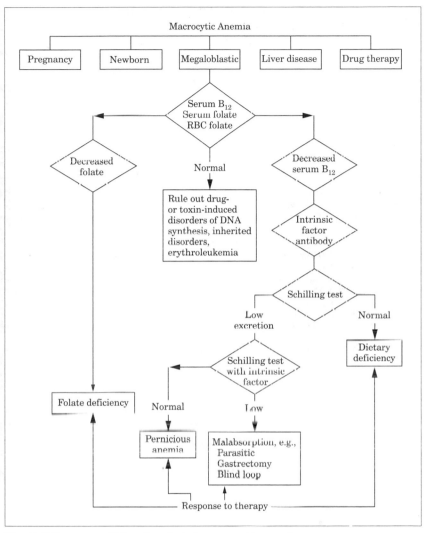

**Fig. 11-5.** Sequence of laboratory tests in macrocytic anemia.

MCV is increased (95–110 fL) with mild to moderate anemia but may also be due to round macrocytes due to nonmegaloblastic causes; 110–150 fL with more severe anemia. MCV increases months before anemia or clinical symptoms. MCV >95 should prompt further study. MCV >120 fL is most likely due to megaloblastic anemia. MCV may be normal if coexisting iron deficiency, inflammatory disease, renal failure, or thalassemia trait. MCV is normal in ~9% of megaloblastic patients. RDW is usually very increased due to marked anisopoikilocytosis or may be normal.

MCH is increased (33–38 pg with moderate anemia; ≤ 56 pg with severe anemia).

**Table 11-9.** Laboratory Tests in Differential Diagnosis of Vitamin $B_{12}$ and Folic Acid Deficiencies

|  | Vitamin $B_{12}$ Deficiency | Folate Deficiency | Vitamin $B_{12}$ and Folate Deficiency |
|---|---|---|---|
| Serum folate | N or I | D | D |
| Serum vitamin $B_{12}$ | D | N or D | D |
| RBC folate | N or D | D | D |
| Methylmalonic acid | I | N | I |
| Homocysteine | I | I | I |

Large hypersegmented neutrophils ($\geq 5$ lobes) are the earliest morphologic sign of megaloblastic anemia; more than two 5-lobed neutrophils is strongly suggestive and any with more than six lobes is considered diagnostic. Blood smear may show various types of abnormal RBCs.

Reticulocyte count is usually decreased.

Thrombocytopenia and leukopenia may be present.

Marrow shows megaloblastic and erythroid hyperplasia and abnormalities of myeloid and megakaryocytic elements.

In PA, serum vitamin $B_{12}$ is very low, usually <100 pg/mL; 100–150 pg/mL usually signifies early vitamin $B_{12}$ deficiency even without neuropathy or macrocytosis. May occur with neurologic symptoms but without anemia in up to one-third of patients with vitamin $B_{12}$ deficiency. RBC folate is low in many patients with vitamin $B_{12}$ deficiency.

## Serum Vitamin $B_{12}$ May Also Be Decreased in
Diet deficient in folic acid

Malabsorption
- Loss of gastric mucosa (e.g., partial or complete gastrectomy, atrophic gastritis, gastric radiation)
- Small bowel disease (e.g., Crohn's disease, scleroderma, lymphoma, ileal resection, chronic pancreatic insufficiency, bacterial overgrowth)
- Primary hypothyroidism
- Parasites—*Diphyllobothrium latum*

Drugs (e.g., chronic PAS or colchicine use, oral contraceptives, alcohol)

Pregnancy—progressive decrease during pregnancy *(normal serum $B_{12}$ in megaloblastic anemia of pregnancy)*

Impaired cell utilization
- Abnormal vitamin $B_{12}$ carrier protein (transcobalamin II deficiency, abnormal protein)
- Enzyme deficiency (e.g., congenital methylmalonicacidemias)
- Prolonged nitrous oxide exposure

One-third of patients with multiple myeloma

Others
- Iron deficiency
- Vegetarian diet
- Smoking
- 15–30% of aged persons
- Cancer
- Aplastic anemia
- Folate deficiency
- Hemodialysis
- Pregnancy
- High doses of vitamin C

## Serum Folic Acid May Be Decreased in
Nutritional (may fall relatively quickly)
- Alcoholism is most common cause.

- Infancy, prematurity, elderly.
- Chronic disease.
- Hemodialysis.
- Anorexia nervosa.

Increased requirements due to marked cellular proliferation
- Pregnancy
- Hyperthyroidism
- Neoplasia (e.g., acute leukemia, metastatic carcinoma)
- Hemolytic anemias
- Ineffective erythropoiesis (PA, sideroblastic anemia)

Exfoliative dermatitis (e.g., psoriasis)

Malabsorption
- Small bowel disease (e.g., celiac disease, tropical sprue, Crohn's disease, lymphoma, amyloidosis, small bowel resection)

Defect in utilization due to certain enzyme deficiencies

Drugs—folic acid antagonists (e.g., methotrexate, trimethoprim, pyrimethamine; anticonvulsants; oral contraceptives; aspirin)

Decreased liver stores (e.g., cirrhosis, hepatoma)

Idiopathic

Artifactual
- Improper specimen storage
- Radioactivity in blood
- Antibiotic therapy

*Serum folate serves to distinguish combined deficiency from vitamin $B_{12}$ deficiency alone. Decreased serum folate indicates only negative folate balance; it is not evidence of tissue deficiency for which RBC folate should be assayed.*

Usual normal range is 5–15 ng/mL; is associated with normal hematologic findings. 3–5 ng/mL is borderline; is associated with variable hematologic findings. <3 ng/mL is associated with positive hematologic findings.

RBC folate reflects folate status at time RBCs were produced. Decreased in folate or vitamin $B_{12}$ deficiency. *RBC folate does not fall below normal until all body stores are depleted. Thus, all three parameters should be measured simultaneously in suspected cases of megaloblastic anemia.*

## Serum Folic Acid May Be Increased in

Pernicious anemia

After folic acid administration or eating

Vegetarians

Blood transfusion

Some cases of blind loop syndrome (due to folate synthesis by bacteria in gut)

False elevation in hemolyzed specimens (due to folate in RBCs)

Falsely increased to normal in some patients with severe iron deficiency

Serum methylmalonic acid (MMA) and homocysteine (HCYS) become elevated very early in course of vitamin $B_{12}$ deficiency. Patients with folate deficiency usually have an increase in only HCYS although some may have mild increase of MMA. MMA and HCYS levels are the most sensitive tests to detect early vitamin $B_{12}$ deficiency and become positive before obvious hematologic evidence of vitamin $B_{12}$ deficiency. Is useful in patients with borderline vitamin $B_{12}$ levels (100–300 pg/mL). Should be positive in acute neurologic disease due to vitamin $B_{12}$ deficiency even when hematologic changes are absent. Will remain positive for at least 24 hrs after onset of vitamin $B_{12}$ therapy in patients for whom therapy is begun before blood was drawn for vitamin $B_{12}$ levels. Urine MMA may be useful when serum MMA is falsely high in renal insufficiency or intravascular volume depletion.

*Iron deficiency is present in one-half of patients with folate deficiency and one-third with vitamin $B_{12}$ deficiency. If iron deficiency is more severe than folate deficiency, results of serum and RBC folate tests are normal, and diagnosis cannot be made from these tests; hypersegmentation of PMNs in blood smear is the only clue.*

Serum antibodies
- Intrinsic factor antibody is present in 75% of patients with PA; high serum $B_{12}$ causes false-positive results. Positive test strongly supports diagnosis of PA and therefore should be performed in patients with low serum $B_{12}$; positive test combined with low serum $B_{12}$ is virtually pathognomonic of PA; however, a negative test does not rule out PA since almost one-fourth of such patients are negative for this antibody.
- Parietal cell antibodies are more sensitive (90%) for PA but occur frequently in chronic gastritis; frequency increases with age and presence of insulin-dependent diabetes mellitus. Occurs in 50–100% of cases of PA but frequency decreases with duration of PA. Intrinsic antibodies are more specific, but sensitivity is only ~50%.

Schilling test is diagnostic of PA. Differentiates pernicious anemia from other causes of vitamin $B_{12}$ deficiency and can establish the functional absence of intrinsic factor before $B_{12}$ deficiency or anemia are present or after patient has received vitamin $B_{12}$ treatment. Infrequently performed.

Serum LD is markedly increased (principally LD-1 and LD-2 with 1>2).

Serum indirect bilirubin is increased (<4 mg/dL).

Serum iron, TIBC, ferritin, and marrow iron are almost always increased during relapse unless there is concomitant iron deficiency.

Achlorhydria even after administration of histamine or betazole; presence of gastric acid rules out PA; rarely found in children.

Increased serum gastrin with low serum vitamin $B_{12}$ suggests PA.

Serum alkaline phosphatase is decreased; increases after treatment.

Serum cholesterol is moderately decreased.

Recently developed deoxyuridine suppression test: May be useful when other test results are masked by recent therapy or are equivocal. Limited availability at present but may become gold standard.

50% of PA patients have thyroid antibodies.

Increased frequency of gastric adenocarcinoma and carcinoids

**Characteristic Response of Laboratory Tests to Specific Treatment of PA or Folate Deficiency**

RBC count reaches normal between week 8 and 12 regardless of severity of anemia. Peripheral blood is normal in 1–2 months.

Reticulocyte response is proportional to severity of anemia: count begins to rise by day 4 after treatment and reaches maximum on day 8 or 9; returns to normal by day 14.

Megaloblasts disappear from marrow 24–48 hrs followed by reversal of changes in myeloid cells a few days later.

Serum folate decreases (in PA) at the same time reticulocytosis takes place. Serum iron decreases to normal or less than normal at the same time reticulocytosis takes place.

Serum uric acid increases.

Other serum chemical abnormalities are reversed.

Achlorhydria persists.

### Anemia, Macrocytic, of Liver Disease

Increased MCV (100–125 fL) in one-third to two-thirds of patients. Indices resemble those in other megaloblastic anemias.

*Uniform round macrocytosis* is the cardinal finding. Hemolytic anemia or true folate deficiency is frequent in alcoholic liver disease.

### Anemia, Macrocytic, of Sprue, Celiac Disease, Steatorrhea

See Chapter 7.

## Anemia, Myelophthisic

Bone marrow demonstrates primary disease

- Metastatic carcinoma of bone marrow (especially breast, lung, prostate, thyroid)
- Hodgkin's disease, leukemia
- Multiple myeloma (5% of patients)
- Gaucher's, Niemann-Pick, and Hand-Schuller-Christian diseases
- Myelofibrosis

Anemia is usually mild; not more than moderate.

Increased nucleated RBCs and normoblasts in peripheral smear, often without reticulocytosis, are out of proportion to the degree of anemia and may be found even in the absence of anemia. Polychromatophilia, basophilic stippling, and increased reticulocyte count may also occur.

WBC may be normal or decreased; occasionally it is increased up to a leukemoid picture; immature WBC may be found in peripheral smear.

Platelets may be normal or decreased, and abnormal forms may occur.

Abnormalities may occur even when WBC is normal.

## Anemia, Pure Red Cell (Aregenerative Anemia; Idiopathic Hypoplastic Anemia; Primary Red Cell Aplasia)

Severe normochromic normocytic anemia is refractory to all treatment except transfusion and sometimes ACTH or corticosteroids.

Reticulocytes are decreased or absent.

WBC and differential blood count are normal.

There is no hemolysis.

Bone marrow usually shows marked decrease in erythroid series but sometimes is normal. Myeloid cells and megakaryocytes are normal.

Increased erythropoietin level

The disease may be related to thymus tumors, leukemia (which develops in 10% of patients), or chemicals.

## Anemia, Sideroblastic
**(miscellaneous group of diseases characterized by increased sideroblasts [erythroblasts containing iron inclusions] in marrow)**

### Hereditary

X-chromosome linked transmission

### Idiopathic Refractory

Dimorphic anemia is usually moderate, normocytic, or macrocytic with a small population of hypochromic RBCs on blood smear.

WBCs are variable but usually normal. WBCs may show morphologic changes.

Platelet counts are variable. Abnormal thrombopoiesis with abnormal morphology.

Bone marrow shows erythroid hyperplasia; 45–95% of normoblasts are ringed sideroblasts; excessive hemosiderin. Megaloblastic changes due to complicating folate deficiency are found in 20% of patients. Dysgranulopoesis and dysmegakaryopoiesis may be evident.

Serum ferritin and iron stores are increased due to ineffective erythropoiesis. Transferrin saturation is increased (>90% in 33% of patients). But some patients may be iron deficient or have normal iron status. Iron overload is principal feature that determines long-term prognosis.

Acute leukemia develops in ~10% of patients.

### Secondary

Due to drugs and toxic agents (e.g., chloramphenicol, antituberculosis drugs, lead poisoning, alcoholism) or associated with other diseases (e.g., neoplasms, inflammatory diseases, hematologic diseases)

## Elliptocytosis, Hereditary
### (autosomal dominant trait)

Blood smear shows 25–100% elliptical RBCs. In normal individuals, ≤ 10% of RBCs may be elliptical. Also seen frequently in thalassemias, hemoglobinopathies, iron deficiency, myelophthisic anemias, megaloblastic anemia; these must be ruled out to establish the diagnosis in a congenital hemolytic anemia with marked elliptocytosis. Only a few abnormal RBCs are present at birth with gradual increase to stable value after ~3 months old.

Severity of disease varies from severe hemolytic disease to asymptomatic carrier.

* Elliptocytes are the only hematologic abnormality seen in ~85% of patients; they are asymptomatic. Spherocytes are present in some forms.
* Mild normocytic normochromic anemia (Hb 10–12 gm/dL) in 10–20% of patients.
* ~12% of patients show a chronic congenital hemolytic anemia (Hb <9 gm/dL).
* Severe in ~5% of patients (homozygous)—transfusion-dependent anemia with misshapen RBCs.

Elliptocytes are found in at least one parent and may be present in siblings.
Mechanical fragility is increased.

## Erythrocytosis, Classification

See Table 11-2.
Polycythemia vera
Hereditary erythrocytosis (rare conditions)

* High-affinity hemoglobinopathies
* Decreased RBC 2,3-diphosphoglycerate (DPG) (due to high-RBC adenosine triphosphate or autosomal recessive DPG mutase deficiency)
* Increased production of erythropoietin (autosomal recessive)
* Erythropoietin-receptor mutations (autosomal dominant)
* Unknown causes

Secondary polycythemia
Relative polycythemia
Neonatal thick blood syndrome
Factitious (due to blood doping or ingestion of steroids by athletes)

## Polycythemia Vera (PV)

See Table 11-2.

### Criteria for Diagnosis

See Fig. 11-6.

A1 + A2 + A3; if A3 is absent then two of four criteria from B must be present.
A1: Increased RBC mass (≥ 36 mL/kg in men; ≥ 32 mL/kg in women)
A2: Normal arterial oxygen saturation (≥ 92%)
A3: Splenomegaly
B1: WBC >12,000/cu mm
B2: Platelet count >400,000/cu mm.
B3: Increased leukocyte alkaline phosphatase score in absence of fever or infection
B4: Increased serum vitamin $B_{12}$ (>900 pg/mL) or $B_{12}$ binding capacity (>2200 pg/mL).

RBC is increased; often = 7–12 million.
Increased Hb is 18–24 gm/dL.
Increased Hct >55%; >60% indicates increased RBC mass, but <60% may be associated with normal RBC mass.
MCV, MCH, and MCHC are normal or decreased.
Increased $^{51}Cr$ RBC mass is essential for diagnosis; blood volume is increased; plasma volume is variably normal or slightly increased.

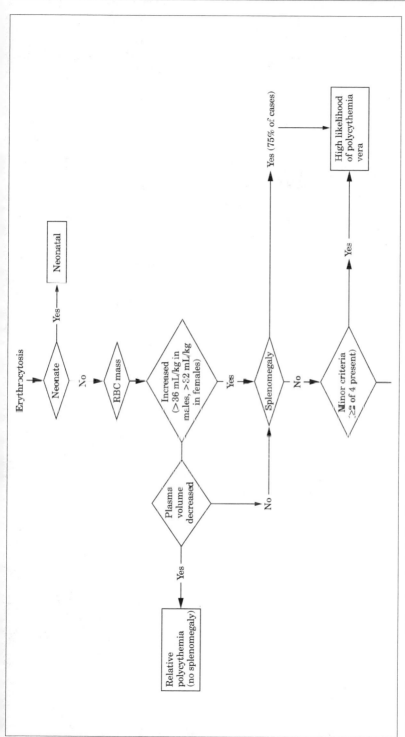

**Fig. 11-6.** Sequence of laboratory tests in the diagnosis of erythrocytosis. Erythropoietin may be assayed before imaging procedures. (CO Hb = carboxyhemoglobin; 2,3-DPG = 2,3-diphosphoglycerate.) (*continues*)

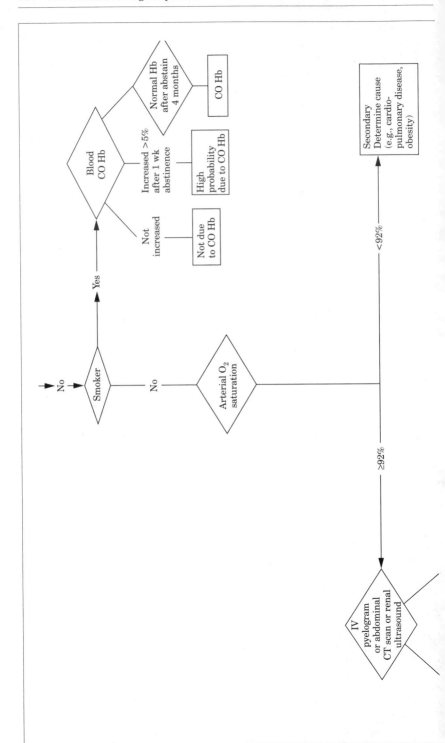

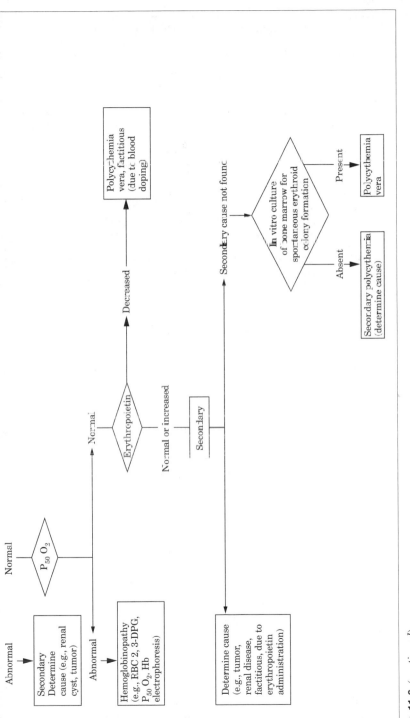

**Fig. 11-6.** (*continued*)

Increased platelet count >400,000/cu mm; often >1 million
Increased PMNs >12,000/cu mm; usually >15,000 cu mm; sometimes there is a
leukemoid reaction. Mild basophilia.
Oxygen saturation of arterial blood is normal.
Increased LAP score >100.
Increased serum vitamin $B_{12}$ >900 pg/mL.
Increased vitamin $B_{12}$–binding capacity >2200 pg/mL.
Erythropoietin level in plasma or serum is usually decreased (but occasionally
normal) in PV; usually remains normal during phlebotomy therapy. Usually
increased in secondary polycythemia; overlap between these. Normal level is
not helpful but *increased level requires search for cause of secondary erythro-
cytosis*. Increases may be intermittent; therefore a single normal level is unre-
liable. Usually normal in relative polycythemia.
ESR is decreased.
Blood viscosity is increased.
Osmotic fragility is decreased (increased resistance).
Reticulocyte count >1.5% in 44% of cases.
Bone marrow shows general hyperplasia of all elements. Cellularity >75%, espe-
cially with megakaryocytic hyperplasia in presence of erythrocytosis is strong evi-
dence for PV. Mild myelofibrosis may be present; iron may be decreased or absent.
Spontaneous erythroid colony formation occurs in in vitro culture of erythroid
progenitors in PV without addition of exogenous erythropoietin but not in sec-
ondary polycythemia or normal persons.
Increased serum uric acid
Serum total bilirubin may be slightly increased.
Serum iron may be decreased.
Laboratory findings due to complications such as thromboses, infection, peptic
ulcer, hemorrhage, myelofibrosis, myeloid metaplasia, leukemia

### Due to

Physiologically appropriate
• Hypoxia with decreased arterial oxygen saturation
Physiologically inappropriate
• Increased erythropoietin secretion e.g., tumors, renal disease
• Increased androgens, e.g., pheochromocytoma, Cushing's syndrome, mas-
culinizing ovarian tumor, factitious (use of androgens by athletes)

## Glucose-6-Phosphate Dehydrogenase Deficiency

Is the most frequent inherited RBC enzyme disorder
After standard dose of primaquine in adult, intravascular hemolysis develops.
• Hemolysis subsides spontaneously even if primaquine is continued.
In vitro tests of Heinz body formation when patients' RBCs are exposed to
acetylphenylhydrazine
Hb varies from 7 gm/dL to normal; is lower when due to exogenous agent; is usu-
ally normochromic, normocytic.
Peripheral smear shows varying amounts of RBC abnormalities.
Diagnosis is established by RBC assay for G6PD; heterozygotes have two RBC
populations and proportion of each determines degree of deficiency. Associated
with several different clinical syndromes.

### Decreased in

American blacks
Some other ethnic groups (e.g., Greeks, Sardinians, Sephardic Jews)
All persons with favism

### Increased in

Pernicious anemia to 3 times normal level
Idiopathic thrombocytopenic purpura (ITP) (Werlhof's disease)

## Hemoglobinuria, Paroxysmal Nocturnal
### (acquired clonal stem cell disorder)

Insidious, slowly progressive hemolytic anemia (mild to moderate, often macrocytic) and cytopenia
Evidence of hemolysis
* Hemoglobinuria (black urine) is evident on arising.
* Hemoglobinemia is present; increases during sleep.

Ham's test (RBC fragility is increased in acid medium and in hydrogen peroxide); amount of change is related to clinical severity. Is most specific test but relatively insensitive.
Sucrose hemolysis test; if positive, should be confirmed by Ham's test.
Autohemolysis is increased.
Negative direct Coombs' test
Bone marrow is not diagnostic.
Leukocyte alkaline phosphatase activity is decreased.
Laboratory findings due to
* Recurrent arterial and venous thromboses, especially of GI tract in ~30% of patients (e.g., hepatic, portal, splenic); cerebral; skin
* Hemorrhage
* Infection
* Renal findings similar to those in SC disease

Diagnosis should be considered in any patient with Coombs'-negative acquired chronic hemolysis, especially if hemoglobinuria, pancytopenia, or thrombosis are present.

## Hemolysis, Intravascular

Anemia varies from mild (Hb = 11.5 gm/dL) to severe (Hb = 2 gm/dL). MCV is usually 80–110 fL; <70 fL in normochromic anemia suggests hemoglobinopathy or paroxysmal nocturnal hemoglobinuria; >115 fL suggests macrocytic anemia.
Peripheral smear shows abnormal RBCs that may be a clue to the cause
Increased reticulocyte count is a major criterion for hemolytic anemia.
Plasma haptoglobin level decreases about 100 mg/dL in 6–10 hrs and lasts for 2–3 days after lysis of 20–30 mL blood. Reliable and very sensitive.
Hemoglobinuria occurs 1–2 hrs after severe hemolysis and lasts ≤ 24 hrs. It is a transient finding and is relatively insensitive.
Schumm's test for methemalbuminemia becomes positive 1–6 hrs after hemolysis of 100 mL blood and lasts 1–3 days. Methemalbuminemia also occurs in hemorrhagic pancreatitis.
Serum bilirubin increases with normal liver function 1 mg/dL in 1–6 hrs to maximum in 3–12 hrs after hemolysis of 100 mL blood.
Increased serum total LD. In compensated hemolysis, there is little or no increase in serum LD, bilirubin, Hb, or urine Hb, as in acute hemolytic anemia.
Bone marrow shows marked normoblastic erythroid hyperplasia.

## Hemoglobin F, Hereditary Persistence

Inherited persistence of Hb F in adult
Decreased MCV and MCHC Hb electrophoresis frequently shows increased Hb F (20–30%) and Hb A (60–70%).

## Hypersplenism

Diagnosis is made by exclusion.
Various combinations of anemia, leukopenia, thrombocytopenia associated with bone marrow showing normal or increased cellularity of affected elements
* Decreased platelet count (100,000–30,000/cu mm).

- Normochromic anemia (Hb = 9.0–11.0 gm/dL) may occur.
- WBCs may be decreased with a normal differential count.
- Bone marrow is normal or shows increased cellularity of all lines with normal maturation.

Peripheral blood smear may reflect the underlying cause. Direct Coombs' test is negative.

## Myelofibrosis, Idiopathic (Agnogenic Myeloid Metaplasia)
**(classified as a myeloproliferative stem cell disease stimulating marrow fibroblasts)**

Bone marrow shows fibrosis without apparent cause. Repeated bone marrow aspiration often produces no marrow elements. Surgical biopsy of bone for histologic examination shows fibrosis of marrow that is usually hypocellular.

Normocytic anemia is usual.

Peripheral smear shows characteristic anisocytosis, and marked poikilocytosis with teardrop (dacrocytes), polychromatophilia, and occasional nucleated RBCs are found. Rarely seen in other hematologic conditions.

Reticulocyte count is increased (10%).

WBC may be normal (50% of patients), increased (usually ≤ 30,000/cu mm) or decreased, and abnormal forms may occur. Immature cells (≤ 15%) are usual. Basophils and eosinophils may be increased.

Platelets may be normal, increased, or decreased, and abnormal and large forms may occur.

Needle puncture of spleen and a lymph node shows extramedullary hematopoiesis involving all three cell lines.

Hypersplenism causes thrombocytopenia in 30% and leukopenia in 15% of these patients.

LAP is usually increased (in contrast to chronic myelogenous leukemia); may be marked.

Serum uric acid is often increased.

Prolonged PT is found in 75% of patients.

Serum vitamin $B_{12}$ is often increased.

Some patients have trisomies of 8, 9, and 21 but Philadelphia chromosome ($Ph^1$) is rare.

*Rule out other myeloproliferative diseases, especially chronic myelogenous leukemia.*

## Sickle-Cell Disease

See Table 11-1.

### Sickling of RBCs

Sickling should be confirmed with Hb electrophoresis and genetic studies.

### Sickle Solubility Test

Does not differentiate between SC anemia, trait, and other Hb S genetic variants
Unreliable for newborn screening because of high Hb F
Inadequate for genetic counseling

### Sickle Cell Anemia (homozygous Hb SC disease)

Hb electrophoresis: Hb S is 80–100%, and Hb F comprises the rest; Hb A is absent.
Normocytic normochromic anemia (Hb = 5–10 gm/dL; normal MCV)
SC preparation is positive; since other Hb variants migrate with Hb S on electrophoresis, it is important to confirm Hb as a sickle type. Sickle solubility test is positive but does not differentiate anemia from other Hb S genetic variants and may be falsely negative if Hb <5 gm/dL.

Blood smear shows a variable number of abnormal RBCs. SCs in smear when RBCs contain >60% Hb S (except in Hb S–persistent Hb F).

WBC is increased (10,000–30,000/cu mm) during a crisis, with normal differential or shift to the left.

Platelet count is increased (300,000–500,000/cu mm), with abnormal forms.

Bone marrow shows hyperplasia of all elements.

Decreased ESR becomes normal after blood is aerated. ESR in normal range may indicate intercurrent illness or crisis.

Laboratory findings of hemolysis
- Hematuria is frequent.
- Renal concentrating ability is decreased, leading to a fixed specific gravity after the first few years of life.
- Serum uric acid may be increased.
- LAP activity is decreased.

Laboratory findings due to complications
- Infections.
- Crises.
- *Anemia and hemolytic jaundice are present throughout life after age 3–6 months; hemolysis and anemia are not increased during crises.*

Newborn screening by Hb electrophoresis on cord blood or filter paper spot
- In newborns with Hb SC, anemia is rarely present. May cause unexplained prolonged jaundice. *In newborn, cellulose agar electrophoresis is useless and acidic citrate agar gel is needed. For exchange transfusion, SC test must be performed on donor blood. Hb solubility tests (e.g., Sickledex [Ortho Diagnostics, Raritan, NJ]) are usually not suitable on cord blood.*

Antenatal diagnosis is possible as early as 7–10 wks gestation. Also detects Hb SC disease.

## Spherocytosis, Hereditary
**(defective RBC membrane due to spectrin deficiency; deficiency ~30% of normal in severe cases to 80% of normal in mildest cases)**

Autosomal dominant form in ~70% of cases have moderately severe disease in which one parent and half the siblings are affected; 20% have mild compensated hemolysis; may be sporadic and occur without a family history or may be recessive inheritance. ~10% have severe debilitating disease with severe anemia that makes them transfusion-dependent.

Abnormal peripheral blood smear is most suggestive finding. Many microspherocytes are present.

Hemolytic anemia is moderate (RBC = 3–4 million/cu mm), microcytic (MCV = 70–80 fL), and hyperchromic (increased MCHC = 36–40 gm/dL). *MCHC ≥ 36% means congenital spherocytic anemia if cold agglutinins and hypertriglyceridemia have been excluded.*

Osmotic fragility is increased; increase generally reflects clinical severity of disease. Diagnosis is not established without abnormal osmotic fragility. Osmotic fragility does not distinguish hereditary spherocytosis from autoimmune hemolytic disease with spherocytosis. Abnormal osmotic fragility and autohemolysis are reduced by 10% glucose; false-negative test may occur with concomitant diabetes mellitus.

Autohemolysis is increased (10–50% compared to normal of <4% of cells); very nonspecific test. Sometimes is found in nonspherocytic hemolytic anemias.

Direct Coombs' test must be negative.

Mechanical fragility is increased.

WBC and platelet counts are usually normal.

Evidence of hemolysis
- Degree of reticulocytosis (usually 5–15%) is greater than in other hemolytic anemias with similar degrees of anemia.
- Bone marrow shows marked erythroid hyperplasia.
- Increased serum LD and indirect bilirubin.

**Table 11-10.** Classification of Beta-Thalassemia Syndromes

| Genotype | Anemia | Microcytosis | Hb Electrophoresis |
|---|---|---|---|
| Normal | | | |
|   Beta/beta | None | None | Hb $A_2$ <3.5%, Hb F <1% |
| Thalassemia minima | | | |
|   Beta/beta$^+$ (mild) | None | None | Hb $A_2$ = N or slightly I<br>Hb F = I |
| Thalassemia minor | | | |
|   Beta/beta$^+$ (severe) | Mild | Mild to moderate | Hb $A_2$ = 3.5–7.5%<br>Hb F = N or slightly I |
|   Beta/beta$^0$ | Mild | Mild to moderate | Hb $A_2$ = 3.5–7.5%<br>Hb F = N or slightly I |
|   Beta/delta beta$^0$ | Mild | Mild to moderate | Hb $A_2$ = N or D<br>Hb F = 5–20% |
|   Beta/beta Lepore | Mild | Mild to moderate | Hb $A_2$ = N or D<br>Hb F = I<br>Hb Lepore up to 8% |
| Thalassemia intermedia | | | |
|   Beta$^+$ (mild)/beta$^+$<br>  (severe) | Moderate to severe | Moderate to severe | Hb $A_2$ = 6–8%<br>Hb F = 20–50%<br>Hb A = remainder |
|   Delta beta$^0$/delta beta$^0$ | Moderate to severe | Moderate to severe | Hb F only |
| Thalassemia major | | | |
|   Beta$^0$/beta$^0$ | Severe | Severe | Hb $A_2$ = 3–11%<br>Hb F = remainder |
|   Beta$^+$ (severe)/beta$^+$<br>  (severe) | Severe | Severe | Hb $A_2$ = 3–11%<br>Hb F = 10–90%<br>Hb A = remainder |
|   Beta$^0$/beta$^+$ (severe) | Severe | Severe | Hb $A_2$ = 3–11%<br>Hb F = 10–90%<br>Hb A = remainder |
|   Beta$^0$/beta Lepore | Severe | Severe | Hb F > 80%<br>Hb Lepore = remainder |

- Haptoglobins are decreased or absent.
- Hemolytic crises usually precipitated by infection (especially parvovirus) cause more profound anemia despite reticulocytosis and increased jaundice and splenomegaly.
- Hemoglobinemia and hemoglobinuria only during hemolytic crises.

*Diagnosis should be questioned if splenectomy does not cause a complete response.*

## Thalassemias

See Tables 11-10 through 11-12.

### *Beta-Thalassemia Trait*

In uncomplicated cases, Hb = 11–12 gm/dL whereas the RBC is increased (5–7 million/cu mm).

Most nonanemic patients with microcytosis have thalassemia minor.

**Table 11-11.** Classification of Alpha-Thalassemia Syndromes

| | Number of Gene Deletions | Anemia | Micro-cytosis | Hb Electrophoresis | |
| --- | --- | --- | --- | --- | --- |
| | | | | At Birth | Adults |
| Alpha-thal trait 2 (silent carrier) | 1 | 0 | 0 | 1–2% Bart | N |
| Alpha-thal trait 1 (heterozygous or homozygous) | 2 | Mild | Mild | 5–10% Bart | N Hb A2 not I |
| Hb H disease (alpha-thal 2 + thal 1) | 3 | Moderate | Marked | 20–40% Bart | Hb H Small amount of Hb A |
| Hydrops fetalis (homozygous) | 4 | Fatal at/ before birth | | >50% Bart | Hb Bart |

Notes: Alpha-thalassemias—decreased or absent synthesis of globin chains; very common in African, Asian, and Mediterranean populations. Most prevalent genetic trait in the world.
Hb Bart disappears by age 3–6 months. Hb Bart acts like very high affinity Hb with marked left-shifted oxygen dissociation curve resembling carbon monoxide poisoning.
Normal Hb electrophoresis and England-Fraser <–6 in the absence of iron deficiency implies alpha-thalassemia minor. Most common deletions of alpha-thalassemia can be screened for using PCR amplification of specific DNA sequences.
Alpha-thal = Alpha-thalassemia.

Microcytic anemia with anemia <9.3 gm/dL is unlikely to be thalassemia minor. MCV <75 fL whereas Hct is >30; may be as low as 55 fL.
Blood smear shows abnormal RBC morphology.
Serum iron is normal or slightly increased, transferrin saturation may be increased. TIBC and serum ferritin are normal.
Cellular marrow contains stainable iron.
Hb electrophoresis shows increased Hb A2 (>4%); normal value does not rule out this diagnosis.

### Thalassemia Major
*(Cooley's anemia, Mediterranean anemia)*

Marked hypochromic microcytic regenerative hemolytic anemia. Often Hb = 2.0–6.5 g/dL, Hct = 10–24%, RBC = 2–3 million, indices are decreased.
Blood smear shows marked RBC abnormalities.
WBCs are often increased, with normal differential or marked shift to left.
Bone marrow is cellular and shows erythroid hyperplasia.
Serum iron and TIBC are increased. After age 5 yrs, iron binding capacity is usually saturated.
Laboratory findings of hemolysis, liver dysfunction, and complications. Prenatal diagnosis is possible at 16 wks gestation.

## Myelodysplastic (Preleukemic) Syndromes

Clonal proliferative disorders of bone marrow that show peripheral blood cytopenias and dysmyelopoiesis; patient may progress to acute nonlymphocytic leukemia, may die of complications or associated diseases, or may die of unrelated causes. Loss of chromosomes 5 and/or 7 and trisomy 8 are very common.

**Table 11-12.** Differentiation of Microcytic Anemias of Iron Deficiency and Thalassemia Minor

| | Iron Deficiency | No Differentiation | Thalassemia Minor | Sensitivity (%)[a] | Accuracy (%)[a] |
|---|---|---|---|---|---|
| Hb (gm/L) | <9.3 M or F | 9.3–13.5 M<br>9.3–12.5 F | >13.5 M<br>>12.5 F | | |
| MCV (fL) | | >68 | <68 | 100 | 65 |
| MCHC (gm/dL) | <30 | >30 | | | |
| RBC (per cu mm) | <4.2 | 4.2–5.5 | >5.5 | | |
| Erythrocytosis | | | | 68 | 90 |
| Mentzer formula[b] (MCV/RBC) | >13 | | <13 | 95 | 65 |
| England-Fraser formula[b]<br>(MCV – [5 × Hb + RBC + K, if K = 3.4]) | | Positive number | Negative number | 69 | 77 |
| Shine-Lal formula[b]<br>(MCV$^2$ × MCH) | | | <1530 | 100 | 86 |
| MCV of 1 parent <79 | | | | 100 | 86 |
| Free erythrocyte protoporphyrin = 25 | | | | 60 | 67 |
| Hb A$_2$ >3.5% | | | | 85 | 90 |
| Microcytic-hypochromic ratio[c] | <0.9 | | >0.9 | | |

M = males; F = females.
[a] Accuracy in distinguishing anemias of thalassemia minor and iron deficiency (%).
[b] In patients with polycythemia vera who develop iron deficiency with microcytosis, a negative number results. These formulas do not account for the indeterminate zone of no differentiation.
[c] Using Technicon H-1 hematology analyzer (Technicon, Tarrytown, NY).

### French, American, British (FAB) Classification

Includes the following conditions:
- Refractory anemia.
- Refractory anemia with ring sideroblasts (same as acquired idiopathic sideroblastic anemia).
- Refractory anemia.
- Refractory anemia with excess blasts (usually progress to acute leukemia).
- Refractory anemia with excess blasts in transformation (from myelodysplasia to overt acute nonlymphocytic leukemia).
- Chronic myelomonocytic leukemia.
- Other clinicopathologic forms include refractory anemias of various types, pure red cell aplasia, paroxysmal nocturnal hemoglobinuria, chronic idiopathic neutropenia, chronic idiopathic thrombocytopenia, etc.

## Leukemia, Acute

In adults, 20% of acute leukemias are lymphocytic (ALL) and 80% are nonlymphocytic (AML). In children, 75% of cases are ALL and 25% are AML or chronic; >80% show clonal chromosomal abnormalities.
Peripheral blood
- WBC is rarely >100,000/cu mm; may be normal and is commonly less than normal. Peripheral smear shows many cells that resemble lymphocytes; it may not be possible to differentiate the very young forms as lymphoblasts or myeloblasts, and special cytochemical stains may be used. Special immunologic markers distinguish T cell, B cell, and non–T, non–B cell types of ALL.
Anemia is almost always present at clinical onset. Usually normocytic, progressive, and may become severe.
Platelet count is usually decreased at clinical onset and becomes progressively severe.
Bone marrow
- Blast cells are present even when none are found in peripheral blood.
- The myeloid:erythroid ratio is increased.
- Erythroid and megakaryocyte elements are replaced.
- Histochemical, phenotypic, and cytogenetic studies are important for classification, prognosis, and therapy.
DIC may be present at onset.
Serum uric acid is frequently increased
Tumor lysis syndrome may occur.
Increased serum creatinine and BUN reflects infiltration of kidneys.
In AML, serum LD, AST, ALT may be increased.
Laboratory findings due to complications
- Meningeal leukemia.
- Urate nephropathy.
- Infection causes 90% of deaths.
- Hemolytic anemia.

## Leukemia, Lymphoblastic, Acute (ALL)

In adults, 80% of ALL are B cell and 20% are T cell lineage.
Classified as L-1, L-2, L-3 (FAB) based on cell morphology; cannot be differentiated by cytochemical stains.
WBC increased; may be >100,000/cu mm but normal or low in some patients. Moderate to severe thrombocytopenia.
Variable degree of anemia
Marrow usually shows >50% lymphoblasts.
High incidence of meningeal involvement
Ph[1] is present in ~20% of adults and <5% of children.

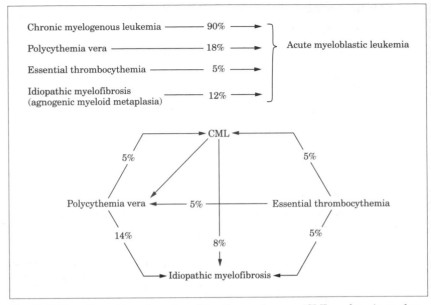

**Fig. 11-7.** Transformation of myeloproliferative syndromes. (CML = chronic myelogenous leukemia.)

Serum LD, uric acid often increased
See Fig. 11-7.

## Leukemia, Nonlymphocytic, Acute

### French, American, British Classification

Based on morphology and cytochemistry. Immunophenotyping and cytogenetics provide additional essential information. Includes the following conditions:
- M-1 Acute myeloid leukemia with minimal maturation
- M-2 Acute nonlymphocytic leukemia with t(8;21)
- M-3 Acute promyelocytic leukemia
- M-4 Acute myelomonocytic leukemia
- M-5 Acute monocytic leukemia with t(9;11)
- M-5a and M-5b variants of M-5
- M-6 Erythroleukemia
- M-7 Acute megakaryocytic leukemia
- M-0 Acute myeloid leukemia without differentiation

Not included in classification are the following:
- Acute undifferentiated leukemia has no evidence of either myeloid or lymphoid lineage.
- Acute mixed-lineage leukemia—myeloid and lymphoid lineages in same clone.
- Therapy-related leukemia occurs after several years. >70% have a preleukemic phase lasting about 11 months. Develop acute myelogenous leukemia.

## Leukemia, Myelogenous, Chronic

See Table 11-13 and Fig. 11-7.
Increased WBC due to increase in myeloid series is earliest change.
- WBC is usually 50,000–300,000/cu mm when disease is discovered.

**Table 11-13.** Differential Diagnosis of Chronic Myelogenous Leukemia

|  | Chronic Myelogenous Leukemia | Acute Myeloblastic Leukemia | Granulocytic Leukemoid Reaction | Myelo-fibrosis |
|---|---|---|---|---|
| WBC >100,000/cu mm | Yes | Rare | No | No |
| Whole spectrum of immature granulocytes | Yes | No (leukemic hiatus) | No | Yes |
| Myeloblasts and pro-myelocytes in blood or marrow | >30% | >30% | 0 | <30% |
| LAP | Usually <10 | 30–150 | >150 | Variable |
| Bone marrow | Granulocytic hyperplasia | >30% myelo-blasts | Granulocytic hyperplasia | Fibrosis |
| Philadelphia chromosome | Yes | No | No | No |

- Decreased number of leukocytes show positive alkaline phosphatase staining reaction.
- Eosinophilic, basophilic leukocytes may be slightly increased at first with more marked increases in later stages.
- Lymphocytes are normal in absolute number but relatively decreased.

Anemia is usually normochromic, normocytic; absent in early stage and severe in late stage. Degree of anemia is a good index of extent of leukemic process, prognosis, and disease progression.

Platelet count is normal or increased; decreased in terminal stages with findings of thrombocytopenic purpura.

Bone marrow findings confirm diagnosis.

Serum uric acid are increased, especially with high WBC and antileukemic therapy. Urinary obstruction may develop because of uric acid crystals.

Serum LD is increased; rises several weeks before relapse and falls several weeks before remission. LD is useful for following course of therapy.

Increased serum AST and ALT in half of patients show less elevation than in acute leukemia.

Ph[1] chromosome is found in 95% of early chronic phase cases; persists in chronic stable phase when marrow and blood appear normal. Persists during blast phase. Ph[1]-negative cases are usually chronic myelomonocytic leukemias. Ph[1] chromosome has also been found in ~20% of adults with ALL, 2% of adults with AML, 5% of children with ALL. Ph[1] is present in granulomonocytic, erythroid, megakaryocytic lines as well as some B-lymphocytes.

Blast crisis diagnosed by >20% blasts in marrow or peripheral blood or both or extramedullary proliferation of blasts, or large foci of blasts in bone marrow biopsy.

Platelet count <15,000 or >1,000,000/cu mm, blasts in peripheral blood, absence of Ph[1], moderate to marked myelofibrosis at time of diagnosis are poor prognostic signs.

Coombs' test is positive in one-third of patients.

Peripheral blood remission due to drugs—decreased WBC to nearly normal levels with only rare immature cells, correction of anemia, control of thrombocytosis; marrow continues to show granulocytic hyperplasia and Ph[1].

## Leukemia, Lymphocytic, Chronic (CLL)

See Table 11-14.

**Table 11-14.** Comparison of CLLs

| | |
|---|---|
| B-lymphocytes | |
| CLL | Autoimmune hemolytic anemia, hypogamma-globulinemia |
| Prolymphocytic leukemia (not a variant of CLL but a separate entity) | B-type lymphocytes derived from medullary cords of lymph nodes show less mature forms than in CLL extreme leukocytosis with >54% prolymphocytes with a typical phenotype, very high blast counts, prominent splenomegaly often without much lymphadenopathy |
| Waldenström's macro-globulinemia | Increased serum IgM |
| Leukemic phase of poorly differentiated lymphoma | Usually is leukemic phase of lymphoma, but up to 50% have marrow involvement lymphoma when first seen; occasionally may present without node involvement |
| Hairy cell leukemia | Pancytopenia and prominent splenomegaly; usually leukopenia with many hairy cells showing characteristic tartrate-resistant acid phosphatase |
| T-lymphocytes | |
| CLL | Causes <5% of cases of CLL |
| Adult T cell leukemia/lymphoma | Hypercalcemia, lytic bone lesions; WBC usually >50,000/cu mm; due to HTLV-1 infection |
| Prolymphocytic | Morphologically identical to B cell type, but lymphadenopathy is more frequent in T cell type leukemia |
| T-gamma–chronic lymphoproliferative disease | Severe granulocytopenia; moderate increase in WBC; recurrent infections are common; usually no lymphadenopathy or skin involvement |
| Cutaneous T cell lymphoma | Sézary syndrome refers to both skin and systemic involvement; mycosis fungoides is cutaneous form, which may be present for years before clinical systemic involvement |

### Diagnostic Criteria

Lymphocyte count >15,000/cu mm in absence of other causes and marrow infiltration >30% for >6 months. Have characteristic immunophenotype.

Demonstration of monoclonality in the proper clinical context confirms the diagnosis regardless of absolute lymphocyte count.

Peripheral blood
- WBC is usually 50,000–250,000/cu mm with 90% lymphocytes producing a monotonous blood picture of small, mature-looking, normal-looking lymphocytes. Blast cells are uncommon. Granulocytopenia. Neutropenia is a late occurrence.
- Autoimmune hemolytic anemia and thrombocytopenia in 25% of patients.
- Platelet count is less likely to increase with therapy than in myelogenous leukemia.

Bone marrow
- Infiltration with earlier lymphocytic cell types increases progressively.
- There is replacement of erythroid, myeloid, and megakaryocyte series that show normal morphology and maturation.

Lymph node biopsy shows pattern of diffuse lymphoma with well-differentiated cells; aspirate or imprint shows increased number of immature leukocytes, predominantly blast cells.

Serum enzyme levels are less frequently elevated and show a lesser increase than in chronic myelogenous leukemia.

Direct Coombs' test is positive in up to one-third of patients.

Hypogammaglobulinemia occurs in two-thirds of cases depending on duration of disease.

Uric acid levels are normal but may increase during therapy.

Ph[1] chromosome is not found.

Chromosomal abnormalities in ~50% of patients, most often chromosomes 12 and 14.

## Lymphomas and Hodgkin's Disease

Diagnosis is established by histologic findings of biopsied lymph node.

Blood findings may vary from completely normal to markedly abnormal.
- Moderate normochromic normocytic anemia.
- Leukopenia, marked leukocytosis, and anemia are bad prognostic signs.
- Eosinophilia occurs in ~20% of patients.
- Relative and absolute lymphopenia may occur; if lymphocytosis is present, look for another disease.

Small lymphocytic and follicular lymphomas have leukemic phase in 5–15% of patients.

Cytopenias occur commonly.

Bone marrow involvement at time of diagnosis.

Increased serum LD, uric acid, and abnormal liver function tests are common in non-Hodgkin's lymphomas.

Hodgkin's disease patients commonly have abnormal T cell function with deficiencies of cell-mediated immunity with increased susceptibility to infections.

Non-Hodgkin's lymphomas are of B-lymphocyte origin with characteristic surface markers.

Patients often have abnormalities of humoral immunity; hypogammaglobulinemia in 50% of cases and monoclonal gammopathy in ~10% of small lymphocytic lymphomas.

Non-Hodgkin's lymphomas occur frequently in AIDS patients.

In follicular lymphomas, bcl-2 gene rearrangement; found in >80% by cytogenic analysis and virtually all by molecular testing; differentiates this from reactive lymph nodes.

## Monoclonal Gammopathies, Classification

See Table 11-15.

Monoclonal gammopathy of unknown significance
- Benign (IgG, IgA, IgD, IgM; rarely free light chains)
- Associated with neoplasms of cells now known to produce M proteins
- Biclonal gammopathies

Malignant
- Multiple myeloma
- Plasmacytoma
  Solitary of bone
  Extramedullary
- Malignant lymphoproliferative diseases
  Waldenström's macroglobulinemia
  Malignant lymphoma
- Heavy-chain diseases
- Amyloidosis
  Secondary to multiple myeloma

**Table 11-15.** Comparison of Diseases with Monoclonal Immunoglobulins

| | Multiple Myeloma | Macroglobulinemia | Benign Monoclonal Gammopathy | Heavy-Chain Diseases | | |
| --- | --- | --- | --- | --- | --- | --- |
| | | | | Gamma | Alpha | Mu |
| Clinical | Bone lesions Anemia Infections | Enlarged LNN, L, S | None | Enlarged LNN, L, S | Intestinal malabsorption | Enlarged LNN, L, S |
| Bone marrow | Sheets of plasma cells | Lymphocytosis or lymphocytoid plasma cells | Up to 10% plasma cells | Plasma cells or lymphocytoid plasma cells | | Lymphocytosis or lymphocytoid plasma cells with vacuoles |
| Monoclonal Ig in serum (electrophoresis) | 80% | Present | Present | Present | Present | Present |
| BJ protein in urine (electrophoresis) | 70–80% | 80–95% | Rare | Common | Rare | Common |
| Serum (immunoelectrophoresis) | 1 type of M chain[a] 1 type of L chain[b] | Mu chain 1 type of L chain[b] | 1 type of M chain[a] 1 type of L chain[b] | Gamma chain No L | Alpha chain No L | Mu chain Free kappa or lambda in two-thirds |
| Urine (immunoelectrophoresis) | Kappa or lambda | Kappa or lambda | Rare kappa or lambda | Gamma chain | | Kappa or lambda in two-thirds |

Notes: Monoclonal proteins (paraproteins, M proteins) are immunoglobulins synthesized by atypical cells of reticuloendothelial system. Each is a homogeneous product of a single clone of proliferating cells and is expressed as a monoclonal gammopathy. Monoclonal proteins consist of two heavy polypeptide chains of the same class (e.g., gamma, alpha, mu) and subclass and two light polypeptide chains of the same type (either kappa or lambda); may be present in serum, urine, and CSF. Heavy-chain disease is production of only heavy chains without accompanying light chains; light-chain disease is the reverse. They are detected by conventional protein electrophoresis and identified by immunoelectrophoresis. Paraproteinemia is due to monoclonal gammopathy of unknown significance (63%), multiple myeloma (14%), primary amyloidosis (9%), indolent non-Hodgkin's lymphoma (5%), extramedullary or solitary bone plasmacytoma (4%), chronic lymphocytic leukemia (3%), Waldenström's macroglobulinemia (2%).

LNN = lymph nodes; L = liver; S = spleen.
[a]M chain is gamma, alpha, mu, delta, or epsilon.
[b]L chain is kappa or lambda.

**Table 11-16.** Comparison of Multiple Myeloma and MGUS

|  | Multiple Myeloma | MGUS |
|---|---|---|
| Paraprotein level | Higher | Lower (rarely <3 gm/dL) |
| Nonparaprotein immunoglobulins suppressed | 96% of cases | 12% of cases |
| BJ proteinuria | 57% of cases | 17% of cases |
| Bone marrow plasmacytosis >20% | 100% of cases | 4% of cases |

MGUS = monoclonal gammopathy of unknown significance.

Primary
* Unknown significance
Idiopathic

# Monoclonal Gammopathy, Idiopathic ("Benign," "Asymptomatic") (Plasma Cell Dyscrasia of Unknown Significance) (MGUS)

See Table 11-16.
The following changes are present for a period of >5 yrs.
* Monoclonal serum protein concentration usually <3 gm/dL and does not increase during follow-up; IgG type in 73% of patients. Multiple myeloma always shows depression of background Ig and monoclonal serum protein >3 gm/dL.
* Normal serum albumin.
* Usually <10% plasma cells in bone marrow.
* Absence of BJ protein, anemia, myeloma bone lesions, lymphoproliferative disease, hypercalcemia, renal insufficiency
* Monoclonal light-chain proteinuria may occur (up to 1 gm/24 hrs).
* May be associated with aging, neoplasms, many chronic diseases (most often RA) and infections (e.g., TB).

Many patients will develop myeloma, macroglobulinemia, or primary amyloidosis within 5 yrs and 25% at 10 yrs; lymphoproliferative disorders develop in 17% at 10 yrs, and 33% of patients at 20 yrs; more likely to become malignant if these criteria are present:
* IgG >200 mg/dL, or either IgA or IgM >100 mg/dL or IgD or IgE paraprotein found at any concentration.
* Ig fragments in urine (usually BJ protein) or serum.
* Progressive increase in paraprotein concentration.
* Low levels of polyclonal Ig.

# Multiple Myeloma

See Tables 11-16 and 11-17.

## *Diagnostic Criteria*

Bone marrow shows sheets or >20% plasma cells *and*
Abnormality of immunoglobulin formation (monoclonal spike >4 gm/dL or BJ proteinuria >0.5 gm/24 hrs)
* If monoclonal spike is <4 gm/dL, then substitute criteria:
Reciprocal depression of normal immunoglobulins *or*

**Table 11-17.** Comparison of Immunoproliferative Disorders

| Disease | Relative Frequency (%) | Ig Heavy Chain | Ig Light Chain | Urine BJ (%) | Complications/Associated Conditions |
|---|---|---|---|---|---|
| Myelomas | | | | | |
| IgG | 75 | Gamma | Kappa or lambda | 60 | Infection |
| IgA | 15 | Alpha | Kappa or lambda | 70 | Infection |
| IgD | <2 | Delta | Usually lambda | 100 | Amyloidosis |
| IgE | Very rare | Epsilon | Kappa or lambda | ? | Plasma cell leukemia |
| Light-chain myeloma | 10 | None | Kappa or lambda | 100 | Amyloid kidney, hypercalcemia |
| Macroglobulinemia | | Mu | Kappa or lambda | 30–40 | Hyperviscosity<br>Hemolytic anemia (cold agglutinin)<br>Bleeding |
| Heavy-chain disease | | | | | |
| Gamma | | | None | Gamma chain | |
| Alpha | | | None | None | GI tract lymphoma<br>Malabsorption |
| Mu | | | None | Kappa chain BJ | Amyloidosis<br>Chronic lymphocytic leukemia |

Panhypogammaglobulinemia and osteolytic bone lesions *or*
No plasmacytosis not due to other causes
Very elevated serum total protein is due to increase in globulins (with decreased
A:G ratio) in one-half to two-thirds of the patients.
Serum protein immunoelectrophoresis or immunofixation characterizes protein
as monoclonal (i.e., one light-chain type) and classifies disease by identifying
specific heavy chain. It reveals abnormal Ig in 80% of patients.

| % of Patients | Immunoelectrophoresis or Immunofixation Shows |
| --- | --- |
| ≤ 99 | Monoclonal protein in serum or urine |
| 90 | Serum monoclonal spike |
| 20 | Both serum and urine monoclonal protein |
| 20 | Monoclonal light chains in urine only |
| <2 | Hypogammaglobulinemia only without serum or urine paraprotein |
| 60 | IgG myeloma protein |
| 20 | IgA myeloma protein |
| 10 | Light chain only (BJ proteinemia) |
| Very rare | IgE myeloma protein |
| <1 | IgD myeloma protein* |

*IgD myeloma is difficult to recognize. BJ proteinuria is almost always present, and TP is
often normal.

BJ proteinuria occurs in 35–50% of patients. >50% of IgG or IgA myeloma and
100% of light-chain myelomas have BJ proteinuria.
  • Dipstick tests for urine protein will miss BJ protein and heat precipitation
    is not reliable.
Electrophoresis/immunofixation of both serum and urine is abnormal in almost
all patients. If only serum electrophoresis is performed, kappa and some
lambda light-chain myelomas will be missed. 10% of patients have hypogam-
maglobulinemia (<0.6 gm/dL).
Bone marrow aspiration usually shows 20–50% plasma cells or myeloma cells,
usually in sheets; abnormal plasma cells may be found.
Hematologic findings
  • Anemia (usually normocytic, normochromic) in 60% of patients.
  • WBC and platelet count usually normal; 40–55% lymphocyte frequently pre-
    sent on differential count, with variable number of immature lymphocytic
    and plasmacytic forms. Decreased WBC and platelet counts with extensive
    marrow replacement.
  • Rouleaux formation in 85% of patients, occasionally causing difficulty in
    cross-matching blood.
  • Increased ESR in 90% of patients and other abnormalities due to serum pro-
    tein changes. ESR >100 is rare in any condition other than myeloma.
  • Cold agglutinins or cryoglobulins.
Hyperviscosity syndrome is characteristic of IgM and occurs in 4% of IgG and
10% of IgA myeloma and may be the presenting feature.
Clinical amyloidosis occurs in 15% of cases of multiple myeloma (especially IgD
myeloma and light-chain disease), but monoclonal spikes are present in urine
in most, if not all, cases of primary amyloidosis.
Chromosome analysis frequently shows translocation t(11;14)(q13;q32).
Serial measurement of serum globulins and/or BJ proteinuria are excellent indi-
cations of efficacy of chemotherapy.
Lowered anion gap in IgG myeloma only (due to cationic IgG paraproteins caus-
ing retention of excess chloride ion)
Increased incidence of other neoplasms
  • Acute myelomonocytic leukemia.
  • 20% of patients develop adenocarcinoma of GI tract, biliary tree, breast.

## Macroglobinemia (Primary; Waldenström's)
(monoclonal proliferation of plasma cells and B-lymphocytes producing an IgM M protein)

Electrophoresis of serum shows an intense sharp peak in globulin fraction, identified as IgM by immunoelectrophoresis. The pattern may be indistinguishable from that in multiple myeloma. IgM protein $\geq 3.0$ gm/dL.

Total serum protein and globulin are markedly increased.

ESR is very high.

Rouleaux formation is marked; positive Coombs' reaction; difficulty in cross-matching blood.

Severe anemia, usually normochromic normocytic

WBC is decreased, with relative lymphocytosis but no evidence of lymphocytic leukemia.

Bone marrow biopsy is always hypercellular and shows >30% involvement by pleomorphic infiltrate with atypical "lymphocytes" and also plasma cells.

Increased number of mast cells

Lymph node may show malignant lymphoma.

Flow cytometry shows $\leq 50\%$ of patients have circulating monoclonal B-lymphocyte population.

50% of patients with Waldenström's macroglobulinemia have hyperviscosity syndrome causing coagulation abnormalities. Causes persistent oronasal hemorrhage (occurs in ~75% of patients), neurologic and visual disturbances, hypervolemia and congestive heart failure.

IgM may also cause cryoglobulinemia.

BJ proteinuria is found in 10% of cases. Monoclonal light chain in 70–80% of cases.

Coagulation abnormalities: There may be decreased platelets, abnormal BT, coagulation time, PT, prothrombin consumption, etc.

Impaired renal function is much less common than in myeloma.

Amyloidosis is rare.

*Differs from multiple myeloma by absence of lytic bone lesions and of hypercalcemia.*

## Immunodeficiency Diseases, Classification

See Fig. 11-8 and Tables 11-18 and 11-19.

### *Primary*

Antibody deficiency disorders
- X-linked agammaglobulinemia
- Common variable immunodeficiency
- Selective IgA deficiency
- Transient hypogammaglobulinemia of infancy
- Selective IgG subclass deficiency

Primary T-cell deficiency
- DiGeorge syndrome
- Chronic mucocutaneous candidiasis
- Hyper-IgE syndrome

Combined T/B-cell deficiency
- Severe combined immunodeficiency disease (SCID)
- Wiskott-Aldrich syndrome
- Ataxia-telangiectasia

Complement deficiencies

Phagocyte disorders

B-cell deficiency should be suspected with recurrent, complicated, or severe pyogenic infections.

Screen by serum protein electrophoresis and immunofixation; anti-A, anti-B iso-hemagglutinins, specific antibody titers (tetanus, diphtheria, rubella).

T cell–deficient patients tend to have chronic recurrent *Candida* infection of scalp, nails, mucous membranes. Screen by skin testing, response to mitogen.

Lymphopenia usually indicates T-cell dysfunction since most circulating lymphocytes are T cells.

Monoclonal antibody phenotyping for specific B and T cells

### Secondary Associated with

Virus infections
Metabolic disorders (e.g., uremia, malnutrition, diabetes mellitus)
Protein deficiency
Immunosuppression
Respiratory tract disorders
Prematurity

## Alpha$_1$-Antitrypsin (AAT) Deficiency
**(autosomal recessive deficiency; the heterozygous state occurs in 10–15% of general population who have serum levels of AAT ~60% of normal; homozygous state occurs in 1:2000 persons who have serum levels ~10% of normal)**

Usually discovered by absent alpha$_1$ peak on serum protein electrophoresis. Should be confirmed by assay of serum AAT and Pi phenotyping; DNA analysis also permits prenatal diagnosis and functional analysis of total trypsin inhibitory capacity (90% is due to AAT activity).

### AAT May Be Decreased in
*(is typically <50 mg/dl )*

Prematurity
Severe liver disease
Malnutrition
Renal losses
GI losses
Exudative dermopathies
*AAT deficiency should be ruled out in children with neonatal hepatitis, giant cell hepatitis, chronically abnormal liver chemistries, or juvenile cirrhosis, and in adults with chronic hepatitis without serologic markers, cryptogenic cirrhosis, hepatoma.*

### AAT May Be Increased in
*(is an acute phase reactant)*

Acute or chronic infections
Neoplasia
Pregnancy
Use of birth control pills
Liver biopsy supports the diagnosis and helps stage extent of liver damage.
Pulmonary emphysema occurs in heterozygotes and homozygotes; occurs in family of 25% of patients. Secondary bronchitis and bronchiectasis may occur.
Liver disease occurs in 10–20% of children with this deficiency. Clinical picture may be neonatal hepatitis, prolonged obstructive jaundice during infancy, cirrhosis, or asymptomatic.

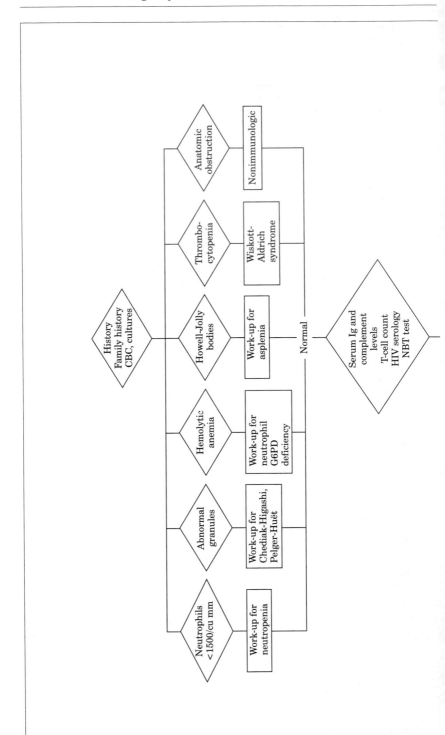

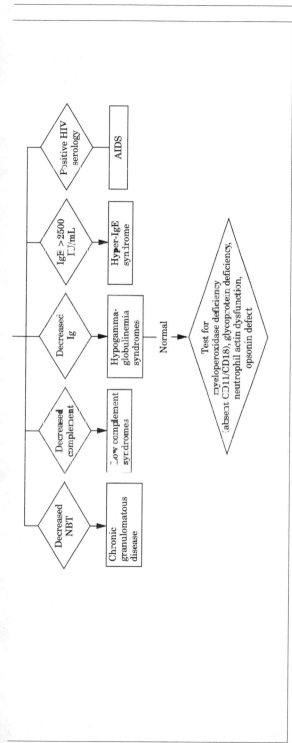

**Fig. 11-8.** Algorithm for work-up for recurrent infections. (CBC = complete blood count; hyper-IgE = hyperimmunoglobulinemia E.)

**Table 11-18.** Tests for Immune Deficiency

| Arm of the Immune System Deficient | Screening Tests | Definitive Tests[a] | Type of Infection[b] | Suggestive Organism | Example of Immunodeficiency Disease |
|---|---|---|---|---|---|
| Antibody | Quantitative IgM, IgG, IgA Pre-existing antibodies to prior immunizations: *Haemophilus influenzae*, rubella Isohemagglutinins | Diphtheria-tetanus titer Antibody response to pneumococcal polysaccharide vaccination B-lymphocytes Plasma cells | Sinusitis, diarrhea, failure to thrive | *Streptococcus pneumoniae*, nontypeable *H. influenzae*, *Giardia lamblia* from gut | Bruton's disease, selective IgA deficiency, hypogammaglobulinemia with normal or increased IgM |
| Complement | Total hemolytic C3, C4, C5 Factor B | Chemotactic factors Opsonins Immunoelectrophoretic analysis | Sinusitis | *S. pneumoniae*, *Neisseria* species | Deficiency of C3, C3b inactivator, Factor B, C6, C7, C8 |
| Phagocytes | WBC and differential count Nitroblue tetrazolium test IgE | Chemotaxis Adhesion Aggregation Chemiluminescence Phagocytosis and killing WBC oxidative metabolism CD11/CD18 Cytochrome b558 | Osteomyelitis, eczema, stomatitis, furunculosis, liver abscess, draining lymphadenitis | *Staphylococcus aureus*, *Staphylococcus epidermidis*, *Candida albicans*, *Serratia marcescens* | Primary or secondary neutropenia, chronic granulomatous disease, Chédiak-Higashi syndrome |
| Cell-mediated immunity | Skin tests (e.g., *C. albicans*) | Flow cytometry Mitogen responses Suppressor or helper cells | Failure to thrive, autoimmune disease, eczema, diarrhea, candidiasis (perineal/oral) | Lungs—cytomegalovirus, *Pneumocystis carinii*, VZV, *Cryptococcus*, *Nocardia*, recurrent *Candida* | Wiskott-Aldrich syndrome, ataxia-telangiectasia, thymic hypoplasia, severe combined immunodeficiency disease |

[a]At special immunologic centers.
[b]Severe or recurrent pneumonia, acute otitis media in all groups.

**Table 11-19.** Classification of Primary Immunologic Defects

| Syndrome | Number of Circulating Lymphocytes | Number of Plasma Cells | Ig Changes | Thymus | Lymph Node Germinal Center | Lymph Node Paracortical Zone | Other Laboratory Findings |
|---|---|---|---|---|---|---|---|
| Infantile gender-linked agammaglobulinemia (Bruton's disease). Probably represents a heterogeneous group of defects. | N | O | Markedly D in all | N | O | N | A, B, C. Inability to make functional antibody is the distinguishing feature; antibody responses to immunization are usually absent. Live virus vaccination may cause severe disease (e.g., paralytic polio). B cells in peripheral blood detected by surface Ig techniques are absent or found in very low numbers. T cell numbers and function are intact. |
| Selective inability to produce IgA | N | IgA-producing plasma cells especially in lamina propria | IgA is O; others are usually N | N | N | N | May have malabsorption syndrome, steatorrhea, bronchitis. Intestinal lamina propria lacks IgA-producing cells. Serum antibodies to IgA in >40% of patients. Peripheral blood lymphocytes bearing IgA, IgM, and IgG are normal. Plasma cells producing IgA are absent in GI and respiratory epithelium. |

**Table 11-19.** (continued)

| Syndrome | Number of Circulating Lymphocytes | Number of Plasma Cells | Ig Changes | Thymus | Lymph Node | | Other Laboratory Findings |
|---|---|---|---|---|---|---|---|
| | | | | | Germinal Center | Paracortical Zone | |
| Transient hypogamma-globulinemia of infancy | N | D | IgG is D | | O or rare | | Symptomatic or recurrent pyogenic respiratory infections; increased incidence of atopic disease, RA, lymphonodular hyperplasia of small intestine. A |
| Non-sex-linked primary immunoglobulin deficiencies (e.g., dysgammaglobulinemias—acquired, congenital) | N | V (Usually D) | Present, but type and amount are V | N | Usually O Reticulum hyperplasia | Often D | A, B, C; increased frequency of autoimmune diseases |
| Agammaglobulinemia with thymoma (Good's syndrome) | Progressively D, often to very low levels | D or O | Markedly D in all | Enlarged (stromal epithelial spindle-cell type); thymoma | D or O | May be D | A, B Pure red cell aplasia may occur; eosinophils O or markedly D |
| Wiskott-Aldrich syndrome (X-linked, recessive immune deficiency with thrombopenia and eczema) | Usually progressively D | N | Usually present, but type and amount are V (frequently IgM) | N | May be D | Progressively D in lymphocytes | A, B; eczema and thrombocytopenia; increased frequency of malignant lymphoma; serum lacks isohemagglutinins; platelets one-half normal size |

| Disease | | | | | | | |
|---|---|---|---|---|---|---|---|
| Ataxia-telangiectasia (Louis-Bar syndrome), autosomal recessive. Progressive cerebellar ataxia; telangiectasia in tissues. Autosomal recessive disorder of humoral and cellular defects. | V (usually slightly D) | V (usually present) | is D and IgA is D; IgG usually N | Usually present, but type and amount are V (frequently IgA and IgE are D or O, and D IgG) | Embryonic type (no Hassall's corpuscles or cortical medullary organization) | May be D | Lymphocytes D | Serum AFP is almost always increased. Decreased total T cells (CD3) and helper cells (CD4) with normal or increased suppressor cells (CD8). Recurrent infections in 80% of cases, usually bacterial sinopulmonary but not viral. Delayed cutaneous anergy indicates impaired cell-mediated immunity. C. Increased frequency of adenocarcinomas. Hepatic and endocrine (e.g., ovarian dysgenesis) abnormalities may be present. |
| Primary lymphopenic immunologic deficiency (Gitlin's syndrome) | V–D | V | | Always present but type and amount are V | Hypoplastic (Hassall's corpuscles and lymphoid cells D) | Marked D in tissue lymphocytes; foci of lymphocytes may be present in spleen and lymph nodes | | B |
| Autosomal recessive alymphocytotic agammaglobulinemia (Swiss type agammaglobulinemia; Glanzmann and Riniker's lymphocytophthisis) | Markedly D | O | | Markedly D in all | Hypoplastic (Hassall's corpuscles and lymphoid cells O) | Lymphocytes O or markedly D | | A, B, C |

**Table 11-19.** (continued)

| Syndrome | Number of Circulating Lymphocytes | Number of Plasma Cells | Ig Changes | Thymus | Lymph Node | | Other Laboratory Findings |
|---|---|---|---|---|---|---|---|
| | | | | | Germinal Center | Paracortical Zone | |
| Autosomal recessive lymphopenia with normal immunoglobulins (Nezelof syndrome) | D | Present | N | Hypoplastic (Hassall's corpuscles and lymphoid cells O) | May be present | Lymphocytes markedly D | B<br>Lymphopenia, neutropenia, eosinophilia. Marked deficiency of total T cells and T-cell subsets; normal helper:suppressor (CD4:CD8) ratio. |
| DiGeorge syndrome (thymic aplasia) Absent parathyroids (tetany of the newborn); frequent cardiovascular malformations | V (usually N) | Present | N | Absent | Present | Rare paracortical lymphocytes present | B<br>Serum Ig are usually near normal for age, but may be decreased, especially IgA. IgE may be increased. Decreased T cells and relative increase in B-cell percentage. Normal ratio of helper and suppressor types. With complete syndrome, susceptible to opportunistic infection and to graft-versus-host disease from blood transfusion. In partial syndrome, growth and response to infection may be normal. |

O = absent; A = recurrent infections with pyogenic organisms; B = frequent virus, fungus, or *Pneumocystis* infection; C = increased frequency of lymphomas.

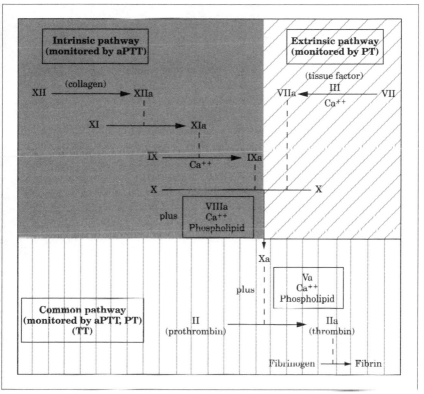

**Fig. 11-9.** Coagulation mechanisms. *Shaded area* encloses the intrinsic coagulation reactions that occur on the surface membrane phospholipids of platelets. *Diagonal lines* enclose the extrinsic coagulation reactions that occur on disrupted tissue cell phospholipoprotein membranes intruded into the circulation. *Vertical lines* enclose the common pathway. (TT = thrombin time.)

# Coagulation Tests

See Fig. 11-9.

## Antithrombin III

### *Use*

To detect hypercoagulable state associated with episodes of venous thrombosis; decreased in ~4.5% of patients with idiopathic venous thrombosis

### *Decreased in*

Hereditary familial deficiency (typically 40–60% of normal); autosomal dominant trait
Chronic liver disease
Protein-wasting diseases (e.g., nephrotic syndrome)
Heparin therapy for >3 days
L-Asparaginase therapy

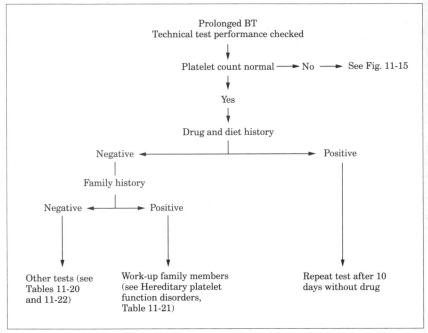

Prolonged BT
Technical test performance checked

↓

Platelet count normal ⟶ No ⟶ See Fig. 11-15

↓

Yes

↓

Drug and diet history

Negative ⟵————————————⟶ Positive

|

Family history

Negative ⟵——|——⟶ Positive

↓

Other tests (see
Tables 11-20
and 11-22)

↓

Work-up family members
(see Hereditary platelet
function disorders,
Table 11-21)

↓

Repeat test after 10
days without drug

**Fig. 11-10.** Algorithm for prolonged BT.

Last trimester of pregnancy (rarely <75% of normal)
Newborns (~50% of adult level which are attained by age 6 months)
Others (e.g., acute leukemia, carcinoma, burns, postsurgical trauma, renal disease, gram-negative septicemia)

## Bleeding Time (BT)

See Fig. 11-10.
Normal = 4–7 mins. Longer in women than men.

### Use

BT is functional test of primary hemostasis.
BT is best single screening test for acquired or congenital functional or structural disorders of platelets. Normal BT without suggestive history usually excludes platelet dysfunction.
May be useful to monitor treatment of active hemorrhage in patients with prolonged BT due to uremia, von Willebrand's disease (vWD), congenital platelet function abnormalities, or severe anemia.
No value in performing BT if platelet count <100,000/cu mm. Prolonged BT with platelet count >100,000/cu mm usually indicates impaired platelet function (e.g., due to aspirin or vWD).

### Usually Prolonged in

Thrombocytopenia
• Platelet count <100,000/cu mm and usually <80,000/cu mm before BT becomes abnormal. May also have a qualitative platelet abnormality.

Platelet function disorders
Vascular disorders

## Clot Retraction

### Use

Reflects platelet number and function
Little value for detection of mild to moderate bleeding disorders

### May Occur in

Various thrombocytopenias
Thrombasthenia

## Coagulation (Clotting) Time (CT) ("Lee-White Clotting Time")

### Use

*It is not a reliable screening test for bleeding conditions because will only detect severe ones.*
*Normal CT does not rule out a coagulation defect.*
Bleeding and coagulation times are of little value for routine preoperative screening.

### Prolonged in

Severe deficiency (<6%) of any known plasma clotting factors except factors XIII and VII
Afibrinogenemia
Presence of a circulating anticoagulant (including heparin)

## Fibrinogen Degradation Products (FDP)
(detects major breakdown products of fibrin or fibrinogen; does not distinguish between fibrinolysis and fibrinogenolysis)

### Use

Aid in diagnosis of DIC

### Increased in Serum

DIC
In association with fibrinolytic therapy
Thromboembolic events

### Increased in Urine

Kidney disease
  • UTI—increased in infection of upper tract but not of bladder
  • Proliferative glomerulonephritis
  • Rejection of renal transplant
Conditions causing increased serum level

## Partial Thromboplastin Time (aPTT), Activated

See Figs. 11-11 through 11-13, and Tables 11-20 through 11-24.

### Use

Monitor heparin therapy.
Screen for hemophilia A and B.

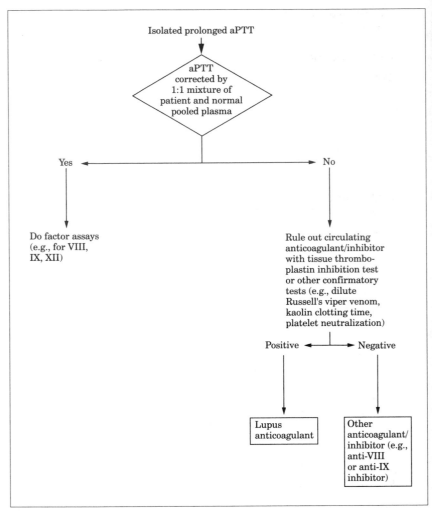

**Fig. 11-11.** Algorithm for isolated prolonged aPTT.

Detect clotting inhibitors.

aPTT is the *best single screening test* for disorders of coagulation; it is abnormal in 90% of patients with coagulation disorders. Screens for all coagulation factors that contribute to thrombin formation except VII and XIII.

May not detect mild clotting defects (25–40% of normal levels). Not recommended for preoperative screening of asymptomatic adult.

### Prolonged by

Defect in factors (assays <30% of normal; intrinsic pathway) I, II, V, VIII, IX, X, XI, XII

Presence of specific inhibitors of clotting factors

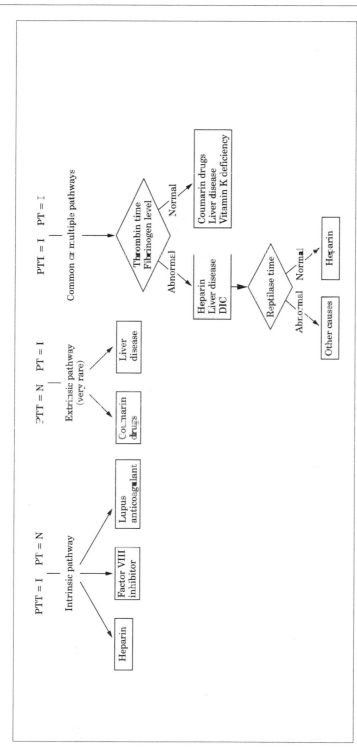

**Fig. 11-12.** Algorithm for acquired coagulation disorders. (PTT = partial thromboplastin time.)

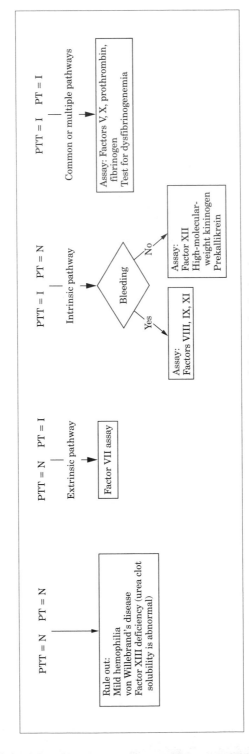

**Fig. 11-13.** Algorithm for hereditary coagulation disorders. (PTT = partial thromboplastin time.)

**Table 11-20.** Screening Tests for Presumptive Diagnosis of Common Bleeding Disorders[a]

| Platelet Count | BT | PT | aPTT[b] | Location of Defect | Most Frequent Causes | |
|---|---|---|---|---|---|---|
| | | | | | Acquired | Hereditary |
| N | N | I | N | Extrinsic pathway[c] | Liver disease, coumarin therapy, vitamin K deficiency, DIC (very rare) | Deficiency of factor VII (very rare) |
| N | N | N | I | Intrinsic pathway[d] | Heparin therapy, inhibitors | Hemophilia A or B, deficiency of XI, XII, prekallikrein, high-molecular-weight kininogen, Passavoy factor |
| N[e] | N | I | I | Common or multiple pathways | Heparin therapy, liver disease, vitamin K deficiency, DIC, fibrinogenolysis (very common) | Deficiency of V, X, prothrombin; dysfibrinogenemias (very rare) |
| D | I | N | N | Thrombocytopenia | ITP, secondary (e.g., drugs) | Aldrich's syndrome, etc. |
| N or I | I | N | N | Disorder of platelet function | Thrombocythemia, drugs, uremia, dysproteinemias | Thrombasthenia, deficient release reaction |
| N | I | N | I | von Willebrand's disease | | |
| N | N | N | N | Vascular abnormality | Allergic purpura, drugs, scurvy, etc | Deficiency of XIII, telangiectasia |

[a]Screening tests may be normal in mild von Willebrand's disease that has borderline or intermittent normal bleeding time, in mild hemophilia, and in factor XIII deficiency.

[b]Concentration of factors must be decreased to ≤30% of normal for these tests to be abnormal.

[c]Extrinsic pathway function depends on factors VII, X, V, II (prothrombin), I (fibrinogen); is assessed by PT.

[d]Intrinsic pathway depends on factors XII, XI, IX, VIII, X, V, II; is assessed by partial thromboplastin time.

[e]May be I in acquired disorders that produce abnormalities of platelets and multiple coagulation factors.

**Table 11-21.** Some Congenital Hemorrhagic Diseases Due to Disorders of Platelet-Vessel Wall

**Platelet defects**

| | |
|---|---|
| Bernard-Soulier syndrome | Moderate thrombocytopenia<br>BT markedly increased<br>Large platelets<br>Decreased ristocetin-induced agglutination not corrected by vWF |
| Glanzmann's thrombasthenia | Normal platelet count and morphology<br>Increased BT<br>Clot retraction absent or much decreased<br>No platelet aggregation with any agonists |
| Pseudo–von Willebrand's disease | Variable mild thrombocytopenia<br>Increased BT<br>Increased ristocetin-induced agglutination<br>Variable plasma immunoreactive vWF |
| Gray-platelet syndrome | Moderate thrombocytopenia<br>Large platelets<br>BT slightly increased<br>Platelets agranular on blood smear<br>Abnormal platelet aggregation with collagen or thrombin |
| Dense-granule deficiency syndrome | Normal platelet count<br>Normal platelet morphology on blood smear<br>BT variably increased<br>Abnormal aggregation with ADP and collagen |
| Deficiency of platelet enzyme (cyclooxygenase or thromboxane synthetase) | Normal platelet count and morphology<br>Abnormal aggregation with ADP, collagen, and arachidonic acid |
| May-Hegglin anomaly | Autosomal dominant trait<br>Moderate thrombocytopenia with huge platelets; normal platelet function<br>Döhle's bodies in granulocytes |

**Plasma defects**

| | |
|---|---|
| von Willebrand's disease | Normal platelet count and morphology<br>Increased BT<br>Abnormal ristocetin-induced agglutination<br>Abnormal plasma vWF |
| Afibrinogenemia | Normal platelet morphology<br>Mild thrombocytopenia occasionally<br>BT variably increased<br>Plasma coagulation abnormalities |

**Vessel wall defects**

| | |
|---|---|
| Genetic disorders of connective tissue | Platelets may be large<br>Collagen-induced aggregation may be abnormal |

ADP = adenosine diphosphate.

## Plasma Protein C

Normal range = 70–130%

### *Use*

Detect hypercoagulable states associated with episodes of venous thrombosis.

### Decreased in

Hereditary (autosomal dominant) deficiency (heterozygote levels are usually
    30–65%; found in screening in 1/300 persons; thrombosis is not usual if level
    >50%). *Establishes the diagnosis of purpura fulminans, which is seen in
    homozygous infants* (usually <1% of normal). *Warfarin-induced skin necrosis
    is almost pathognomonic for protein C deficiency.*
Liver disease
Malignancy
Acute respiratory distress syndrome
Pregnancy
High loading dose of warfarin causes transient rapid drop in protein C levels.
L-Asparaginase therapy

## Plasma Protein S

### Use

Detect hypercoagulable states associated with episodes of venous thrombosis.
Should be assayed whenever protein C is assayed. Heterozygotes with levels of
    30–60% may have episodes of recurrent thrombosis. Functional rather than
    immunologic tests are preferred.

### Decreased in

Pregnancy
First month of life
Oral anticoagulants or contraceptives
Acute phase reaction
Nephrotic syndrome
Liver disease
L-Asparaginase therapy
Some patients with deep venous thrombosis

## Plasminogen
(normal adults = 76–124% males; 65–153% females; infants = 27–59%)

### Use

Is one indicator of fibrinolytic activity
Monitor fibrinolytic therapy with streptokinase or urokinase

### May Be Decreased in

Some familial or isolated cases of idiopathic deep venous thrombosis
Diabetics with thrombosis
DIC and systemic fibrinolysis
Behçet's disease
Cirrhosis of the liver

## Platelet Count

See Tables 11-20 and 11-21 and Fig. 11-14.

### May Be Increased (>450,000/cu mm; <1,000,000/cu mm in 97% of patients) in

Myeloproliferative disease
Malignancy. *Approximately 50% of patients with "unexpected" increase of platelet
    count are found to have a malignancy.*
Patients recently having surgery
Infections

**Table 11-22.** Summary of Coagulation Studies in Hemorrhagic Conditions

| Condition | Screening Tests | | | | Accessory Tests | | | | |
|---|---|---|---|---|---|---|---|---|---|
| | Platelet Count | BT | PT | aPTT | Capillary Fragility (tourniquet test) | Coagulation Time | Clot Retraction | Prothrombin Consumption Time | Factor Assay |
| Thrombocytopenic purpura | D | I | N | N | + | N | Poor | I | |
| Nonthrombocytopenic purpura | N | N | N | N | V | N | N | N | |
| Glanzmann's thrombasthenia | N[a] | N or I | N | | + or N | N | Poor | I Corrected by platelet substitute | |
| von Willebrand's disease | N | I or N | N | N or I | N, + in severe | V | N | I | + |
| AHF (factor VIII) deficiency (hemophilia) | N | N | N | I | N | I N in mild | N | I | + |
| PTC (factor IX) deficiency (hemophilia B; Christmas disease) | N | N | N | I[c] | N | I N in mild | N | I | + |
| Factor X (Stuart) deficiency | N | N | I[b] | I[b] | N | N or slightly I | N | I | + |

| | | | | | | | | |
|---|---|---|---|---|---|---|---|---|
| PTA (factor XI) deficiency | N | N | N | I[c] | N | I | N | I | + |
| Factor XII (Hageman) deficiency | N | N / I in severe | N | I[c] | N | I | N | I | + |
| Factor XIII deficiency | N | N | N | N | N | N | N | N | + |
| Fibrinogen deficiency | N | N / I in severe | I | I | N | I | N | N |
| Hypoprothrombinemia | N | N or I | I | I | N | I | N | N |
| Excess dicumarol therapy | N | N | I | I | + in severe | I | N | N |
| Heparin therapy | N | N to I | May be I | I | N in mild | I | N | N |
| Vascular purpura (e.g., Schönlein-Henoch, hereditary hemorrhagic telangiectasia) | N | N | N | N | N | N | N | N |
| Increased antithromboplastin | N | | I | | | I | | I |
| Increased antithrombin | N | N | I | | N | May be I in severe / N or I | N | N[d] |
| Increased fibrinolysin | N | N or I | N | | N | N or I | Lysis of clot | N[d] |

+ = positive; PTC = plasma thromboplastin components; PTA = plasma thromboplastin antecedent; AHF = antihemophilic factor.

[a] Platelets appear abnormal.
[b] Corrected by serum.
[c] Corrected by serum or plasma.
[d] Not useful; may be difficult to do.

**Table 11-23.** DIC (Consumption Coagulopathy)

| Determination | % of Cases Abnormal | Abnormal Level for DIC | Mean Values for DIC | Response to Heparin Therapy | Tests |
|---|---|---|---|---|---|
| Decreased platelet count (per cu mm) | 93 | <150,000 | 52,000 | None or may take wks* | Platelet count, PT, fibrinogen level are performed first as screening tests; if all three are positive, diagnosis is considered established. If only two of these are positive, diagnosis should be confirmed by at least one of the tests for fibrinolysis. |
| Increased PT (secs) | 90 | >15 | 18.0 | Becomes normal or falls >5 secs in few hrs to 1 day | |
| Decreased fibrinogen level (mg/dL) | 71 | <160 | 137 | Rises significantly (>40 mg) in 1–3 days | |
| Latex test for fibrinogen degradation products (titer) | 92 | >1:16 | 1:52 | Begins to fall in 1 day; if very high, may take >1 wk to become normal | Tests for fibrinolysis |
| Prolonged thrombin time (secs) | 59 | >25 | 27 | | |
| Euglobulin clot lysis time (mins) | 42 | <120 | 27 | Returns to normal | |

*Platelet count is not a satisfactory indicator of response to heparin therapy.

**Table 11-24.** Differential Diagnosis of DIC

| | DIC | Chronic Liver Disease | Primary Fibrinolysis | TTP | Hemolytic-Uremic Syndrome | Multiple Transfusion |
|---|---|---|---|---|---|---|
| Platelet count | D | D | N | N–D | D | D |
| PT | I | I | I | N | N | I |
| aPTT | I | N–I | I | N | N | I |
| FDP | I | N–I | I | N–I | N–I | N |
| D-Dimer assay | I | N | I | N | N | N |
| Fibrinogen | D | V | D | N | N | I |
| Schistocytes | + | O | + | + | + | O |
| BUN | I | N | N | I | I | N |
| Liver function tests | N | I | N | N | N | N |
| Protamine sulfate | I | N–I | I | N–I | N | N |
| Euglobulin clot lysis | N | N | D | N | N | N |

+ = present; O = absent; FDP = fibrin degradation products; TTP = thrombotic thrombocytopenic purpura.

Chronic inflammation
Iron deficiency anemia
Miscellaneous disease states

***Decreased In***
*(thrombocytopenia)*

Acquired
- Decreased platelet production (e.g., aplastic anemia, myelophthisis)
- Increased platelet destruction
    Drug-induced immune thrombocytopenia *Antiplatelet antibodies* may be found in most patients. Negative results are strongly against an immune etiology of thrombocytopenia.
    ITP
    SLE
    Lymphoproliferative disorders
    Post-transfusion
    Extracorporeal circulation
- Increased platelet consumption
    TTP
    DIC
    Septicemia
    Toxemia of pregnancy
    Massive blood loss
- Hypersplenism (e.g., cirrhosis)
- Dilutional (e.g., after massive transfusion)
- Renal insufficiency
- Paroxysmal nocturnal hemoglobinuria
Inherited

# Prothrombin Consumption

See Table 11-22.

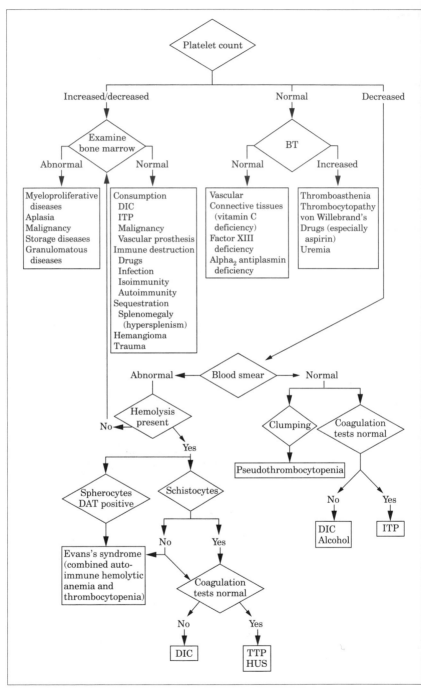

**Fig. 11-14.** Evaluation of hemostatic abnormalities. (PT and aPTT—see Figs. 11-11 and 11-12.) (DAT = direct antiglobulin test [Coombs']; HUS = hemolytic-uremic syndrome; TTP = thrombotic thrombocytopenic purpura.)

### Impaired by

Any defect in phase I or phase II of blood coagulation
- Thrombocytopathies
- Thrombocytopenia
- Hypoprothrombinemia
- Hemophilias
- Circulating anticoagulants

## Prothrombin Time

See Figs. 11-9 and 11-12 and Tables 11-22 through 11-24.

### Use

Primarily used for three purposes
- Control of long-term oral anticoagulant therapy
- Evaluation of coagulation disorders—screen for abnormality of extrinsic pathway factors
- Evaluation of liver function

### Prolonged by Defect in
### (assays <30% of normal)

Factors I, II, V, VII, X (extrinsic pathway)

### Prolonged in

Inadequate vitamin K in diet
Premature infants
Newborn infants of vitamin K–deficient mothers
Poor fat absorption
Severe liver damage
Drugs
Factitious ingestion of warfarin
Idiopathic familial hypoprothrombinemia
Circulating anticoagulants
Hypofibrinogenemia

## Thrombin Time

### Use

Detects abnormal fibrinogen

### Increased in

Fibrinogen level very low (<80 mg/dL) or high (>400 mg/dL)
Interference with polymerization of fibrin
Dysfibrinogenemia
Heparin contamination of specimen is common cause in hospital patients.

## Tourniquet Test

### Use

Differential diagnosis of purpura

### Positive in

Thrombocytopenic and nonthrombocytopenic purpuras
Thrombocytopathies
Scurvy

# Hemorrhagic Disorders

## Anticoagulants, Circulating
**(usually antibodies that inhibit function of specific coagulation factors, especially VIII or IX; occasionally V, XI, XIII, vWF)**

May be acquired (antibodies) due to multiple transfusion for congenital deficiency of a coagulation factor or spontaneous

Abnormal PT or aPTT is not corrected by equal mixtures of patient and normal plasma but is corrected if due to deficient coagulation factor.

Rosner index >15 indicates an inhibitor:

$$\frac{\text{(Clotting time of mixture of patient + normal plasma)} - \text{Normal plasma clotting time}}{\text{Normal plasma clotting time}}$$

Antiphospholipid-thrombosis syndrome comprised of two syndromes that usually occur separately with anticardiolipin antibodies or lupus anticoagulant on two occasions at least 12 wks apart, associated with arterial and venous thrombosis, recurrent fetal wastage, thrombocytopenia. Either antibody may also be associated with drugs, non-autoimmune diseases (e.g., syphilis, acute infection, malignancy, HIV infection), and elderly persons; majority are in otherwise healthy persons. See Fig. 11-15.
* Anticardiolipin antibodies present in 44% of SLE patients and ≤ 7.5% of normal persons.
* Lupus anticoagulant syndrome—heterogeneous group of antibodies directed against phospholipids rather than against a specific factor.

Arterial thrombosis is uncommon.

Criteria for diagnosis of lupus anticoagulant
* Abnormal dilute Russell's viper venom time (dRVVT) (is best test) and tissue thromboplastin inhibition test. Heparin or warfarin can prolong dRVVT and most other tests.
* Modified kaolin clotting time is increased; less sensitive than dRVVT.
* Increased aPTT (not reliable for screening); 1:1 mixture with normal plasma is >4 secs longer than control aPTT.
* Decrease in ≥ 2 factors (VIII, IX, XI, or XII) by one-stage assay but normal by two-stage assay.
* Low factor activity increases toward normal with further dilution of test plasma.
* Prolonged incubation with normal plasma does not increase inhibitor effect.
* Platelet neutralization procedure (addition of platelets will shorten the prolonged aPTT and dRVVT due to lupus anticoagulants but not due to Factor VIII inhibitors).
* Thrombocytopenia is often present.
* Slightly increased PT in 10%.

Clinical conditions associated with lupus anticoagulant
Autoimmune diseases (e.g., SLE, RA)
Drugs
Infections (e.g., bacterial, viral, *Pneumocystis carinii*)
Lymphoproliferative diseases (e.g., malignant lymphoma, hairy cell leukemia, Waldenström's macroglobulinemia)
Others (e.g., epithelial cancers)
Causes 6–8% of thrombosis in apparently healthy persons.

## Disseminated Intravascular Coagulation (DIC)

See Tables 11-23 and 11-24.
Clinical picture and laboratory findings are very variable.
*Criteria for specific diagnosis are not well defined. No single test is diagnostic and diagnosis usually depends on combination of findings. Single normal*

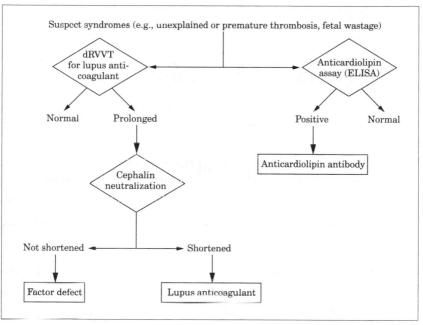

**Fig. 11-15.** Laboratory diagnosis of antiphospholipid syndromes. (dRVTT = dilute Russell's viper venom time.)

*value does not rule out DIC and a repeat test screen should be done a few hours later for changes in platelet count and fibrinogen.*
Repeated PT's (if initially prolonged) and fibrinogen levels are particularly useful. Normal or supernormal in 25% of acute DIC.
Most sensitive and specific tests
- Test for fibrin degradation products (FDP) in serum may be >100 μg/mL (normal = 0–10 μg/mL).
- Declining serial fibrinogen levels (normal = 200–400 μg/dL).
- D-Dimer assay is specific for fibrin and is a more reliable indicator of DIC than FDP assay.
- Antithrombin III is useful for diagnosis and to monitor therapy but immunologic assay should not be used.
- Fibrinopeptide A is increased.
- Protamine sulfate or ethanol gelation. A negative protamine is against ongoing DIC; ethanol test is less sensitive.
Less sensitive and specific tests
- PT (should be done serially if prolonged)
- aPTT (increased in 50–60% of acute DIC)
- Thrombin time
- Decreased platelet counts and abnormal platelet function tests (e.g., BT, platelet aggregation)
Least sensitive and specific tests
- Euglobulin clot lysis measures fibrinolytic activity in plasma.
- Peripheral blood smear examination.
In addition, the following abnormalities often occur:
- Evidence of microangiopathic hemolytic anemia may be present.
- Cryofibrinogen may be present.
- Observation of the blood clot may show abnormal clot.
Clotting time determinations are used to monitor heparin therapy.

*Suspect clinically in patients with underlying conditions who show bleeding (frequently acute and dramatic), purpura or petechiae, acrocyanosis, arterial or venous thrombosis*

## Factor IX (Plasma Thromboplastin Components [PTC]) Deficiency (Christmas Disease; Hemophilia B)
**(inherited recessive X-linked deficiency)**

In more severe cases, increased coagulation time, BT, prothrombin consumption time, and aPTT are found.
Defect is corrected by frozen plasma just as well as by bank blood.

## Hemophilia (Factor VIII [AHG] Deficiency)
**(X-linked recessive deficiency or abnormal synthesis of Factor VIII)**

Classic hemophilia (Factor VIII assay <1%) shows increased coagulation time, prothrombin consumption time, and aPTT; prolonged BT in ~20% of patients.
Moderate hemophilia (Factor VIII assay 1–5%) shows normal coagulation time and normal prothrombin consumption time but increased aPTT.
In mild hemophilia (Factor VIII assay <16%) and "sub-hemophilia" (Factor VIII assay 20–30%), these tests may be normal; seldom bleed except after surgery.
Screening tests for Factor VIII deficiency: normal PT and platelet count, prolonged aPTT, thrombin time, BT
Secondary tests: Factor VIII:C, Factor VIIIR:Ag, platelet aggregation, platelet agglutination, ristocetin cofactor
Specific factor assay is required to differentiate from Factor IX deficiency (hemophilia B).
"Acquired" hemophilia may occur when an inhibitor (autoantibody) is present. Antibodies develop in ~20% of patients receiving repeated transfusion of Factor VIII products.
Prenatal diagnosis during week 8–10 of pregnancy by DNA analysis of amniocytes or chorionic villus material or by analysis of fetal blood at 12–14 wks for VIII:C and VIII:Ag

## Hemorrhagic Disorders, Classification

See Figs. 11-12 and 11-13, and Tables 11-20 through 11-22.
Vascular abnormalities
 • Congenital (e.g., hereditary hemorrhagic telangiectasia)
 • Acquired (see Purpura, Nonthrombocytopenic)
   Infection (e.g., bacterial endocarditis, rickettsial infection)
   Immunologic (e.g., Schönlein-Henoch, allergic purpura, drug sensitivity)
   Metabolic (e.g., scurvy, uremia, diabetes mellitus)
   Miscellaneous (e.g., neoplasms, amyloidosis, angioma serpiginosum)
Connective tissue abnormalities
 • Congenital (e.g., Ehlers-Danlos syndrome)
 • Acquired (e.g., Cushing's syndrome)
Platelet abnormalities (thrombocytopenic purpura, thrombocythemia, thrombocytopathies)
 • Most useful tests are platelet count, peripheral smear examination, BT, platelet aggregation, platelet lumi-aggregation (release), platelet antibodies, other special platelet studies.
Plasma coagulation defects
 • Causing defective thromboplastin formation
   Factor VIII IX, XI deficiency
   vWD
 • Causing defective thrombin formation
   Vitamin K deficiency
   Congenital deficiency of Factor II, V, VII, X

- Decreased fibrinogen due to intravascular clotting and/or fibrinolysis
- Circulating anticoagulants
  Heparin therapy
  Dysproteinemias, SLE, postpartum state, some cases of hemophilia, etc.

## Hypercoagulable States

### Due to

Primary
- Protein C deficiency
- Protein S deficiency
- Antithrombin deficiency
- Plasminogen defects
- Dysfibrinogenemia
- Hypo- or dysplasminogenemia
- Homocystinuria
- SC anemia

Secondary
- Antiphospholipid antibody syndrome
- Pregnancy
- Oral contraceptives
- Neoplasia
- Surgery/trauma
- Sepsis
- Protein loss (e.g., nephrotic syndrome)
- Myeloproliferative disorders
- DIC
- Antineoplastic drugs

### Indications for Screening

Recurrent venous thrombosis or at unusual site (e.g., mesenteric, portal) or older
  than age 45 yrs
Familial thrombosis
Arterial thrombosis older than age 30 yrs
Unexplained neonatal thrombosis
Recurrent fetal loss

## Purpura, Allergic
### (called Henoch's purpura when abdominal symptoms are predominant and Schönlein's purpura when joint symptoms are predominant)

No pathognomonic laboratory findings
Platelet count, BT, coagulation time, and clot retraction and bone marrow are
  normal.
Renal biopsy shows minimal change pattern in mild cases and diffuse proliferative glomerulonephritis in severe cases with IgA deposition.

## Purpura, Thrombocytopenic

See Platelet Count, Decreased in.

## Purpura, Idiopathic Thrombocytopenic (Werlhof's Disease) (ITP)

Diagnosis by low platelet count, bone marrow normal or increased number and
  volume of megakaryocytes but without marginal platelets, and absence of
  other causes such as SLE or leukemia

Decreased platelet count (<100,000/cu mm)
Normal blood count and blood smear except for decreased number of platelets;
platelets may appear abnormal.
Positive tourniquet test
Increased BT
Poor clot retraction
Normal PT, aPTT, and coagulation time
Platelet antibodies are not important for diagnosis or treatment.

### Due to

Acute usually in children after viral infections
Chronic usually in adults is idiopathic or with immune disorders (e.g., SLE, lymphomas).
Neonatal in infants of mothers with ITP
Post-transfusion
Extracorporeal circulation (hemodialysis, cardiopulmonary bypass)

## Purpura, Nonthrombocytopenic

### Due to

Abnormal platelets (e.g., thrombocytopathies, thrombasthenia, thrombocythemia)
Abnormal serum globulins (e.g., multiple myeloma, macroglobulinemia)
Infections (e.g., meningococcemia, subacute bacterial endocarditis, typhoid)
Other diseases (e.g., amyloidosis, Cushing's syndrome, polycythemia vera, hemochromatosis, diabetes mellitus, uremia)
Drugs and chemicals (e.g., mercury, phenacetin, salicylic acid)
Allergic reaction (e.g., Schönlein-Henoch purpura, serum sickness)
Diseases of the skin (e.g., Osler-Weber-Rendu disease, Ehlers-Danlos syndrome)
vWD
Avitaminosis (e.g., scurvy)
Miscellaneous (e.g., mechanical, orthostatic)
Blood coagulation factors (e.g., hemophilia)

## Purpura, Thrombotic Thrombocytopenic (TTP)

Classic pentad: thrombocytopenia, microangiopathic hemolytic anemia, neurologic involvement, acute renal failure, fever
Diagnosis by excluding other known causes of these features
  • Diarrhea-associated form: related commonly to a verocytotoxin-producing strain of *Escherichia coli* O157:H7 and to *Shigella* with gastroenteritis and bloody diarrhea
  • Non–diarrhea-associated form is associated with
      Complications of pregnancy (e.g., eclampsia, abruptio placenta)
      Drugs (e.g., oral contraceptives, phenylbutazone, cyclosporin)
      Underlying systemic diseases (e.g., primary glomerulopathies, rejection of renal transplant, hypertension, adenocarcinoma)
      Inherited disorder
      Nonenteric pathogens
Severe thrombocytopenic purpura with normal or increased megakaryocytes in bone marrow. Platelet count usually <50,000/cu mm; usually becomes normal in a few weeks.
Microangiopathic hemolytic normochromic, normocytic anemia is present at onset or within a few days.
  • Hb usually <10 gm/dL; often <6 gm/dL.
  • Numerous fragmented and misshapen RBCs on blood smear are virtually required for this diagnosis.
  • Increased reticulocytes, nucleated RBCs, basophilic stippling and polychromatophilia.

- Increased serum Hb, indirect bilirubin, LD, and decreased haptoglobin.
- Negative Coombs' test.

Increased or normal WBCs and neutrophils.

In contrast to DIC, PT and aPTT are usually normal or may be mildly increased, clotting and fibrinogen are normal or only slightly increased; fibrin split products are usually present in low levels. Must also be differentiated from hemolytic-uremic syndrome.

Acute renal failure. BUN may rise 50 mg/dL/day; is often >100 mg/dL. Urine may show blood, protein, casts or anuria. Progressive renal disease or recovery. Oliguria and acute renal failure are uncommon.

## Thrombocytosis, Primary (Essential Thrombocythemia)
**(myeloproliferative disorder involving the thrombocytes)**

See Fig. 11-14.

### Diagnostic Criteria

Platelet count >600,000/cu mm on two occasions (>1,000,000/cu mm in 90% of cases)

No cause for reactive thrombocytosis

Platelets appear normal early in disease; later abnormal size, shape; changes in structure occur. Aggregation may be abnormal.

Mild anemia (10–13 gm/dL) in one-third of patients due to blood loss.

WBC usually >12,000/cu mm without cells earlier than myelocyte forms in ≤ 40% of patients; LAP is usually normal or may be increased.

Increased serum LD, uric acid

Artifactual increase in serum potassium, calcium, oxygen

Thrombohemorrhagic disease (bleeding—skin, GI tract, nose, gums in 35% of patients but normal BT) and thromboses of major vessels, usually arterial in ≤ 40% of patients

## Thrombocytosis, Reactive

See Platelet Count, Increased in

## Von Willebrand's Disease

See Table 11-25.

Most common inherited hemostatic abnormality. Hereditary deficiency (types I and III) or qualitative defect (type II) of a high-molecular-weight plasma protein (vWF) that mediates adherence of platelets to injured endothelium. Type I: decreased amount of vWF without qualitative abnormality; mild to moderate bleeding. Type III: vWF completely or almost completely absent from plasma and platelets; severe mucocutaneous and deep tissue bleeding. Type II: qualitative abnormalities of vWF due to loss of various multimers. vWF circulates complexed to (carrier for) factor VIII:C, which also responds as an acute phase protein. Acquired vWD due to formation of autoantibodies or other mechanisms (e.g., myeloproliferative, vascular and congenital heart diseases) or idiopathic.

Many patients do not have the classic laboratory findings; five clinical variants have been described.

BT is prolonged using a calibrated template; in a few patients, may only be prolonged after administration of 300 mg of aspirin.

aPTT is prolonged.

Platelet adhesiveness to glass beads is decreased. Ristocetin-induced aggregation of platelets is abnormal if ristocetin cofactor activity <30%; thus may be normal in mild vWD. May not identify some mild cases in which activity is >30% but less than normal of 50–150%.

**Table 11-25.** Types of von Willebrand's Disease (vWD)

| | Type of vWD | | | | | |
| --- | --- | --- | --- | --- | --- | --- |
| | I (classic) | IIA | IIB | IIC | III | Platelet Type |
| Frequency | 70% | 15–20% | | | 10% | |
| Platelet count | N | N | N or D | N | N | D or low N |
| BT | I or N | I | I | I | Marked I | I |
| Factor VIII:C | D or N | D or N | D or N | N | Marked D | D or N |
| vWF:Ag | D | D or N | D or N | D or N | O or tiny amounts | D or N |
| vWF:RCoF | D | D | D or N | D | O | D or N |
| RIPA | D or N | O or D | I | D | O | I |
| Plasma SDS multimers | All present; HMW may be D | Large and intermediate A | Large A | Large A; doublet structure | May be A | Large A |
| Platelet SDS multimers | All present; HMW may be D | Large and intermediate A | N | Large A; doublet structure | A | N |
| Response to desmopressin | Hemostasis becomes N | | Platelets D | Little benefit | No response | Platelets D; contraindicated |
| Genetics | AD | AD | AD | AR | AR, homozygous or doubly heterozygous | AD |

O = absent; A = abnormal; RCoF = ristocetin cofactor; RIPA = ristocetin-induced platelet aggregation; SDS = sodium dodecyl sulfate; HMW = high molecular weight; AD = autosomal dominant; AR = autosomal recessive.

Platelet count is usually normal but may be mildly decreased in type IIB or platelet-type vWD.

PT and clot retraction are normal.

Factor VIII coagulant activity (VIII:C) may range from normal to severely reduced.

Factor VIII-related antigen is decreased. May be increased in endothelial cell injury (e.g., trauma, surgery, surgical graft failure, clotting).

Transfusion of normal plasma (or of hemophiliac plasma, cryoprecipitate, serum) causes a rise in Factor VIII activity greater than the amount of Factor VIII infused, which does not peak until 8–10 hrs and slowly declines for days; in contrast, hemophilia shows rapid peak and fall after infusion of normal plasma or cryoprecipitate. This response to transfusion is a good diagnostic test in patients in whom diagnosis is equivocal.

Screening of family members may be useful in difficult diagnostic cases even if they are asymptomatic and have no history of unusual bleeding.

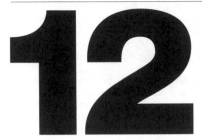

# Metabolic and Hereditary Disorders

## Acid-Base Disorders

See Fig. 12-1 and Tables 12-1 and 12-2.

### Acidosis, Metabolic

#### With Increased Anion Gap (AG) (>15 mEq/L)

Lactic acidosis—commonest cause of metabolic acidosis with increased AG (frequently >25 mEq/L)
Renal failure (AG <25 mEq/L)
Ketoacidosis
* Diabetes mellitus (AG frequently >25 mEq/L)
* Associated with alcohol abuse (AG frequently 20–25 mEq/L)
* Starvation (AG usually 5–10 mEq/L)
Drugs
* Salicylate poisoning (AG frequently 5–10 mEq/L; higher in children)
* Methanol poisoning (AG frequently >20 mEq/L)
* Ethylene glycol poisoning (AG frequently >20 mEq/L)
* Paraldehyde (AG frequently >20 mEq/L)

#### With Normal Anion Gap (Hyperchloremic Acidosis)

Decreased serum potassium
* Renal tubular acidosis
    Acquired (e.g., drugs, hypercalcemia)
    Inherited (e.g., cystinosis, Wilson's disease)
* Carbonic anhydrase inhibitors (e.g., acetazolamide, mafenide)
* Increased loss of alkaline body fluids (e.g., diarrhea, loss of pancreatic or biliary fluids)
* Ureteral diversion (e.g., ileal bladder or ureter, ureterosigmoidostomy)
Normal or increased serum potassium
* Hydronephrosis
* Early renal failure
* Administration of HCl (e.g., ammonium chloride)
* Hypoadrenalism (diffuse, zona glomerulosa, or hyporeninemia)
* Renal aldosterone resistance
* Sulfur toxicity
*In lactic acidosis, the increase in AG is usually > decrease in $HCO_3^-$, in contrast to diabetic ketoacidosis in which the increase in AG = decrease in $HCO_3^-$.*

#### Laboratory Findings

Serum pH is decreased (<7.3).
Total plasma $CO_2$ content is decreased; <15 mEq/L almost certainly rules out respiratory alkalosis.

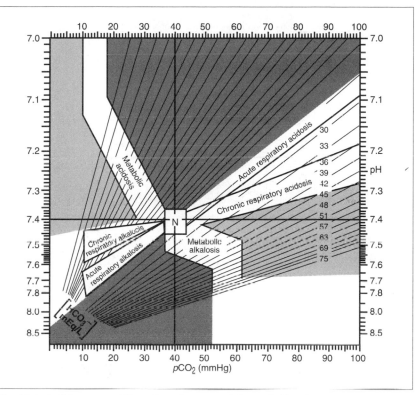

**Fig. 12-1.** Acid-base map. The values demarcated for each disorder represent a 95% probability range for each *pure* disorder. Coordinates lying outside these zones suggest mixed acid-base disorders.

Serum potassium is frequently increased; it is decreased in renal tubular acidosis, diarrhea, or carbonic anhydrase inhibition.

Azotemia suggests metabolic acidosis due to renal failure.

Urine is strongly acid (pH = 4.5-5.2) if renal function is normal.

In evaluating acid-base disorders, calculate the anion gap.

## Anion Gap Classification
(calculated as $Na - [Cl + HCO_3^-]$; normal = 8–16 mEq/L [if K is included, normal = 10–20 mEq/L])

### *Increased in*

Increased "unmeasured" anions
- Organic (e.g., lactic acidosis, ketoacidosis)
- Inorganic (e.g., administration of phosphate, sulfate)
- Protein (e.g., hyperalbuminemia, transient)
- Exogenous (e.g., salicylate, formate, nitrate, penicillin, carbenicillin)
- Not completely identified (e.g., hyperosmolar hyperglycemic nonketotic coma, uremia, poisoning by ethylene glycol, methanol, salicylates)
- Artifactual
  Falsely increased serum sodium

**Table 12-1.** Illustrative Serum Values in Acid-Base Disturbances

| Condition | Sodium (mEq/L) | Chloride (mEq/L) | HCO$_3$$^-$ (mEq/L) | $p$CO$_2$ (mm Hg) | pH |
|---|---|---|---|---|---|
| Normal | 140 | 105 | 25 | 40 | 7.40 |
| Metabolic acidosis | 140 | 115 | 15 | 31 | 7.30 |
| Chronic respiratory alkalosis | 136 | 102 | 25 | 40 | 7.44 |
| Mixed metabolic acidosis and chronic respiratory alkalosis (e.g., sepsis: addition of respiratory alkalosis to metabolic acidosis further decreases HCO$_3$$^-$ but pH may remain normal; lactic acidosis plus respiratory alkalosis due to severe liver disease, pulmonary emboli, or sepsis) | 136 | 108 | 14 | 24 | 7.39 |
| Metabolic alkalosis | 140 | 92 | 36 | 48 | 7.49 |
| Chronic respiratory acidosis | 140 | 100–102 | 28–30 | 50–55 | 7.37 |
| Mixed metabolic alkalosis and chronic respiratory acidosis (e.g., patient with COPD receiving glucocorticoids or diuretics; $p$CO$_2$ and HCO$_3$$^-$ are increased by both conditions, but pH is neutralized) | 140 | 90 | 40 | 67 | 7.40 |

| Condition | | | | | |
|---|---|---|---|---|---|
| Metabolic alkalosis | 129 | 89 | 35 | 47 | 7.49 |
| Respiratory alkalosis | 136 | 102 | 20 | 30 | 7.44 |
| Mixed alkalosis, mild | 139 | 92 | 32 | 39 | 7.53 |
| Mixed alkalosis, severe (e.g., postoperative patient with severe hemorrhage stimulating hyperventilation [respiratory alkalosis] plus massive transfusion and nasogastric drainage [metabolic alkalosis]) | 139 | 92 | 32 | 30 | 7.63 |
| Mixed chronic respiratory acidosis and acute metabolic acidosis (e.g., COPD [chronic respiratory acidosis] with severe diarrhea [metabolic acidosis]. pH is too low for $pCO_2$ of 55 mm Hg in chronic respiratory acidosis, indicating low pH due to mixed acidosis, but $HCO_3^-$ effect is offset.) | 133 | 102 | 22 | 55 | 7.22 |
| Mixed metabolic acidosis and metabolic alkalosis (e.g., gastroenteritis with vomiting [metabolic alkalosis] and diarrhea [metabolic acidosis due to loss of $HCO_3^-$]; surprisingly normal findings with marked volume depletion) | 140 | 103 | 25 | 40 | 7.40 |

**Table 12-2.** Illustrative Serum Electrolyte Values in Various Conditions

| Condition | pH | HCO$_3^-$ | Potassium | Sodium | Chloride |
|---|---|---|---|---|---|
| Normal | 7.35–7.45 | 24–26 | 3.5–5.0 | 136–145 | 100–106 |
| Metabolic acidosis | | | | | |
| Diabetic acidosis | 7.2 | 10 | 5.6 | 122 | 80 |
| Fasting | 7.2 | 16 | 5.2 | 142 | 100 |
| Severe diarrhea | 7.2 | 12 | 3.2 | 128 | 96 |
| Hyperchloremic acidosis | 7.2 | 12 | 5.2 | 142 | 116 |
| Addison's disease | 7.2 | 22 | 6.5 | 111 | 72 |
| Nephritis | 7.2 | 8 | 4.0 | 129 | 90 |
| Nephrosis | 7.2 | 20 | 5.5 | 138 | 113 |
| Metabolic alkalosis | | | | | |
| Vomiting | 7.6 | 38 | 3.2 | 150 | 94 |
| Pyloric obstruction | 7.6 | 58 | 3.2 | 132 | 42 |
| Duodenal obstruction | 7.6 | 42 | 3.2 | 138 | 49 |
| Respiratory acidosis | 7.1 | 30 | 5.5 | 142 | 80 |
| Respiratory alkalosis | 7.6 | 14 | 5.5 | 136 | 112 |

Falsely decreased serum chloride or bicarbonate
• Decreased unmeasured cations (e.g., hypokalemia, hypocalcemia, hypomagnesemia)
*When AG >12–14 mEq/L, diabetic ketoacidosis is the most common cause, uremic acidosis is the second most common cause, and drug ingestion (e.g., salicylates, methyl alcohol, ethylene glycol, ethyl alcohol) is the third most common cause; lactic acidosis should always be considered when these three causes are ruled out.*

### Decreased in

Decreased unmeasured anions (e.g., hypoalbuminemia is probably the most common cause of decreased AG)
Artifactual
• "Hyperchloremia" in bromide intoxication (if chloride determination by colorimetric method)
• Hyponatremia due to viscous serum
• False decrease in serum sodium; false increase in serum chloride or HCO$_3^-$
Increased "unmeasured" cations
• Hyperkalemia, hypercalcemia, hypermagnesemia
• Increased proteins in multiple myeloma, paraproteinemias, polyclonal gammopathies (abnormal proteins are positively charged and lower the AG)

• Increased lithium, tris(hydroxymethyl)-aminomethane buffer

*AG >30 mEq/L almost always indicates organic acidosis even in presence of uremia.*

*AG = 20–29 mEq/L occurs in absence of identified organic acidosis in 25% of patients.*

AG is rarely >23 mEq/L in chronic renal failure.

*AG may provide a clue to the presence of a mixed rather than simple acid-base disturbance.*

## Acidosis, Lactic

Should be considered in any metabolic acidosis with increased AG (>15 mEq/L).

Diagnosis is confirmed by exclusion of other causes of metabolic acidosis and serum lactate ≥ 5 mEq/L (upper limit of normal = 1.6 for plasma and 1.4 for whole blood).

Exclusion of other causes by

• Normal serum creatinine and BUN *(Increased acetoacetic acid [but not beta-hydroxybutyric acid] will cause false increase of creatinine by colorimetric assay.)*
• Osmolar gap <10 mOsm/L
• Negative nitroprusside reaction *(Nitroprusside test for ketoacidosis measures acetoacetic acid but not beta-hydroxybutyric acid; thus blood ketone test may be negative in diabetic ketoacidosis.)*
• Urine negative for calcium oxalate crystals
• No known ingestion of toxic substances

Associated or compensatory metabolic or respiratory disturbances (e.g., hyperventilation or respiratory alkalosis may result in normal pH)

### Due to

Type A due to clinically apparent tissue hypoxia (e.g., acute hemorrhage, severe anemia, shock, asphyxia; marathon running, seizures)

Type B without clinically apparent tissue hypoxia

• Common disorders (e.g., diabetes mellitus, uremia, liver disease, infections, malignancies, alkaloses)
• Drugs and toxins (e.g., ethanol, methanol, ethylene glycol, salicylates)
• Hereditary enzyme defects (e.g., methylmalonic aciduria, propionicaciduria, defects of fatty acid oxidation, pyruvate-carboxylase deficiency, multiple carboxylase deficiency, glycogen storage disease [GSD] Type I).

With a typical clinical picture (acute onset after nausea and vomiting, altered state of consciousness, hyperventilation, high mortality), the following laboratory findings occur:

• Decreased serum bicarbonate.
• Low serum pH, usually 6.98–7.25.
• Increased serum potassium, often 6–7 mEq/L.
• Serum chloride normal or low with increased AG.
• WBC is increased (occasionally to leukemoid levels).
• Increased serum uric acid is frequent (up to 25 mg/dL in lactic acidosis).
• Increased serum phosphorus. Phosphorus:creatinine ratio >3 indicates lactic acidosis either alone or as a component of other metabolic acidosis.
• Increased AST and LD in serum.

## Acidosis, Respiratory

Laboratory findings differ in acute and chronic conditions.

### Acute

Due to decreased alveolar ventilation impairing $CO_2$ excretion

• Cardiopulmonary (e.g., pneumonia, pneumothorax, pulmonary edema, foreign body aspiration, bronchospasm, mechanical ventilation, cardiac arrest)

- CNS depression (e.g., general anesthesia, drugs, brain injury, infection)
- Neuromuscular (e.g., Guillain-Barré syndrome, hypokalemia, myasthenic crisis)

Acidosis is severe (pH 7.05–7.10), but $HCO_3^-$ concentration is only 29–30 mEq/L.
Severe mixed acidosis is common in cardiac arrest when respiratory and circulatory failure cause marked respiratory acidosis and severe lactic acidosis.

### Chronic

Due to chronic obstructive or restrictive conditions
- Nerve disease (e.g., poliomyelitis)
- Muscle disease (e.g., myopathy)
- Central neurologic disorder (e.g., brain tumor)
- Restriction of thorax (e.g., musculoskeletal, scleroderma)
- Pulmonary disease (e.g., prolonged pneumonia, alveolar hypoventilation)

Acidosis is not usually severe.
Beware of commonly occurring mixed acid-base disturbances (e.g., chronic respiratory acidosis with superimposed acute hypercapnia resulting from acute infection, such as pneumonia).
Superimposed metabolic alkalosis (e.g., due to diuretics or vomiting) may exacerbate the hypercapnia.

## Alkalosis, Metabolic

### Due to

Loss of acid
- Vomiting, gastric suction, gastrocolic fistula
- Diarrhea in mucoviscidosis (rarely)
- Villous adenoma of colon
- Aciduria secondary to potassium depletion

Excess of base due to administration of
- Absorbable antacids (e.g., sodium bicarbonate; milk-alkali syndrome)
- Salts of weak acids (e.g., sodium lactate, sodium or potassium citrate)
- Some vegetarian diets

Potassium depletion (causing sodium and $H^+$ to enter the cells)
- GI loss (e.g., chronic diarrhea)
- Lack of potassium intake (e.g., anorexia nervosa, IV fluids without potassium supplements for treatment of vomiting or postoperatively)
- Diuresis (e.g., mercurials, thiazides, osmotic diuresis)
- Extracellular volume depletion and chloride depletion
- All forms of mineralocorticoid excess (e.g., primary aldosteronism, Cushing's syndrome, administration of steroids)
- Glycogen deposition
- Chronic alkalosis
- Potassium-losing nephropathy

Hypoproteinemia per se may cause a nonrespiratory alkalosis. Decreased albumin of 1 gm/dL causes an average increase in standard bicarbonate of 3.4 mmol/L, an apparent base excess of +3.7 mEq/L and a decrease in AG of ~3 mEq/L.

### Laboratory Findings

Serum pH is increased.
Total plasma $CO_2$ is increased (bicarbonate >30 mEq/L).
$pCO_2$ is normal or slightly increased.
Serum pH and bicarbonate above those predicted by the $pCO_2$ (by nomogram)
Serum potassium is usually decreased; this condition is the chief danger in metabolic alkalosis.
Decreased serum chloride is relatively lower than sodium.
BUN may be increased.

Urine pH is >7.0 (≤ 7.9) if potassium depletion is not severe and concomitant sodium deficiency (e.g., vomiting) is not present.

When the urine chloride is low (<10 mEq/L) and the patient responds to chloride treatment, the cause is more likely loss of gastric juice, diuretic therapy, or rapid relief of chronic hypercapnia. Chloride replacement is completed when urine chloride remains >40 mEq/L. When the urine chloride is high (>20 mEq/L) and the patient does not respond to NaCl treatment, the cause is more likely hyperadrenalism or severe potassium deficiency.

## Alkalosis, Respiratory
(decreased $pCO_2$ of <38 mm Hg)

### Due to

Hyperventilation
- CNS disorders (e.g., infection, tumor, trauma, cerebrovascular accident)
- Salicylate intoxication
- Fever
- Gram-negative bacteremia
- Liver disease
- Pulmonary disease (e.g., pneumonia, pulmonary emboli, asthma)
- Mechanical overventilation
- Congestive heart failure
- Hypoxia (e.g., decreased barometric pressure, ventilation-perfusion imbalance)

### Laboratory Findings

Acute hypocapnia—usually only a modest decrease in plasma $HCO_3^-$ concentrations and marked alkalosis

Chronic hypocapnia—usually only a slight alkaline pH

## Mixed Acid-Base Disturbances
(must always be interpreted with clinical data and other laboratory findings)

### Respiratory Acidosis with Metabolic Acidosis

Examples: Acute pulmonary edema, cardiopulmonary arrest (lactic acidosis due to tissue anoxia and $CO_2$ retention due to alveolar hypoventilation)

Acidemia may be extreme with
- pH <7.0 ($H^+$ >100 mEq/L)
- $HCO_3^-$ <26 mEq/L. Failure of $HCO_3^-$ to increase ≥ 3 mEq/L for each 10-mm Hg rise in $p(a)CO_2$ suggests metabolic acidosis with respiratory acidosis.

*Mild metabolic acidosis superimposed on chronic hypercapnia causing partial suppression of $HCO_3^-$ may be indistinguishable from adaptation to hypercapnia alone.*

### Metabolic Acidosis with Respiratory Alkalosis

Examples: Rapid correction of severe metabolic acidosis, salicylate intoxication, gram-negative septicemia, initial respiratory alkalosis with subsequent development of metabolic acidosis. *Primary metabolic acidosis with primary respiratory alkalosis with an increased AG is characteristic of salicylate intoxication in absence of uremia and diabetic ketoacidosis.*

pH may be normal or decreased. Hypocapnia remains inappropriate to decreased $HCO_3^-$ for several hours or more.

### Respiratory Acidosis with Metabolic Alkalosis

Examples: Chronic pulmonary disease with $CO_2$ retention developing metabolic alkalosis due to administration of diuretics, severe vomiting, or sudden improvement in ventilation ("posthypercapnic" metabolic alkalosis)

Decreased or absent urine chloride indicates that chloride-responsive metabolic alkalosis is a part of the picture.

### Respiratory Alkalosis with Metabolic Alkalosis

Examples: Hepatic insufficiency with hyperventilation plus administration of diuretics or severe vomiting; metabolic alkalosis with stimulation of ventilation (e.g., sepsis, pulmonary embolism, mechanical ventilation) that causes respiratory alkalosis
Marked alkalemia with decreased $pCO_2$ and increased $HCO_3^-$ is diagnostic.

### Acute and Chronic Respiratory Acidosis

Example: Chronic hypercapnia with acute deterioration of pulmonary function causing further rise of $pCO_2$
May be suspected when $HCO_3^-$ in intermediate range between acute and chronic respiratory acidosis (similar findings in chronic respiratory acidosis with superimposed metabolic acidosis or acute respiratory acidosis with superimposed metabolic alkalosis)

### Coexistence of Metabolic Acidoses of Hyperchloremic Type and Increased AG Type

Examples: Uremia and proximal renal tubular acidosis, lactic acidosis with diarrhea, excessive administration of NaCl to patient with organic acidosis
May be suspected by plasma $HCO_3^-$ that is lower than is explained by the increase in anions (e.g., AG = 16 mEq/L and $HCO_3^- = 5$ mEq/L)

### Coexistence of Metabolic Alkalosis and Metabolic Acidosis

Examples: Vomiting causing alkalosis plus bicarbonate-losing diarrhea causing acidosis
May be suspected by acid-base values that are too normal for clinical picture

## Inherited Metabolic Conditions, Classification

*(deficient enzyme is shown in parentheses; PD = prenatal diagnosis is possible)*

Disorders of carbohydrate metabolism
    Diabetes mellitus
    Pentosuria
    Fructose
        Fructosuria (aldolase B)
        Fructose 1,6-bisphosphatase deficiency
    Lactose
        Familial lactose intolerance
    Galactose
        Galactosemia (galactose-1-phosphate-uridyltransferase)    PD
        Galactokinase deficiency    PD
    Glycogen storage diseases    PD for some
Disorders of amino acid metabolism
    Phenylalanine
        Phenylketonuria (phenylalanine hydroxylase)    PD
    Methionine
        Homocystinuria (cystathionine synthase)    PD
    Tyrosine
        Tyrosinemia II (tyrosine aminotransferase)
    Valine, leucine, isoleucine
        Maple syrup urine disease (branched-chain ketoacid
            dehydrogenase)    PD
    Glycine
        Nonketotic hyperglycinemia (glycine cleavage system)    PD
    Lysine
        Hyperlysinemia (aminoadipic semialdehyde synthase)

Proline
    Hyperprolinemia I (proline oxidase)
    Hyperprolinemia II (pyrroline-5-carboxylate dehydrogenase)
    Hyperimidodipeptiduria (prolidase)
Urea cycle disorders
    Citrullinemia (argininosuccinic acid synthetase)          PD
    Argininemia (arginase)                                     PD
    Argininosuccinic aciduria (argininosuccinate lyase)        PD
    Ornithine carbamoyltransferase deficiency                  PD
    N-acetylglutamate synthetase deficiency
    Carbamoyl phosphate synthetase deficiency
Organic acidurias
    Propionate and methylmalonate metabolism
        Propionicacidemia (propionyl–coenzyme A (CoA)
            carboxylase)                                       PD
        Methylmalonic acidemia (methylmalonyl-CoA mutase,
            adenosylcobalamin synthesis)                       PD
        Multiple carboxylase deficiency (holocarboxylase
            synthetase, biotinidase)
    Pyruvate and lactate metabolism
        Lactate dehydrogenase deficiency
        Pyruvate dehydrogenase deficiency
        Pyruvate carboxylase deficiency                        PD
        Phosphoenolpyruvate carboxykinase deficiency
    Branched chain organic acidemias
        Isovaleric acidemia (isovaleryl-CoA dehydrogenase)     PD
        Mevalonicaciduria (mevalonate)                         PD
    Other organic acid disorders
        Alkaptonuria (homogentisic acid oxidase)
        Hyperoxaluria Type I, glycolic aciduria (alanine-glyoxylate
            aminotransferase)
        Hyperoxaluria Type II, glyceric aciduria (glyceric
            dehydrogenase)
        Glycerol kinase deficiency
Lysosomal enzyme defects
    Mucopolysaccharidoses                                      PD
    Mucolipidosis II and III (UDP-N-acetylglucosamine-lysosomal
        enzyme, N-acetylglucosamine-L-phosphotransferase)      PD
    Glycoproteinoses
        Alpha- and beta-mannosidosis (alpha- and beta-
            mannosidase)                                       PD
        Sialidosis type I, II (neuraminidase)                  PD
        Fucosidosis (alpha-fucosidase)                         PD
    $GM_2$ gangliosidoses
        Tay-Sachs disease (hexosaminidase alpha-subunit)       PD
        Sandhoff's disease (hexosaminidase beta-subunit)       PD
        $GM_2$ activator deficiency
    Other lysosomal storage disorders
        Metachromatic leukodystrophy (arylsulfatase A)         PD
        Multiple sulfatase deficiency (multiple lysosomal
            sulfatases)                                        PD
        Niemann-Pick disease (sphingomyelinase)                PD
        Farber's disease (ceramidase)                          PD
        Gaucher's disease (glucocerebrosidase)                 PD
        Pompe's disease (GSD II) (alpha-1,4-glucosidase
            deficiency)
        Krabbe's disease (galactocerebrosidase)                PD
        Fabry's disease (alpha-galactosidase)                  PD
        $GM_1$ gangliosidosis (beta-galactosidase)             PD
        Wolman's disease (acid lipase)                         PD

| | |
|---|---|
| Cholesteryl ester storage disease (acid lipase) | PD |
| Mucolipidosis Type IV | |
| Peroxisomal disorders | |
|   Acatalasia (catalase) | |
|   Refsum's disease (phytanic acid alpha-hydroxylase) | PD |
|   Zellweger syndrome (peroxisome biogenesis) | PD |
| Purine and pyrimidine metabolism disorders | |
|   Lesch-Nyhan syndrome (hypoxanthine phosphoribosyl-transferase) | PD |
|   Xanthinuria (xanthine oxidase) | |
| Disorders of metal metabolism | |
|   Wilson's disease | |
|   Hemochromatosis | |
|   Menkes' disease | PD |
| Disorders of lipid metabolism | |
|   Abetalipoproteinemia | |
|   Familial hypercholesterolemia (hyperlipidemia IIA) | PD |
|   Dysbetalipoproteinemia (hyperlipidemia type III) | |
|   Lipoprotein lipase deficiency | |
| Disorders of heme proteins | |
|   Porphyrias | PD for some |
|   Bilirubin metabolism | |
|     Crigler-Najjar syndromes I, II (UDP-glucuronyltransferase) | |
|     Gilbert syndrome (UDP-glucuronyltransferase) | |
|     Dubin-Johnson syndrome | |
|     Rotor's syndrome | |
| Membrane transport disorders | |
|   Cystinuria | |
|   Hartnup disease | |
|   Cystinosis | PD |
| Disorders of serum enzymes | |
|   Hypophosphatasia (alkaline phosphatase) | PD |
|   Hyperphosphatasia | |
|   Alpha$_1$-antitrypsin deficiency | |
| Disorders of plasma proteins | |
|   Analbuminemia | |
|   Agammaglobulinemia | |
| Disorders of blood | |
|   Coagulation diseases (e.g., hemophilias) | PD |
|   RBC G6PD deficiency | PD |
|   Hemoglobinopathies and thalassemias | PD |
|   Hereditary spherocytosis | PD |
|   Hereditary nonspherocytic hemolytic anemia | PD |
| Others | |
|   Congenital adrenal hyperplasia | |

# Tests of Lipid Metabolism

Blood lipid tests should not be performed during stress or acute illness (e.g., recent myocardial infarction, use of certain drugs); *should not be performed on hospitalized patients or until 2–3 months after illness.*

Abnormal lipid test results should always be confirmed with a new specimen before beginning or changing therapy.

## Cholesterol, Total, Serum

### Use

Monitoring for increased risk factor for coronary artery disease (CAD)

Screening for primary and secondary hyperlipidemias
Monitoring treatment of hyperlipidemias

## Interferences

Intra-individual variation may be ~4–10% for serum total cholesterol.
Repeat cholesterol values should be within 30 mg/dL.
Cholesterol values are up to 8% higher in winter than summer, 5% lower if bled
   when sitting compared to when standing and 10–15% different when recumbent compared to when standing.
*Note effect of illness, intra-individual variation, drugs, etc., when these values are
   used to diagnose and treat hyperlipidemias.*

## Increased in

Idiopathic hypercholesterolemia
Hyperlipoproteinemias
Biliary obstruction
 • Stone, carcinoma of duct
 • Cholangiolitic cirrhosis
 • Biliary cirrhosis
 • Cholestasis
von Gierke's disease
Hypothyroidism
Nephrosis (due to chronic nephritis, renal vein thrombosis, amyloidosis, SLE,
   periarteritis, diabetic glomerulosclerosis)
Pancreatic disease
 • Diabetes mellitus
 • Total pancreatectomy
 • Chronic pancreatitis
Pregnancy
Certain drugs (e.g., progestins, anabolic steroids, corticosteroids)
Total fasting that induces ketosis leads to a rapid increase.
*Secondary causes should always be ruled out.*

## Decreased in

Severe liver cell damage (e.g., due to chemicals, drugs, hepatitis)
Hyperthyroidism
Malnutrition (e.g., starvation, neoplasms, uremia, malabsorption)
Myeloproliferative diseases
Chronic anemia
 • Pernicious anemia in relapse
 • Hemolytic anemias
 • Marked hypochromic anemia
Hypobeta- and abetalipoproteinemia
Infection
Inflammation
Certain drugs (e.g., cortisone and ACTH therapy)

# Cholesterol High-Density Lipoprotein (HDL), Serum

Intra-individual variation may be ≤ 12.4%.

## Use

Assessment of risk for CAD
Diagnosis of various lipoproteinemias

## Increased in
*(>60 mg/dL is negative risk factor for CAD)*

Vigorous exercise

Increased clearance of triglyceride (VLDL)
Moderate consumption of alcohol
Insulin treatment
Oral estrogens
Familial lipid disorders with protection against atherosclerosis (illustrates impor-
tance of measuring HDL to evaluate hypercholesterolemia)
- Hyperalphalipoproteinemia (HDL excess)
  1 in 20 adults with mild increased total cholesterol (240–300 mg/dL) sec-
  ondary to increased HDL (>70 mg/dL)
  LDL not increased
  Triglycerides are normal
  Inherited as simple autosomal dominant trait in families with longevity
  or may be caused by alcoholism, exogenous estrogens, etc.
- Hypobetalipoproteinemia

### Decreased in
*(<32 mg/dL in men, <38 mg/dL in women)*

*Is inversely related to risk of CAD. For every 1 mg/dL decrease in HDL, risk for
CAD increases by 2–3%.*
Secondary causes
- Stress and recent illness (e.g., AMI, surgery)
- Starvation
- Obesity
- Lack of exercise
- Cigarette smoking
- Diabetes mellitus
- Hypo- and hyperthyroidism
- Acute and chronic liver disease
- Nephrosis
- Uremia
- Various chronic anemias and myeloproliferative disorders
- Certain drugs (e.g., anabolic steroids, progestins, antihypertensive beta
  blockers, thiazides, neomycin, phenothiazines)
Genetic disorders
- Familial hypertriglyceridemia.
- Familial hypoalphalipoproteinemia—common autosomal dominant condi-
  tion with premature CAD and stroke. One-third of patients with premature
  CAD may have this disorder.
  HDL <10th percentile (<30 mg/dL in men and <38 mg/dL in women of
  middle age).
- Non-neuropathic Niemann-Pick disease.
- HDL deficiency with planar xanthomas.

## Cholesterol, Low-Density Lipoprotein (LDL), Serum

### Use

Assess risk and decide about treatment of CAD.

### Increased in
*(is directly related to risk of CAD)*

Familial hypercholesterolemia
Familial combined hyperlipidemia
Diabetes mellitus
Hypothyroidism
Nephrotic syndrome
Chronic renal failure
Diet high in cholesterol and total and saturated fat
Pregnancy
Multiple myeloma, dysgammaglobulinemia

Porphyria
Pregnancy
Anorexia nervosa
Certain drugs (e.g., anabolic steroids, antihypertensive beta blockers, progestins, carbamazepine)

### Decreased in

Severe illness
Abetalipoproteinemia
Oral estrogens
Can estimate LDL using the following formula:

$$LDL = total\ cholesterol - (HDL\ cholesterol - VLDL)$$

$$VLDL = triglycerides/5$$

Formula underestimates LDL (e.g., chronic alcoholism), is unsuitable for monitoring, misclassifies 15–40% of patients when triglycerides = 200–400 mg/dL, and fails if fasting triglycerides >400 mg/dL.
Some laboratories also report various total cholesterol:HDL ratios:

| | |
|---|---|
| Low risk | 3.3–4.4 |
| Average risk | 4.4–7.1 |
| Moderate risk | 7.1–11.0 |
| High risk | >11.0 |

## Cholesterol Decision Levels

| | Cholesterol (in mg/dL) | | | |
|---|---|---|---|---|
| | LDL | HDL | Total | LDL:HDL Ratio |
| Desirable level/low risk | <130 | >60 | <200 | 0.5–3.0 |
| Borderline level/moderate risk | 130–159 | 35–60 | 200–239 | 3.0–6.0 |
| Elevated level/high risk | ≥ 160 | <35 | ≥ 240 | >6.0 |

Definite CAD: Definite myocardial infarction or definite angina pectoris
Other CAD risk factors:
• HDL cholesterol <35 mg/dL (not part of initial screen)
• Diabetes mellitus
• Family history of premature CAD
• Hypertension
• Cigarette smoking
• Male gender
• Extreme obesity (>30% above ideal body weight)
• History of stroke or peripheral vascular disease

## Lipoproteins, Serum

### Decreased in

Hypobetalipoproteinemia

### Increased in

Hyperbetalipoproteinemia
Hyperalphalipoproteinemia

## Apolipoproteins, Serum
(protein component of lipoproteins and regulate their metabolism)

### Use

Assess risk of coronary heart disease
Classify hyperlipidemias

Apo A-I:B ratio showed greater sensitivity and specificity for CAD than LDL:HDL cholesterol ratio or HDL cholesterol:triglyceride ratio or any of the individual components.

## Lipoprotein Electrophoresis

### Use

Identify rare familial disorders (e.g., types I, III, V hyperlipidemias) to anticipate problems in children. Shows a specific abnormal pattern in <2% of Americans (usually type II, IV).
May be indicated if
- Serum triglycerides >300 mg/dL.
- Fasting serum is lipemic.
- Significant hyperglycemia, impaired glucose tolerance, or glycosuria.
- Increased serum uric acid.
- Strong family history of premature congestive heart disease (CHD).
- Clinical evidence of CHD or atherosclerosis in patient < age 40.

If lipoprotein electrophoresis is abnormal, tests should be performed to rule out secondary hyperlipidemias.

## Triglycerides, Serum
**(80% in VLDL, 15% in LDL)**

### Interferences

Serum for triglycerides and for calculating LDL should follow a 12-hr fast.
Diurnal variation causes triglycerides to be lowest in the morning and highest around noon. Intra-individual variation in serum triglycerides is 12–40%; analytical variation is 5–10%.

### Increased in

Genetic hyperlipidemias (e.g., lipoprotein lipase deficiency, apo C-II deficiency, familial hypertriglyceridemia, dysbetalipoproteinemia)
Liver diseases
Nephrotic syndrome
Chronic renal failure
Hypothyroidism
Diabetes mellitus (higher values correlate with hyperglycemia and poorer control of diabetes; reduced by insulin therapy)
Alcoholism
Gout
Pancreatitis
von Gierke's disease
AMI (rise to peak in 3 wks; increase may persist for 1 yr)
Acute illness (e.g., cold, flu)
Certain drugs (e.g., oral contraceptives, high-dose estrogens, beta blockers, hydrochlorothiazide, anabolic steroids, corticosteroids). See Chapter 18.
Pregnancy
Certain concentrations are associated with certain disorders
- <250 mg/dL: Not associated with any disease state.
- 250–500 mg/dL: Associated with peripheral vascular disease; may be a marker for patients with genetic forms of hyperlipoproteinemias who need specific therapy.
- >500 mg/dL: Associated with high risk of pancreatitis.
- >1000 mg/dL: Associated with hyperlipidemia, especially type I or type V substantial risk of pancreatitis.
- >5000 mg/dL: Associated with eruptive xanthoma, corneal arcus, lipemia retinalis, enlarged liver and spleen.

### Decreased in

Abetalipoproteinemia
Malnutrition
Dietary change (within 3 wks)
Recent weight loss
Certain drugs (e.g., alpha$_1$ receptor blockers)
*Total and HDL cholesterol levels are similar in fasting and nonfasting but triglycerides should be measured after 12–14 hrs fasting. Serum levels are about 5% higher than plasma levels.*
*Triglyceride levels are not a strong predictor of atherosclerosis or CAD and are not an independent risk factor. Triglyceride levels are inversely related to HDL cholesterol levels.*

# Disorders of Lipid Metabolism

See Figs. 12-2 and 12-3.

## Hyperlipidemias, Primary

See Table 12-3.

## Hyperlipidemias, Secondary

Occur in
- Poorly controlled diabetes mellitus
- Hypothyroidism
- Nephrotic syndrome
- Other renal disorders (chronic uremia, hemodialysis)
- Hepatic glycogenoses
- Obstructive liver disease
- Chronic alcoholism
- Hyperlipoproteinemia of "affluence" (dietary)

# Disorders of Amino Acid Metabolism

## Maple Syrup Urine Disease (Ketoaciduria)
**(due to autosomal recessive deficiency of branched-chain keto acid-decarboxylase; characteristic maple syrup or curry odor in urine, sweat, hair, and cerumen)**

Chromatography of urine and plasma shows greatly increased urinary excretion of ketoacids of leucine, isoleucine, and valine. Presence of alloisoleucine (stereoisomeric metabolite of isoleucine) is characteristic.
Metabolic acidosis and ketoacidosis occur.
Ferric chloride test of urine produces green-gray color.
Hypoglycemia is usual.
Measurement of amount of defective enzyme in leukocytes and fibroblasts shows classic (enzyme level 0–2% of normal), intermittent (enzyme level 2–8% of normal), and intermediate (enzyme level 8–16% of normal) forms. Blood levels are normal in intermittent forms except during acute episodes caused by infection, surgery, vaccination, or sudden increased intake of protein during which the disease resembles classic form. Intermediate form shows persistent elevation of blood amino acids, which can be kept in normal range by diet protein <2g/kg/day.
Prenatal diagnosis by measuring enzyme concentration in amniocytes

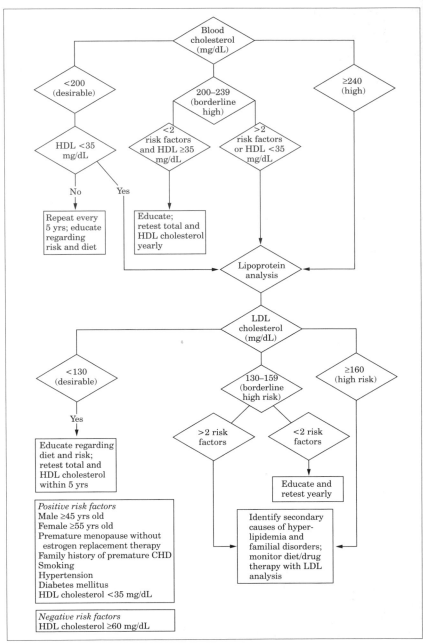

**Fig. 12-2.** Algorithm of recommended testing and treatment of increased serum total and HDL cholesterol in adults without evidence of coronary heart disease. Measure serum total cholesterol, HDL cholesterol, and triglycerides after 12- to 14-hr fast. Average of two to three tests; if difference 30 mg/dL repeat 1–8 wks apart and average three tests. Use total cholesterol for initial case finding and classification and to monitor diet therapy. Do not use age- or gender-specific cholesterol values as decision levels. Always rule out secondary and familial causes. (CHD = congestive heart disease.)

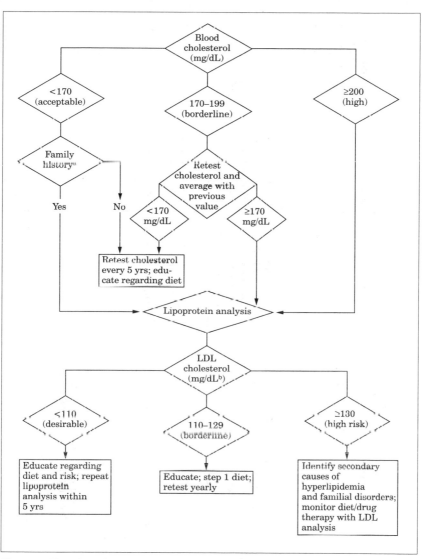

**Fig. 12-3.** Algorithm of recommended testing and treatment of increased serum cholesterol in children and adolescents. [a]Cardiovascular disease before age 55 yrs in a parent or grandparent, or parental total cholesterol ≥ 240 mg/dL. [b]Measure serum total cholesterol, HDL cholesterol, and triglycerides after 12- to 14-hr fast. Average of two to three tests.

## Phenylketonuria (PKU)
**(inherited autosomal recessive [due to various mutations on chromosome 12]; absence of phenylalanine hydroxylase activity in liver causes increased phenylalanine and its metabolites [phenylpyruvic acid, orthohydroxyphenylacetic acid] in blood, urine, and CSF; tyrosine and the derivative catecholamines are deficient)**

See Fig. 12-4.

**Table 12-3.** Comparison of Classic Types of Hyperlipoproteinemia

| Point of Comparison | Type I (rarest) | Type IIa (relatively common) | Type IIb (relatively common) | Type III (relatively uncommon) | Type IV (most common) | Type V (uncommon) |
|---|---|---|---|---|---|---|
| Origin | Exogenous hyperlipidemia due to deficient lipoprotein lipase | | Overindulgence lipidemia | | Endogenous hyperlipidemia | Mixed endogenous and exogenous hyperlipidemia (combined types I and IV) |
| Definition | Familial fat-induced hyperglyceridemia | Hyperbetalipoproteinemia (hypercholesterolemia) | Combined hyperlipidemia (mixed hyperlipidemia) | Carbohydrate-induced hyperglyceridemia with hypercholesterolemia | Carbohydrate-induced hyperglyceridemia without hypercholesterolemia | Combined fat and carbohydrate-induced hyperglyceridemia |
| Age | Usually younger than age 10 years | | | Not known younger than age 25 years | Only occasionally seen in children | |
| Gross appearance of plasma | On standing: supernatant creamy, infranatant clear | Clear (no cream layer on top) | No cream layer on top; clear to turbid infranatant | Clear, cloudy, or milky | Slightly turbid to cloudy On standing: unchanged | Markedly turbid On standing: supernatant creamy, infranatant milky |
| Serum cholesterol | N or slightly I | Markedly I (300–600 mg/dL) | Markedly I (300–600 mg/dL) | Markedly I (300–1000 mg/dL) | N or slightly I | I (250–500 mg/dL) |
| LDL cholesterol | N | I | I | I | N | N |
| HDL cholesterol | N to D | N to D | N to D | N to D | N to D | N to D |

| Apolipoprotein | I (B-48) I (A-IV) V (CII) | I (B-100) | I (B-100) | I (E-II) D (E-III) D (E-IV) | V (CII) I (B-100) | V (CII) I (B-48) I (B-100) |
|---|---|---|---|---|---|---|
| Increased lipoprotein | Chylomicrons | LDL | LDL, VLDL | IDL | VLDL | VLDL, chylomicrons |
| Serum triglycerides | Markedly I (usually >2000 mg/dL) | N | I ≤ 400 mg/dL | Markedly I (200–1000 mg/dL) | Markedly I (500–1500 mg/dL) | Markedly I (500–1500 mg/dL) |
| Appearance of lipoprotein components visualized by electrophoresis | | | | | | |
| Chylomicron[a] | Marked I | 0 | 0 | 0 | 0 | I |
| Beta-lipoprotein[b] | N or D | I | I | I, floating beta | N or I | N or I |
| Prebeta-lipoprotein[c] | N or D | N | I | I | I | I |
| Alpha-lipoprotein[d] | | | | | | |
| Other laboratory abnormalities | Glucose tolerance usually N | | | Hyperglycemia; glucose tolerance often abnormal; serum uric acid I | Glucose tolerance often abnormal; serum uric acid often I | Glucose tolerance usually abnormal; serum uric acid usually I |
| Triglyceride:cholesterol ratio | 8 | 1 | Variable | <2 | 1–5 | >5 |

**Table 12-3.** (*continued*)

| Point of Comparison | Type I (rarest) | Type IIa (relatively common) | Type IIb (relatively common) | Type III (relatively uncommon) | Type IV (most common) | Type V (uncommon) |
|---|---|---|---|---|---|---|
| Lipid changes resembling primary hyperlipidemias | | | | | | |
| Diet | | Very high cholesterol diet | Same as type IIa | | Caffeine or alcohol before testing | |
| Drugs | | Triglyceride-lowering drugs in types III and IV | Same as type IIa | Triglyceride-lowering drugs in type IV | Cholesterol-lowering drugs, chlorothiazide, birth control pills or estrogens | |
| Primary disease | | Myxedema, nephrosis, obstructive liver disease, stress, porphyria, anorexia nervosa, idiopathic hypercalcemia | Same as type IIa | Myxedema, dysgammaglobulinemia, liver disease | Nephrotic syndrome, hypothyroidism, pregnancy, glycogen storage disease | Myeloma, macroglobulinemia, nephrosis |

0 = absent.

| | [a]Chylomicrons | [b]LDL (beta-lipoprotein) | [c]VLDL (prebeta-lipoprotein) | [d]HDL (alpha-lipoprotein) |
|---|---|---|---|---|
| Triglycerides | 90% | 5% | 60% | 5% |
| Cholesterol | 5% | 50% | 15% | 20% |
| Phospholipids | 4% | 25% | 15% | 25% |
| Protein | 1% | 20% | 10% | 50% (Apo A-1, II) |

Because apo B is the only protein in LDL and apo A-I is the major protein constituent of HDL and VLDL, the ratio apo-B:apo A-I reflects the ratio LDL:HDL and may be a better discriminator of coronary artery disease than the individual components, but data on apolipoproteins are still limited.

Obtain blood only after at least 12- to 14-hr fast and when patient has been on usual diet for at least 2 wks.

Rule out diabetes and pancreatitis in all groups.

Increased susceptibility to coronary artery disease occurs in types II, III, and IV; accelerated peripheral vascular disease in type III.

Xanthomas appear in types I, II, III.

Abdominal pain occurs in types I, V.

If dietary or drug treatment has begun, it may not be possible to classify the lipoproteinemia or the classification may be erroneous.

Type IIb is overindulgence hyperlipidemia; shows increased cholesterol and triglycerides, with increased beta and prebeta; can only be distinguished from type III by detecting abnormal beta-migrating lipoprotein in serum fraction with density >1.006.

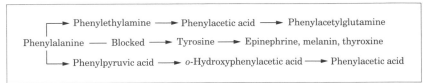

**Fig. 12-4.** Pathways of phenylalanine metabolism.

Unrestricted protein diet
- Normal blood phenylalanine level = 2 mg/dL.
- Classic PKU: Patients have high blood phenylalanine levels (usually >30 mg/dL and always >20 mg/dL in infancy) with phenylalanine and its metabolites in urine; normal or decreased tyrosine concentration.
- Less severe variant form of PKU: Blood phenylalanine levels are 15–30 mg/dL and metabolites may appear in urine.
- Mild persistent hyperphenylalaninemia: Blood phenylalanine levels may be 2–12 mg/dL and metabolites are not found in urine. Diet restriction is not required for this form.

For screening of newborns, urine amounts of phenylpyruvic acid may be insufficient for detection by colorimetric methods when blood level is <15 mg/dL. May not appear in urine until 2–3 wks of age.

Preliminary blood screening tests detect levels >4 mg/dL. Screening should be performed after protein-containing feedings have begun.

When repeat screening test is positive, quantitative blood phenylalanine and tyrosine are performed to confirm phenylalaninemia and exclude transient tyrosinemia of newborn, which is most common cause of positive screening. Diagnosis requires serum phenylalanine ≥ 20 mg/dL. Urine $FeCl_3$ is positive and chromatography confirms o-hydroxyphenylacetic acid.

Serial determinations should be performed on untreated borderline cases because blood levels may change markedly with time or due to stress.

Diagnosis of PKU may be confirmed by giving 100 mg of ascorbic acid and collecting blood and urine 24 hrs later.

### In PKU

Serum phenylalanine is >15 mg/dL.
Serum tyrosine is <5 mg/dL (is never increased in PKU).
Urine phenylalanine is >100 $\mu$g/mL.
o-Hydroxyphenylacetic acid is present in urine.
Phenylpyruvic acid in urine is significant (gives positive $FeCl_3$ test), but may not be present in some patients.

### Abnormalities of Tyrosine Metabolism
### (e.g., incomplete development of tyrosine oxidizing system, especially in premature or low-birth-weight infants)

Serum phenylalanine is >4 mg/dL (5–20 mg/dL).
Serum tyrosine is between 10 mg/dL and 75 mg/dL.
Tyrosine metabolites in urine are ≤ 1 mg/mL (parahydroxyphenyllactic and parahydroxyphenylacetic acids can be distinguished from o-hydroxyphenylacetic acid by paper chromatography).
o-Hydroxyphenylacetic acid is absent from urine.
Without administration of ascorbic acid, 25% of premature infants may have increased serum phenylalanine and tyrosine for several weeks (but reversed in 24 hrs after ascorbic acid administration) and increased urine tyrosine and tyrosine derivatives.
Similar blood and urine findings not reversed by administration of ascorbic acid may occur in untreated galactosemia, tyrosinemia, congenital cirrhosis, and giant-cell hepatitis; jaundice occurs frequently.

Serum serotonin (5-hydroxytryptophan) is decreased.

Urine 5-hydroxyindoleacetic acid excretion is decreased.

Blood levels of phenylalanine deficiency should be monitored frequently during treatment.

Adjust diet by monitoring blood phenylalanine.

In women with untreated PKU and increased serum phenylalanine, there is greatly increased frequency of mental retardation, microcephaly, and congenital heart disease in offspring.

Detection of heterozygotes of 75% of families and prenatal diagnosis are now possible using DNA probe.

# Porphyrias

See Figs. 12-4 through 12-6 and Table 12-4.

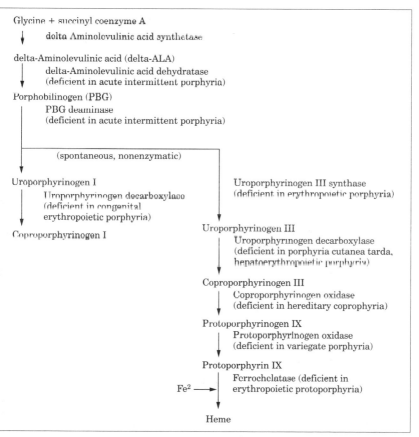

**Fig. 12-5.** Heme biosynthesis pathway showing site of enzyme action and disease caused by enzyme deficiency. Accumulation of porphyrins and their precursors preceding the enzyme block are responsible for the clinical and laboratory findings in each syndrome. PBG and ALA cause abdominal pain and neuropsychiatric symptoms. Increase porphyrins (with or without increased PBG or ALA) cause photosensitivity. Thus, deficiencies near end of metabolic path cause more photosensitivity and fewer neuropsychiatric findings.

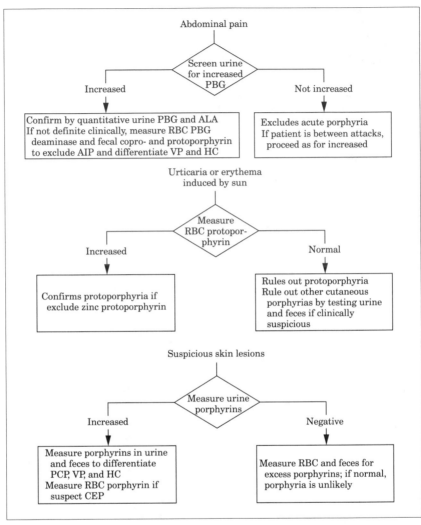

**Fig. 12-6.** Diagnostic strategy (algorithm) for suspected porphyria according to symptoms. Excess production of porphyrins is associated with cutaneous photosensitivity. Excess production of only porphyrin precursors is associated with neurologic symptoms. Excess production of both is associated with both types of clinical symptoms. (PBG = porphobilinogen; PCT = porphyria cutanea tarda; VP = variegate porphyria; HC = hereditary coproporphyria; CEP = congenital erythropoietic porphyria.)

# Other Genetic Diseases

## Down Syndrome (Trisomy 21; Mongolism)

Karyotyping shows 47 chromosomes with trisomy 21 in most patients; due to translocation, usually to chromosome 14; due to other D group chromosome in <5% of cases. 2% have mosaicism with one cell population trisomic.

Increased LAP staining reaction

Leukocytes show decreased incidence of drumsticks and mean lobe counts.

Serum acid phosphatase may be decreased.

Incidence of leukemia is increased (~1%).

Increased susceptibility to infection (e.g., hepatitis is common)

Laboratory findings due to associated congenital abnormalities

### Prenatal Screening and Diagnosis

Decreased maternal serum AFP
* <0.5 multiple of median (MoM) in 5% of unaffected pregnancies and ~20% of Down syndrome.
* In midtrimester, usual range is 10–150 ng/mL; is usually reported as MoM (normal 0.4–2.5 MoM), which must be adjusted for obesity (≤ 2 times greater), race (10–15% higher in blacks), insulin-dependent diabetes mellitus (>1.5 MoM), twin pregnancy (>4.5 MoM), or gestational age. Increase >2.5 MoM for gestational age may occur in fetal neural tube defects (e.g., 80% of open spina bifida or 90% of anencephaly cases; <5% of closed spina bifida cases). May also be increased in omphalocele, gastroschisis, cystic hygroma, congenital nephrosis, interference with fetal swallowing, GI tract obstruction, dead fetus, fetal hemorrhage, fetal teratomas, placental defects (e.g., cystic changes, tumor, placental lakes), or large placenta. *Increased blood level of AFP in pregnancy is a valuable screening test, but diagnosis should be confirmed by finding increased levels in amniotic fluid and sonography; serum should be drawn after week 15 of gestation.* If both are elevated, contamination of amniotic fluid with fetal or maternal blood is ruled out by assay for fetal Hb and acetylcholinesterase. If only maternal serum AFP is elevated without demonstrable defect, pregnancy is at increased risk (e.g., premature delivery, low-birth-weight baby, or fetal death).

### Decreased Maternal Serum AFP in

Down syndrome (trisomy 21) and trisomy 18; useful for screening

Long-standing death of fetus

Overestimation of gestational age

Choriocarcinoma, hydatidiform mole

Maternal diabetes mellitus

Increased maternal weight

Pseudopregnancy, nonpregnancy

Asian women

Various drugs (therefore no medications for at least 12 hrs before test)

Other unknown factors

Increased maternal serum human chorionic gonadotropin (hCG) ≥ 2.5 times MoM at 18–25 wks' gestation will detect ~56% of cases.

Decreased maternal serum unconjugated estriol level (reflects fetal adrenal, liver, and placental function) detects 45% of cases with a 5.2% false-positive rate. ≤ 0.6 MoM in 5% of unaffected pregnancies and 26% of Down syndrome

Optimum screening combines maternal age >35 yrs with hCG, AFP, and unconjugated estriol levels in maternal serum; detects 60% of cases; ultrasound to confirm gestational age reduces false positive to 3.8%.

Chromosomal analysis of amniotic fluid detects ~20% of cases because 80% of Down syndrome babies are born to women <35 yrs old.

## Tay-Sachs Disease (GM₂ Gangliosidosis)
**(autosomal recessive trait [chromosome 15])**

See Table 12-5.

Diagnosis is established by absence of hexosaminidase A activity in serum (also absent in all tissues of body and tears). Electron microscopy shows characteristic cytoplasmic bodies in brain. (In Sandhoff's disease [a variant of Tay-Sachs

**Table 12-4.** Comparison of Porphyrias

| Type | Enzyme Defect | Inheritance | Age at Onset | Frequency | Urine |
|---|---|---|---|---|---|
| Congenital erythropoietic porphyria | Uroporphyrinogen III cosynthase | AR | Infancy | Very rare | **Uro I**; Watson-Schwartz negative[a]; Copro |
| Erythropoietic protoporphyria[1] | Ferrochelatase | AD | Childhood | Common | Negative |
| Porphyria cutanea tarda[2] | Uroporphyrinogen decarboxylase | AD | Middle age | Commonest type in United States and Europe | **Uro > Copro constant**; PBG not increased; ALA may be slightly increased |
| Acute intermittent porphyria | Porphobilinogen deaminase | AD | Adolescence | Uncommon | **ALA[b] and PBG constant; Watson-Schwartz positive** |
| Variegate porphyria[3] | Protoporphyrinogen oxidase | AD | Young adult | | ALA and PBG during attack[a] |
| Hereditary coproporphyria[4] | Coproporphyrinogen oxidase | AD | Young adult | Rarest | Copro; ALA and PBG during attack[a] |
| Hepatoerythropoietic porphyria[5] | Heme synthetase; uroporphyrinogen decarboxylase deficiency more severe than in porphyria cutanea tarda | AR | Early infancy | Rarest | Resembles findings in porphyria cutanea tarda |
| ALA dehydrase deficiency[6] | delta-ALA dehydrase | AR | | Very rare | **ALA; Copro** |

AR = autosomal recessive; AD = autosomal dominant; PBG = porphobilinogen; Uro = uroporphyrin; Proto = protoporphyrin; Iso = isocoproporphyrin; Copro = coproporphyrin; + through ++++ = present in increasing amounts; − = not present.
[a]Present during acute attack; may be absent during remission.
[b]ALA may be increased even more in chronic lead poisoning.
[1]Erythropoietic protoporphyria: Three chemical patterns consist of increased free RBC and stool protoporphyrin alone or with each other.
[2]Porphyria cutanea tarda (PCT): Most common porphyrin disorder. Inherited form (expressed in ~20% of patients with this gene) due to deficiency of uroporphyrinogen decarboxylase in liver in toxic/sporadic

| Feces | RBCs | Comment | Chief Site of Porphyrin Overproduction | Skin Lesions | Neuropsychiatric Symptoms | Liver Disease |
|---|---|---|---|---|---|---|
| **Copro** | **Uro**; fluorescent under UV light | Hemolytic anemia; red teeth; pink/red urine stain on diapers | Bone marrow | ++++ | – | – |
| **Proto** | **Proto** | Gallstones | Bone marrow; liver variable | ++ | – | ↑ |
| Iso > Copro | Negative | Siderosis; precipitated by iron overload, alcoholism | Liver | + | – | + |
| Negative | Negative | Abdominal pain; SIADH with low sodium and osmolarity | Liver | – | + | – |
| **Proto con stant** | Negative | Abdominal pain | Liver | ‖ ‖ | + | – |
| **Copro con stant** | Negative | Abdominal pain | Liver | + | + | – |
| | **Increased Zn-proto** | | Bone marrow, liver | ++++ | – | + |
| Negative | Negative | Acute porphyria symptoms | Liver | – | + | – |

forms and in all tissues in familial form. Associated with alcoholic liver disease and hepatic siderosis. Acquired form (inhibitor of uroporphyrinogen decarboxylase may be generated in liver) may be due to hepatoma, cirrhosis, chemicals. May be activated by increased ingestion of iron, alcohol, estrogens.

[3]Variegate porphyria (VP): Precipitated by same factors as in AIP.

[4]Hereditary coproporphyria (HC): Two-thirds of patients are latent. Precipitated by same factors as in AIP.

[5]Hepatoerythropoietic porphyria: Decarboxylase 5–10% of normal; 50% of normal in parents.

[6]ALA dehydrase deficiency: With 98% deficiency of enzyme; 50% of normal activity in parents.

Boldface type indicates body material used for diagnosis.

**Table 12-5.** Classification of Lipidoses and Gangliosidoses

| Clinical Name | Enzyme Defect Specimen for Assay | Major Lipid Accumulation | Signs/Symptoms |
|---|---|---|---|
| Gaucher's disease | Beta-glucosidase in L, F | Glucosylceramide | Enlarged spleen and liver; erosion of long bones and pelvis; mental retardation only in infantile form |
| Niemann-Pick disease | Sphingomyelinase in F | Sphingomyelin | Enlarged liver and spleen; mental retardation; ~30% have cherry-red spot in retina |
| Krabbe's disease (globoid cell leukodystrophy) | Galactosylceramidase in F, L, A | Galactosylsphingosine | X-linked; mental retardation; almost total absence of myelin; globoid bodies in brain white matter; increased CSF protein |
| Metachromatic leukodystrophy | Arylsulfatase A in L, U, F | Lactosylsulfatide | Mental retardation; psychologic disturbances in adult form |
| Multiple sulfatase deficiencies | Arylsulfatase A, B, C in F, L | | Resembles metachromatic leukodystrophy; dermatan sulfate and heparan sulfate increased in urine |
| Ceramide lactoside lipidosis | Beta-galactosidase in L, S | Ceramide lactoside | Slowly progressive brain damage; enlarged liver and spleen |

| | | | |
|---|---|---|---|
| Fabry's disease (angiokeratoma corporis diffusum universale) | Alpha-galactosidase in S, L, F | Trihexosylceramide | Skin lesions; loss of renal function; involvement of heart and brain vessels; pain in lower limbs; cherry-red spot in retina |
| $GM_2$ gangliosidosis | Beta-galactosidase | | |
| Tay-Sachs disease | Hexosaminidase A in S, L, A, F | Ganglioside $GM_2$ | Mental retardation; cherry-red spot in retina; blindness; muscle weakness |
| Sandhoff's disease | Hexosaminidase A, B in S, L, A, F | Ganglioside $GM_2$ and globoside | Clinical picture same as in Tay-Sachs disease but mild peripheral neuropathy and organomegaly |
| Landing's disease ($GM_1$ gangliosidosis) | Acid-beta-galactosidase in L, F | Ganglioside $GM_1$ | Psychomotor deterioration; cherry-red spot in retina; enlarged liver and spleen; dysostosis multiplex |
| Farber's lipogranulomatosis | Ceramidase in L, F | | Granulomas of dermis and viscera; joint disease in infancy |

Note: Molecular techniques are now available for diagnosis of Gaucher's, Niemann-Pick, Tay-Sachs, Sandhoff's, Fabry's, and Wolman's diseases and for generalized gangliosidosis.

L = leukocytes; F = fibroblasts; A = amniocytes; U = urine; S = serum.

disease] both hexosaminidase A and B are defective and globoside is accumulated in other tissues as well as brain.)

Heterozygotes can be identified by plasma assay showing 50% decrease in activity of hexosaminidase A; screening should be performed before pregnancy, which may cause false-positive results; oral contraceptives, diabetes mellitus, liver disease may also cause false-positive results; in these cases WBC is used for hexosaminidase A assay.

Prenatal diagnosis using cultured amniotic cells

PCR for specific DNA mutations in WBCs or fibroblasts is more specific than enzyme assay, can detect various mutations, can predict severity of disease in affected child.

There is early marked increase of serum LD and AST that return to normal if patient survives 3–4 yrs.

Decreased serum fructose-1-phosphate aldolase; also decreased in *heterozygotes* CSF AST parallels serum AST.

Liver function tests are normal.

Serum acid phosphatase is normal.

# Glycogen Storage Diseases (GSD)

See Table 12-6.

# Lysosomal Storage Disorders

| Disorder | Deficient Enzyme | Major System, Organ, or Tissue Involved |
|---|---|---|
| Glycoprotein degradation | | |
| Fucosidosis | Alpha-fucosidase | CNS, high sweat electrolytes |
| Mannosidosis | Alpha-mannosidase | CNS, mild bone changes, hepatosplenomegaly |

**Table 12-6.** Classification of Glycogen Storage Diseases*

| Type | Frequency (%) | Clinical Name | Deficient Enzyme |
|---|---|---|---|
| I | 20 | von Gierke's disease | Liver glucose-6-phosphatase |
| II | 20 | Pompe's disease | Lysosomal alpha-1,4-glucosidase |
| III | 30 | Forbes' disease | Amylo-1,6-glucosidase (debranched enzyme) |
| IV | <1 | Andersen's disease | Amylo-$(1,4\rightarrow1,6)$-transglucosidase (branched enzyme) |
| V | 5 | McArdle syndrome | Muscle phosphorylase |
| VI | {25% for | Hers' disease | Liver phosphorylase |
| VII | {VI + VII | Tarui's disease | Muscle phosphofructokinase |
| VIII | Very rare | Hug, Huijing | Phosphorylase kinase |
| X | | | Muscle phosphoglycerate kinase |
| XI | | | Muscle phosphoglycerate mutase |
| XII | | | Muscle lactate dehydrogenase |

*All are autosomal recessive except type VIII, which is X-linked recessive.

| Sialidosis (mucolipidosis I) | Alpha-N-acetyl neuraminidase | CNS, bone, liver, spleen |
| Glycogen storage disease | Alpha-glucosidase | Muscle, heart |
| Aspartylglycosaminuria | Aspartylglucosa-minidase | CNS, bone marrow, connective tissue |

Prominent inclusions in leukocytes
Enzyme localization

| Mucolipidosis II (I-cell disease; formerly MPS VII) | N-Acetylglucosaminyl-phosphortransferase | CNS, bone, connective tissue |
| Mucolipidosis III (Pseudo-Hurler tissue poly-dystrophy) | N-Acetylglucosamine-1-transferase | Predominantly joint and connective tissue |

Lysosomal efflux

| Cystinosis | ? | Kidney |
| Salla disease | ? | CNS |

Mucopolysaccharidoses (see Table 12-7)
Sphingolipidoses
Lipidoses (see Table 12-5)

| Chédiak-Higashi syndrome | | WBC |

# Genetic Mucopolysaccharidoses (MPS)

See Table 12-7.

## Hurler's Syndrome (MPS IH)

Initial diagnosis by quantitative increase of MPS in urine; confirmed by assay of alpha-L-iduronidase in cultured fibroblasts or leukocytes.
Similar enzyme assay detects carriers who have ~50% activity but the wide range with overlap between normal and carriers may make the diagnosis difficult in individual cases.
Prenatal diagnosis by assay of enzyme or MPS in amniocytes

## Hunter's Syndrome (MPS II)

Initial diagnosis by quantitation of total glucosaminoglycans in urine and accumulation of keratan sulfate in tissues is confirmed by enzyme assay in fibroblasts.
Heterozygous female carriers recognized by MPS in fibroblasts or enzyme assay in individual hair roots.
Prenatal diagnosis by enzyme assay of amniotic fluid should be confirmed by assay of cultured cells.
Maternal serum shows increased activity of iduronate sulphate sulfatase with a normal or heterozygous fetus but no increase if fetus has Hunter's syndrome.

## Sanfilippo's Type A Syndrome (MPS III)

Only MPS in which finding only heparan sulfate in urine confirms diagnosis.
Assay of fibroblasts shows deficiency of enzyme in patient and decrease in normal activity in carrier, who also shows MPS accumulation.
Metachromatic inclusion bodies in lymphocytes are coarser and sparser than in Hurler's syndrome and may be seen in bone marrow cells. Severe cerebral changes with relatively mild changes in other body tissues.
The four types of Sanfilippo's syndrome cannot be distinguished clinically.

**Table 12-7.** Classification of Mucopolysaccharidoses

| Type of Mucopolysaccharidosis (clinical name) | Deficient Enzyme | Mucopolysaccharide Excreted in Urine | Signs/Symptoms |
|---|---|---|---|
| IH (Hurler's syndrome) | Alpha-L-iduronidase | Dermatan sulfate and heparan sulfate in 7:3 ratio | Progressive mental/physical disability from 1 yr of age; hyperplastic gums; coarse face; stiff joints (clawhands); organomegaly; dwarfing; dysostosis multiplex |
| IS (Scheie's syndrome) | Alpha-L-iduronidase | Dermatan sulfate and heparan sulfate | Mild form of MPS I; mild or no mental retardation; clawhands; aortic stenosis |
| IH/S (Hurler-Scheie syndrome) | Alpha-L-iduronidase | | Features intermediate between Hurler's and Scheie's syndromes |
| II (Hunter's syndrome) | Iduronate sulfatase | Dermatan sulfate and heparan sulfate | Dysostosis multiplex; mild to severe mental retardation; no corneal opacity; longer life compared with MPS I |
| IIIa (Sanfilippo's syndrome, type A) | Heparan N-sulfatase (sulfamidase) | Heparan sulfate | Mild or no connective tissue abnormalities; marked hirsutism; behaviorism progresses to severe mental retardation; no corneal opacity |
| IIIb (Sanfilippo's syndrome, type B) | Alpha-N-acetylglucosaminidase (alpha-hexosaminidase) | Heparan sulfate | Same as MPS IIIa |
| IIIc (Sanfilippo's syndrome, type C) | Acetyl CoA: alpha-glucosaminide N-acetyltransferase | Heparan sulfate | Same as MPS IIIa |

| | | Heparan sulfate | Same as MPS IIIa |
|---|---|---|---|
| IIId (Sanfilippo's syndrome, type D) | N-acetylglucosamine-6-sulfatase | | |
| IVa (Morquio's syndrome, type A) | N-acetylgalactosamine-6-sulfatase | Keratan sulfate | Marked skeletal abnormalities; small stature; short neck; prominent lower ribs; normal intellect; coma |
| IVb (Morquio's syndrome, type B) | Beta-galactosidase | Keratan sulfate | |
| V | This class is vacant now (formerly was Scheie's syndrome). | | |
| VI (Maroteaux-Lamy syndrome) | N-acetylgalactosamine-4-sulfatase (aryl-sulfatase B) | Dermatan sulfate | Severe dysostosis multiplex and corneal opacity; retarded growth; normal intellect; cardiac abnormalities; a mild form also occurs |
| VII (Sly's syndrome) | Beta-glucuronidase | Dermatan sulfate, heparan sulfate, chondroitin 4,6-sulfate | Mild mental retardation; organomegaly; corneal opacity may occur; coarse facies; gingivitis; very heterogeneous clinical appearances |

Notes: All MPSs show metachromatically staining inclusions of mucopolysaccharides in circulating polynuclear leukocytes (Reilly granulations) or lymphocytes, cells of inflammatory exudate, and bone marrow cells (most consistently in plasmacytes). Detection of deficiency of lysosomal enzyme in cultured fibroblasts establishes the diagnosis and makes prenatal diagnosis possible. Serum can be used for diagnosis in MPS II, IIIB, and VI. Leukocytes can be used for diagnosis in MPS IH, IS, IIIA, IIIC. RBCs can be used for diagnosis in III, IV, VI. Enzyme deficiency is demonstrable in liver in all except V; VII; demonstrable in muscle in all except IH, II. Increased glycogen in affected organs except in IV; glycogen structure is normal except in III, IV; Carrier state detection of IH, III, IV, VI is not reliable due to overlapping with normal persons of enzymatic activity values.

Inheritance in Hunter's syndrome is X-linked recessive; others are autosomal recessive.

Cloudy cornea in IH, IS, IVA, IVB, VI, VII.

Mental retardation in IH, II, IIIA, IIIB, IIIC, IIID, VII.

Hepatosplenomegaly in IH, II, IIIA, IIIB, IIIC, IIID, IVB, VI, VII.

Skeletal defects in all.

MPS = mucopolysaccharidosis; CoA = coenzyme A.

## Morquio's Syndrome (MPS IV)

Keratan sulfate is increased in urine (often 2–3 times normal).
Metachromatic granules may be seen in PMNs.
Diagnosis by enzyme assay in fibroblasts and leukocytes
Prenatal diagnosis by assay of enzymes in cultured amniocytes

## Maroteaux-Lamy Syndrome (MPS VI)

Metachromatic cytoplasmic inclusions (Alder granules) may be seen in 50% of
    lymphocytes and 100% of granulocytes are more marked than other MPSs.
Large amount of dermatan sulfate occurs in urine.
Diagnosis is established by deficiency of specific enzyme in cultured fibroblasts.
Enzyme assay also allows diagnosis of heterozygotes and prenatal diagnosis.

**Endocrine Diseases**

# Tests of Thyroid Function

See Fig. 13-1 and Table 13-1.

Thyroid function tests may only be indicated for *screening* of thyroid disease in certain populations, such as newborns (mandatory), patients with a strong family history of thyroid disease, elderly patients, 4–8 wks' postpartum women, and patients with autoimmune diseases (e.g., Addison's disease).

## Thyroid-Stimulating Hormone, Sensitive (S-TSH; Thyrotropin)
**(hormone secreted by anterior pituitary)**

### Use

Screening for euthyroidism—normal level in stable, ambulatory patient not on interfering drugs excludes thyroid hormone excess or deficiency. Is recommended initial test.

Initial screening and diagnosis for hyperthyroidism and hypothyroidism

Especially useful in early or subclinical hypothyroidism before the patient develops clinical findings, goiter, or abnormalities of other thyroid tests. In very early cases with only marginal elevation, the TRH stimulation test may be preferred.

Differentiation of primary (increased levels) from central (pituitary or hypothalamic) hypothyroidism (decreased levels)

Monitor adequate thyroid hormone replacement therapy in primary hypothyroidism, although $T_4$ may be mildly increased; may take up to 6–8 wks before TSH becomes normal. Serum TSH suppressed to normal level is the best monitor of dosage of thyroid hormone for treatment of hypothyroidism, but it does not indicate overtreatment.

Monitor adequate thyroid hormone therapy to suppress thyroid carcinoma (should suppress to <0.1 mU/L) or goiter or nodules (should suppress to subnormal levels).

Help differentiate euthyroid sick syndrome from primary hypothyroid patients.

Replace TRH stimulation test in hyperthyroidism because most patients with euthyroid TSH level will have a normal TSH response, and patients with undetectable TSH level almost never respond to TRH stimulation.

### Interferences

Dopamine or high doses of glucocorticoids may cause false normal values in primary hypothyroidism and may suppress TSH in nonthyroid illness.

### Increased in

Primary untreated hypothyroidism

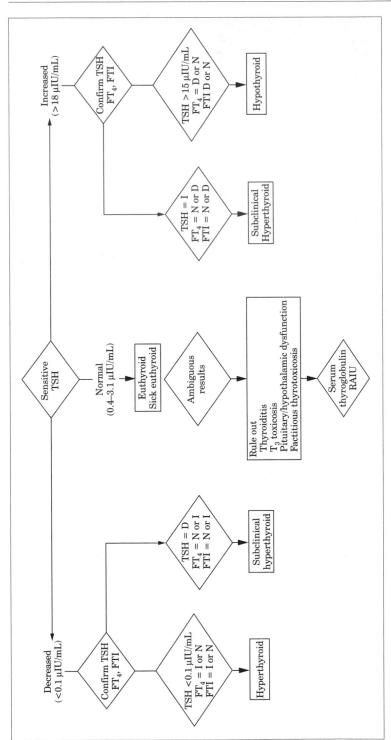

**Fig. 13-1.** Algorithm for thyroid function testing.

**Table 13-1.** Free $T_4$ and TSH in Various Conditions

| | | Sensitive-TSH | | |
|---|---|---|---|---|
| | | **Normal** | **Decreased** | **Increased** |
| $T_4$ | **Normal** | Euthyroid | Subclinical/early hyperthyroidism[a] <br> Nonthyroidal illness <br> Drugs <br>   L-Dopa <br>   Glucocorticoids <br>   Excess $T_4$ therapy <br>     for hypothyroidism | Subclinical/early hypothyroidism <br> Nonthyroidal illness <br> Drugs <br>   Iodine <br>   Lithium <br>   Antithyroid drugs <br>   Amiodarone <br> Insufficient $T_4$ therapy <br>   for hypothyroidism |
| | **Decreased** | Secondary hypothyroidism[h] <br> Nonthyroidal illness <br> Drugs <br>   $T_3$ <br>   Phenytoin <br>   Androgens <br>   Salicylates <br>   Carbamazepine <br>   Rifampin | Secondary hypothyroidism[b] <br> Drugs <br>   Dopamine[c] <br>   Corticosteroids[c] <br>   $T_3$ | Primary hypothyroidism <br> Drugs <br>   Iodine <br>   Lithium <br>   Antithyroid drugs <br> Insufficient $T_4$ therapy <br>   for hypothyroidism |
| | **Increased** | Nonthyroidal illness <br> Acute and psychiatric illness <br> Abnormal binding (excess TBG, familial dysalbuminemic hyperthyroxinemia, transthyretin-associated hyperthyroxinemia, some monoclonal proteins) <br> Thyroid hormone resistance <br> Drugs <br>   Estrogen <br>   Amiodarone <br>   Iodine (drugs, contrast media) <br>   $T_4$ (factitious) | Nonthyroidal illness <br> Acute psychiatric illness <br> Primary hyperthyroidism[d] | TSH-secreting tumor <br> Thyroid hormone resistance |

[a]Confirm with $T_3$ suppression test or lack of serum TSH response to TRH.
[b]Pituitary TSH deficiency shows deficient response to exogenous TRH. Hypothalamic TRH deficiency shows normal TSH response but may be prolonged for >30 mins.
[c]Serial monitoring or testing of serum TSH response to TRH may be needed.
[d]95% of cases; serum $T_3$ needed for diagnosis of $T_3$ thyrotoxicosis.

Hypothyroidism receiving insufficient thyroid hormone replacement therapy
Hashimoto's thyroiditis, including those with clinical hypothyroidism and about one-third of those patients who are clinically euthyroid
Various drugs (e.g., amphetamine abuse)
• Iodine-containing (e.g., iopanoic acid, ipodate, amiodarone)
• Dopamine antagonists (e.g., metoclopramide, domperidone, chlorpromazine, haloperidol)
Thyrotoxicosis due to pituitary tumor or pituitary resistance to thyroid hormone
Some patients with euthyroid sick syndrome
TSH antibodies
Increased in first 2–3 days of life due to postnatal TSH surge

### Decreased

Hyperthyroidism due to
• Toxic multinodular goiter
• Autonomously functioning thyroid adenoma
• Ophthalmopathy of euthyroid Graves' disease
• Treated Graves' disease
• Thyroiditis
• Extrathyroidal thyroid hormone source
Over-replacement of thyroid hormone in treatment of hypothyroidism
Secondary pituitary or hypothalamic hypothyroidism
Euthyroid sick patients
Drug effect, especially large doses
• Glucocorticoids and other endocrine drugs
• Antithyroid drugs
• Assay interference (e.g., antibodies to mouse IgG, autoimmune disease)
• First trimester of pregnancy

### May Be Normal by Immunoradiometric Assay (IRMA) in

Central hypothyroidism
Recent rapid correction of hyperthyroidism or hypothyroidism
Pregnancy
Phenytoin therapy
*In absence of hypothalamic or pituitary disease, normal TSH excludes primary hypothyroidism.*

## Thyroxine, Free (FT$_4$) Assay

### Use

Gives corrected values in patients in whom the total T$_4$ is altered on account of changes in serum proteins or in binding sites:
• Pregnancy
• Drugs (e.g., androgens, estrogens, birth control pills, phenytoin)
• Altered levels of serum proteins (e.g., nephrosis)
Monitoring restoration to normal range is only laboratory criterion to estimate appropriate replacement dose of levothyroxine.

### Increased in

Hyperthyroidism
Hypothyroidism treated with thyroxine
Euthyroid sick syndrome
Occasional patients with hydatidiform mole or choriocarcinoma

### Decreased in

Hypothyroidism
Hypothyroidism treated with triiodothyronine
Euthyroid sick syndrome

# Thyroxine, Total ($T_4$) Assay

## Use

Diagnosis of hyperthyroidism

## Increased in

Hyperthyroidism
Pregnancy
Certain drugs (estrogens, birth control pills, dextrothyroxine, thyroid extract, TSH, amiodarone, heroin, methadone, amphetamines)
Euthyroid sick syndrome
Increase in TBG or abnormal thyroxine-binding prealbumin
• Familial dysalbuminemic hyperthyroxinemia.
• Serum $T_4$ >20 μg/dL usually indicates true hyperthyroidism rather than increased TBG.
• May be found in euthyroid patients with increased serum TBG.

## Decreased in

Hypothyroidism
Hypoproteinemia (e.g., nephrosis, cirrhosis)
Certain drugs (phenytoin, $T_3$, testosterone, ACTH)
Euthyroid sick syndrome
Decrease in TBG

## Normal Levels May Be Found in Hyperthyroid Patients with

$T_3$ thyrotoxicosis
Factitious hyperthyroidism due to $T_3$ (liothyronine [Cytomel])
Decreased binding capacity due to hypoproteinemia or ingestion of certain drugs (e.g., phenytoin, salicylates)

## Interferences

Various drugs

## Not Affected by

Nonthyroidal iodine

# Triiodothyronine ($T_3$) Assay

## Use

$T_3$ thyrotoxicosis (serum $T_4$ is normal)
Serum $T_3$ parallels $FT_4$ and may be helpful
• When serum $FT_4$ is borderline elevated
• When serum $FT_4$ is normal in presence of symptoms of hyperthyroidism
• When overlooking diagnosis of hyperthyroidism is very undesirable (e.g., unexplained atrial fibrillation)
• Monitoring the course of hyperthyroidism
May decrease by up to 25% in healthy older persons while $FT_4$ remains normal
Free $T_3$ gives corrected values in patients in whom the total $T_3$ is altered on account of changes in serum proteins or in binding sites.
• Pregnancy
• Drugs (e.g., androgens, estrogens, birth control pills, phenytoin)
• Altered levels of serum proteins

# Triiodothyronine ($T_3$) Resin Uptake

## Use

Measures unoccupied binding sites on TBG. Is not a measure of $T_3$.

Only with simultaneous measurement of serum $T_4$ to calculate free thyroxine index (FTI) to exclude the possibility that an increased $T_4$ is due to an increase in TBG.

### Increased in

Patients with *decreased* serum TBG

### Decreased in

Patients with *increased* serum TBG

### Normal in

Pregnancy with hyperthyroidism
Nontoxic goiter
Carcinoma of thyroid
Diabetes mellitus (DM)
Addison's disease
Anxiety
Certain drugs (mercurials, iodine)

### Variable in

Liver disease

## Free Thyroxine Index (FTI)

American Thyroid Association now recommends the term *thyroid hormone–binding ratios.*

### Use

This is the calculated product of $T_3$ resin uptake and serum $T_4$. It permits correction of misleading results of $T_3$ and $T_4$ determinations caused by conditions that alter the thyroxine-binding protein concentration (e.g., pregnancy, estrogens, birth control pills).

## Thyroid-Releasing Hormone Stimulation Test

Serum TSH is measured before and after IV administration of TRH.
Now largely replaced by serum-sensitive TSH

## Thyroid Autoantibody Tests
(antimicrosomal [also called *thyroid peroxidase*] and antithyroglobulin autoantibodies)

### Use

Positive in >85% of Hashimoto's disease and ~80% of Graves' disease. Very high titer is pathognomonic of Hashimoto's thyroiditis, but absence does not exclude Hashimoto's thyroiditis. >1:1000 occurs virtually only in Graves' disease or Hashimoto's thyroiditis. Significant titer of microsome antibodies indicates Hashimoto's thyroiditis or postpartum thyroid dysfunction.
To distinguish subacute thyroiditis from Hashimoto's thyroiditis, as antibodies are more common in the latter
Hashimoto's thyroiditis is very unlikely cause of hypothyroidism in the absence of thyroglobulin and microsomal antibodies.
Significant titer of thyroglobulin and microsome antibodies in euthyroid patient with unilateral exophthalmos suggests the diagnosis of euthyroid Graves' disease.
Occasionally useful to distinguish Graves' disease from toxic multinodular goiter when physical findings are not diagnostic

Graves' disease with elevated titers of antimicrosomal antibodies should direct surgeon to perform a more limited thyroidectomy to avoid late post-thyroidectomy hypothyroidism.

### Increased in

Occasionally positive in papillary-follicular carcinoma of thyroid, subacute thyroiditis (briefly), lymphocytic (painless) thyroiditis (in ~60% of patients).
Primary thyroid lymphoma often shows very high titers.
Positive in 7% of normal population, reaching peak of 15% in females in sixth decade
Other autoimmune diseases (e.g., PA, RA, SLE, myasthenia gravis)

## Thyroid Uptake of Radioactive Iodine (RAIU)

After a tracer dose of radioactive iodine ($^{131}I$ or $^{123}I$), the radioactivity over the thyroid is measured. The percent of administered iodine in the thyroid is an index of thyroid trapping and organification of iodide.

### Use

Detection of hyperthyroidism associated with low RAIU (e.g., factitious hyperthyroidism, subacute thyroiditis, struma ovarii)
Evaluate use of radioiodine therapy.
Determine presence of an organification defect in thyroid hormone production.
$T_3$ suppression test. Administration of $T_3$ causes less suppression of RAIU in the hyperthyroid patient than in the normal person; has been replaced by the TRH stimulation test.

### Contraindications

Pregnancy, lactation, childhood

## Thyroxine-Binding Globulin (TBG)

### Use

Diagnosis of genetic or idiopathic excess TBG
To distinguish factitious hyperthyroidism from lymphocytic painless thyroiditis
Sometimes used to detect recurrent or metastatic differentiated thyroid carcinoma, especially follicular type and when patient has had an increased level due to carcinoma
To distinguish increased/decreased total $T_3$ or $T_4$ concentrations due to changes in TBG from normal free $T_3$ or $FT_4$. Same purpose as $T_3$ resin uptake and $FT_4$ index.

### Increased in

Pregnancy
Certain drugs (estrogens, birth control pills, perphenazine, clofibrate, heroin, methadone)
Estrogen-producing tumors
Acute intermittent porphyria
Acute or chronic active hepatitis
Lymphocytic painless subacute thyroiditis
Neonates

### Decreased in

Marked hypoproteinemia, such as nephrosis, liver disease, severe illness, stress ($T_4$-binding prealbumin also decreased)
Deficiency of TBG, genetic or idiopathic
Acromegaly ($T_4$-binding prealbumin also decreased)

Severe acidosis
Certain drugs
• Androgens, anabolic steroids
• Glucocorticoids ($T_4$-binding prealbumin is increased)
Testosterone-producing tumors

### Decreased Binding of Triiodothyronine and Thyroxine Due to Drugs

Salicylates
Phenytoin
Tolbutamide (Orinase), chlorpropamide
Penicillin, heparin, barbital
*An increased TBG is associated with increased serum $T_4$ and decreased $T_3$ resin uptake; a converse association exists for decreased TBG.*

# Diseases of the Thyroid

See Table 13-2.

## Carcinoma of Thyroid

Medullary carcinoma
• Sporadic (noninherited) accounts for 80% of cases
• Familial accounts for 20% of cases
    MEN I
    Most are MEN II
    Familial non-MEN

### Basal Fasting Calcitonin Is Increased

In patients with medullary carcinoma of the thyroid even when there is no palpable mass in the thyroid
Circadian rhythm with peak after lunchtime
Basal level is normal in approximately one-third of cases.
• >2000 pg/mL are always associated with medullary carcinoma of thyroid with rare cases due to obvious renal failure or ectopic production of calcitonin.
• 500–2000 pg/mL generally indicate medullary carcinoma, renal failure, or ectopic production of calcitonin.
• 100–500 pg/mL should be interpreted cautiously with repeat assays and provocative tests; if these and repeat tests in 1–2 months are still abnormal, some authors recommend total thyroidectomy.
• Normal basal levels: Males ≤ 19 pg/mL; females ≤ 14 pg/mL.
Calcium infusion and/or pentagastrin injection are used as provocative tests in patients with normal basal levels who have a family history of thyroid carcinoma, a calcified thyroid mass, pheochromocytoma, hyperparathyroidism (HPT), hypercalcemia, amyloid-containing metastatic carcinoma of unknown origin.
Detects recurrence of medullary carcinoma or metastases after the primary tumor has been removed or confirms complete removal of the tumor if basal calcitonin has been previously increased.
Serum calcitonin may also be increased in some patients with
• Carcinoma of lung, breast, islet cell, or ovary and carcinoid due to ectopic production
• Hypercalcemia of any etiology stimulating calcitonin production
• Z-E syndrome
• PA

- Acute or chronic thyroiditis
- Chronic renal failure

Serum thyroglobulin levels are increased in most patients with differentiated thyroid carcinoma but not in undifferentiated or medullary carcinoma. May not be increased with small occult differentiated carcinoma. May be useful to detect presence and possibly the extent of residual, recurrent, or metastatic follicular or papillary thyroid carcinoma. In patients with carcinomas treated with total thyroidectomy or radioiodine and taking thyroid hormone therapy, thyroglobulin is undetectable if functional metastases are absent but present if functional metastases are present. *Increased levels may be found in patients with nontoxic nodular goiter; presence of autoantibodies interferes with the test.* Is not useful for screening high-risk groups (e.g., neck radiation in childhood).

Serum CEA may be increased in medullary carcinoma and may correlate with tumor size or extent of disease.

Serum LD and CEA may be increased in advanced follicular carcinoma.

Serum $T_3$, $T_4$, TSH are almost always normal in untreated patients.

Laboratory findings due to MEN syndrome and to production of additional substances (e.g., ACTH, serotonin, histaminase) by medullary carcinoma

RAIU is almost always normal.

Radioactive scan of thyroid

Needle biopsy of thyroid nodule

## Euthyroid Sick Syndrome
**(wide variety of nonthyroidal acute and chronic conditions may be associated with abnormal thyroid function tests in euthyroid patients, especially in aged; artifactual changes are not included in euthyroid sick syndrome)**

*No single test is clearly diagnostic, especially in elderly and acutely or severely ill patients.*

### Increased T$_4$ Syndrome

Is most common ($\leq 20\%$) in acute psychiatric admissions, especially in the presence of certain drugs (e.g., amphetamines, phencyclidine) and old age ($< 15\%$ of elderly patients); increased values tend to decrease during first 2 wks after admission as patient improves. Is rarer in acutely ill patients (e.g., acute hepatitis).

- Increased serum $T_4$, FTI, and $T_3$.
- TSH is usually normal in mild to moderate illness.
- 50% of patients with hyperemesis gravidarum show elevated total and sometimes $FT_4$ that persists until hyperemesis abates.

### Decreased T$_4$ Syndrome

- Occurs in >50% of severe or chronic illness.
- TSH is transiently increased during recovery.

### Low T$_3$ Syndrome

Is the most common. Occurs in most illnesses, starvation, and after surgery or trauma. $T_3$ is decreased in ~70% of hospitalized patients without intrinsic thyroid disease and is normal in 20–30% of hypothyroid patients; therefore $T_3$ is not indicated.

- Increased reversed $T_3$.
- With progressive illness, tendency is for fall in total $T_4$ and TBG with increase of $FT_4$. Thus, $T_3$ uptake increases, and FTI tends to remain normal. There is a strong correlation with low $T_4$ ($<3 \mu g/dL$).
- Serum TSH is typically normal or slightly increased.

**Table 13-2.** Thyroid Function Tests in Various Conditions

| Disease | Serum Total $T_4$ | Serum $T_3$ (concentration) | Serum $T_3$ Uptake | Free $T_4$ Index (FTI) | Serum TBG | RAIU | Serum TSH | TRH Test |
|---|---|---|---|---|---|---|---|---|
| Hypothyroidism | D | D | D | D | N or I | D | I[a] | A[b] |
| Euthyroid sick (low $T_3$) syndrome | N or D | D | I | I, N, or D | N | N | N, I, or D | N or D |
| Hyperthyroidism | I | I | I | I | N | I | D | A |
| $T_3$ thyrotoxicosis | N | I | N or slightly I | N | N | N or I | D | A |
| Administration of | | | | | | | | |
| $T_4$ (factitious hyperthyroidism)[c] | I | V | I | I | N | D | D | A |
| Inorganic iodine | N | N | N | N | N | D | I | A |
| Radiopaque contrast media[d] | N | N | N | N | N | D | N | |
| Estrogen and antiovulatory drugs | I | I | D | N | I | I | N | N |
| Testosterone | D | D | I | N | D | D | N | N |
| ACTH and corticosteroids | D | N or D | I | N | D | D | N or D | |

| Dilantin or large doses of salicylates | | | | | | | |
|---|---|---|---|---|---|---|---|
| Pregnancy | I | I | D | N | I | X | N or D | N |
| With hyperthyroidism | I | I | N | I | I | X | N | A |
| With hypothyroidism | D | D or N | D | D | I | X | I | A |
| Hereditary increase of TBG in euthyroid state | I | I | D | N | I | I | N | N |
| Hereditary decrease of TBG in euthyroid state | D | D | I | N | D | D | N | N |
| Granulomatous thyroiditis | V or I | V or D | V or I | V or I | N | D | V or I | |
| Adenomatous thyroid goiter | N | N | N | N | N | N | N | |
| Thyroid neoplasm (nonfunctional) | N | N | N | N | N | N | N | |
| Nephrosis[e] | D | D | I | N | D | May be I | N | |

(Dilantin or large doses of salicylates: D, D, I, N, D, —, N, N)

A = abnormal; X = contraindicated in pregnancy.

[a] Increased serum TSH is diagnostic of primary hypothyroidism; TSH is decreased in secondary and tertiary hypothyroidism.

[b] TRH stimulation test is normal in euthyroid state, increased response in primary hypothyroidism, blunted or no response in pituitary hypothyroidism, delayed response in hypothalamic etiology.

[c] RAIU is decreased when all other thyroid function tests indicate hyperfunction.

[d] Invalidates RAIU results.

[e] Thyroid function tests are altered due to loss of TBG in urine.

## Goiter

See Fig. 13-2.

Isotope scanning of thyroid may show decreased ("cold") or increased ("hot") uptake.

Functioning solitary adenoma may produce hyperthyroidism.

In multinodular goiter, TSH level is rarely increased.

Fine-needle aspiration biopsy will produce a definitive diagnosis in 85% of cases of thyroid nodules.

$T_4$, $T_3$, TBG, and thyroglobulin do not differ in benign and malignant cyst fluid.

## Hyperthyroidism

See Fig. 13-3.

### Causes of Hyperthyroidism

Diffuse toxic goiter (Graves' disease)
Toxic adenoma
Toxic multinodular goiter
Thyroiditis
• Hashimoto's
• Lymphocytic (painless)
• Subacute granulomatous
Iodide-induced (Jod-Basedow)
Metastatic functioning thyroid carcinoma
Factitious
Struma ovarii with hyperthyroidism
TRH-induced hyperthyroidism
• With pituitary tumor
• Without pituitary tumor
Neoplasms that secrete thyroid stimulators
• Choriocarcinoma, hydatidiform mole
• Embryonal carcinoma of testis
In neonate, is usually due to transplacental maternal TSH receptor-stimulating antibodies that mimic TSH action.

Serum TSH is decreased in all forms of thyrotoxicosis except the very rare cases of pituitary neoplasms that secrete TSH; sensitive TSH as initial screening test for thyrotoxicosis will detect virtually all hyperthyroid patients but a number of euthyroid patients are also included.

Serum total and $FT_4$ are increased. With a typical clinical picture of hyperthyroidism, serum $T_4$ >16 μg/dL confirms the diagnosis. Normal in ~10% of patients, although TSH is low.

Serum $T_3$ concentration on RIA and $T_3$ resin uptake are increased in up to 85% of patients. $T_3$ is usually elevated to a greater degree than $T_4$. Ratio $T_3$:$T_4$ >20:1 in $T_3$-dependent Graves' disease.

Serum TBG is normal.

Technetium-99m pertechnetate uptake parallels hormone production and may be useful when $T_4$ and TSH results are discordant.

Microsomal antibodies are found in moderate to high titers in most patients with Graves' disease; may be helpful in confirming diagnosis in a hyperthyroid patient without ocular findings or an euthyroid patient with ocular findings.

Other thyroid autoantibodies are TSIs and TSH-binding inhibitory immunoglobulins found only with Graves' disease that are sometimes helpful in diagnosis and management. TSH-receptor antibody (formerly called *long-acting thyroid stimulator* [LATS]) is present in 80–100% of untreated Graves' disease patients.

Serum cholesterol is decreased, and total lipids are usually decreased.

Normal serum creatine almost excludes hyperthyroidism.

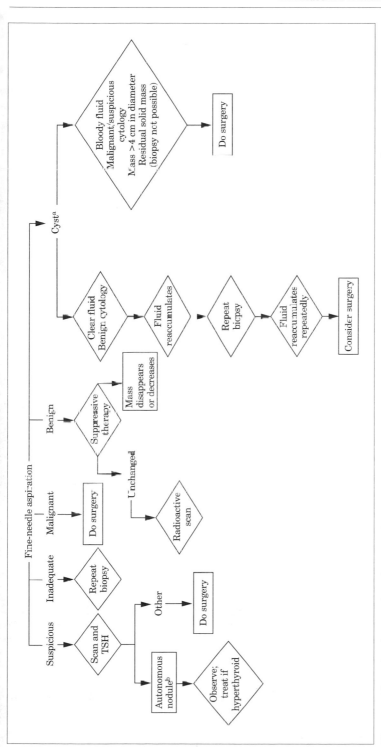

**Fig. 13-2.** Algorithm for tests for solitary nodule of thyroid. [a]Contrary to common belief, cystic lesions may be malignant. [b]Autonomous nodules are rarely malignant; thus, a "hot" nodule on scan avoids surgery.

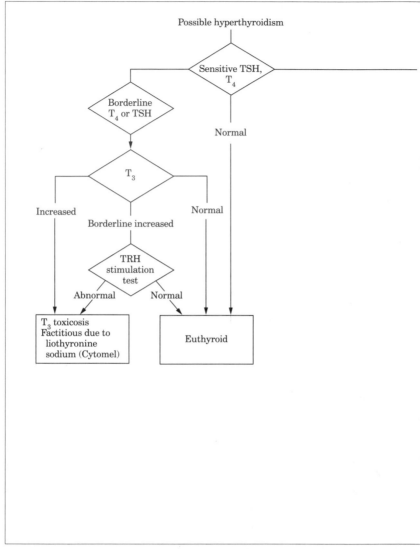

**Fig. 13-3.** Algorithm for diagnosis of hyperthyroidism.

Serum total and ionized calcium are increased in >10% of patients. Serum phosphorus is high normal or increased. Parathormone level is decreased. Serum 1,25-dihydroxyvitamin D is decreased.
Increased serum ALP in 75% of patients

### $T_3$ Toxicosis

Causes 5% of cases of hyperthyroidism
Should be suspected in patients with clinical thyrotoxicosis in whom usual laboratory tests are normal but serum $T_3$ is increased.
RAIU is autonomous (not suppressed by $T_3$ administration).
TSH may be increased.

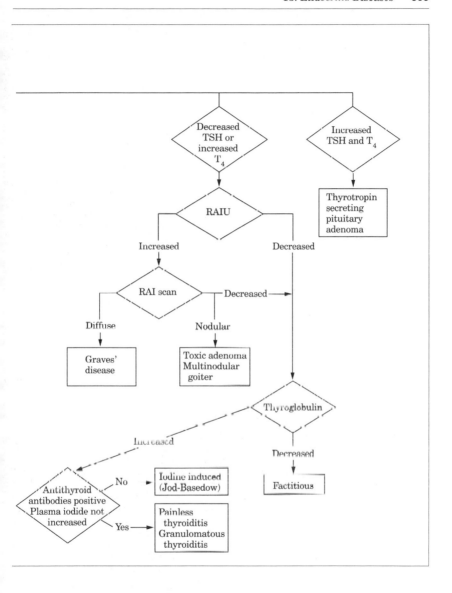

## Hypothyroidism

See Fig. 13-4.

### *Due to*

Treatment of preceding hyperthyroidism (surgery, drugs, radioiodine)
Radiation (e.g., treatment of head and neck cancer)
Autoimmune disease, thyroiditis
Pituitary disease (e.g., tumors, granulomas, cysts, vascular)
Hypothalamic disease (e.g., granulomas, TRH deficiency, pituitary-stalk section)
Iodine deficiency

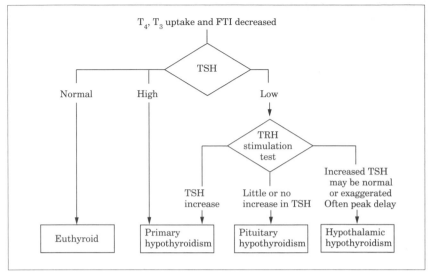

**Fig. 13-4.** Algorithm for diagnosis of hypothyroidism. Sensitive TSH test is the preferred primary screening test for thyroid disease. Low TSH obviates need for the TRH stimulation test in most patients.

Drugs (e.g., iodides, propylthiouracil, methimazole, phenylbutazone, amiodarone, lithium)
Congenital developmental defects
Organification defect (diagnosis by perchlorate washout test)

Serum TSH is increased in proportion to degree of hypofunction; is at least 2 times and often 10 times normal value. A single determination is usually sufficient to establish the diagnosis. Because increased serum TSH is earliest evidence of hypothyroidism, it should be measured to document subclinical hypothyroidism and begin early therapy in patients with Graves' disease. TSH is especially useful in cases in which $T_4$ and FTI are not diagnostic; and is essential when the diagnosis of hypothyroidism must be confirmed. Serum TSH should always be measured before treatment of all patients with hypothyroidism to distinguish primary from secondary (pituitary) or tertiary (hypothalamic) types. Serum TSH is increased in primary hypothyroidism but undetectable or inappropriately low in relationship to degree of thyroid hormone deficiency in secondary or tertiary hypothyroidism.

Serum $T_4$ and $FT_4$ concentrations are decreased; $T_4 > 7\ \mu g/dL$ almost certainly excludes hypothyroidism. Serum $FT_4$ and TSH together is diagnostic method of choice.

Serum $T_3$ concentration is decreased; has little role in this diagnosis.

$FT_4$ index is decreased.

Serum $T_3$:$T_4$ ratio is increased.

Serum TBG is normal.

Serum cholesterol is increased (may be useful to follow effect of therapy, especially in children).

Serum myoglobin is significantly increased in 90% of untreated, long-term hypothyroid patients.

Increased serum CK and CK-MM, AST, LD

Serum ALP is decreased.

Laboratory findings indicative of other autoimmune diseases

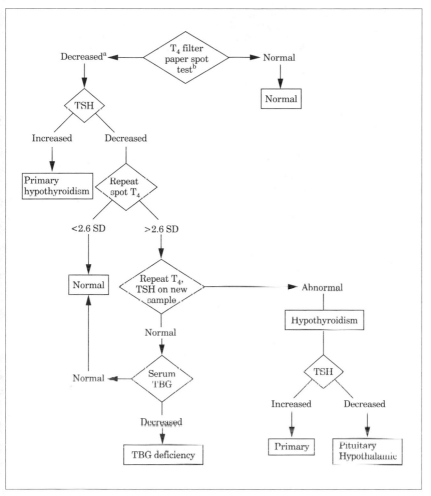

**Fig. 13-5.** Algorithm for neonatal screening for hypothyroidism. [a]Cases with lowest 2–3% of concentrations. $T_4$ alone for screening has false-positive rate = 2–3%. [b]Serum from infant age 3–5 days, combined with phenylketonuria program.

### *Myxedema Coma*

Hypoglycemia, hyponatremia, and findings due to adrenocortical insufficiency may be found.
Serum creatinine may be increased.

## Hypothyroidism, Neonatal

See Fig. 13-5.
Neonatal screening is usually performed on same filter paper specimen of blood used for phenylketonuria screening at age 3–5 days. *Do not test $T_4$ or TSH during first few days of life when levels may surge.*

RAIU ($^{123}$Iodine) scan should be performed on babies with confirmed hypothyroidism to differentiate thyroid agenesis/dysgenesis from dyshormonogenesis.
If mother has autoimmune thyroid disease, baby should be checked for TSH receptor–blocking antibodies since this type of hypothyroidism cannot be distinguished clinically from thyroid agenesis/dysgenesis and RAIU may be absent. Hypothyroidism is transient.

### Due to

### Primary Hypothyroidism
Aplasia and hypoplasia (63%)
Ectopic gland (23%)
Inborn errors of thyroid hormone synthesis or metabolism (14%)
* Increased serum TSH is most sensitive test for primary hypothyroidism
* Decreased serum $T_4$
* Normal or decreased serum $T_3$
* Normal serum TBG
* Increased serum CK

### Deficiency of TBG
Hereditary
Drug effect
Hypoproteinemia
* Decreased serum $T_4$ (e.g., 3.2 $\mu$g/dL)
* Normal serum TSH

### Secondary Hypothyroidism
Pituitary aplasia, septo-optic dysplasia
Idiopathic hypopituitarism
Hypothalamic disease
* Serum TSH is low or not detectable.
* Decreased serum $T_4$.
* TSH response to TRH differentiates pituitary from hypothalamic cause of hypothyroidism.
* Normal serum TBG.

### Transient
Prematurity
Euthyroid sick syndrome
Small for gestational age
Maternal ingestion of iodides or antithyroid drugs
Idiopathic

## Thyroiditis Syndromes

### Hashimoto's Thyroiditis (Chronic Lymphocytic Thyroiditis)

Thyroid function may be normal; occasionally, a patient passes through a hyperthyroid stage. 15–20% of patients develop hypothyroidism, but Hashimoto's disease is a very unlikely cause of hypothyroidism in the absence of thyroglobulin and microsomal antibodies.
Antimicrosomal antibodies are 99% sensitive and 90% specific. Antithyroglobulin antibodies are 36% sensitive and 98% specific and are seldom positive if microsomal antibodies are negative. Thus, antimicrosomal antibody alone is sufficient for diagnosis. High titers are pathognomonic.
Radioiodine scan may show involvement of only a single lobe (more common in younger patients); "salt and pepper" pattern is classic.
RAIU is variable; may be higher than expected in hypothyroidism.
Biopsy of thyroid may be diagnostic.

### Lymphocytic (Painless) Thyroiditis; Silent Thyroiditis

This is a form of hyperthyroidism that comprises ≤ 25% of all cases of hyperthyroidism; resolves spontaneously in weeks to months and is often followed by a transient hypothyroidism during recovery period. Hashimoto's thyroiditis cannot be ruled out in biopsy specimens.

## Hyperthyroid Phase

- Increased serum $T_4$, $T_3$, FTI. $T_3$:$T_4$ ratio <20:1. Levels become normal in 10 days with prednisone therapy.
- RAIU is very low (<3%); not increased after TSH administration.
- Serum TSH is low and fails to respond to TRH.
- Antithyroglobulin antibodies are increased in most patients; antimicrosomal antibodies are increased in about 60% of patients. High titers are rarely in the very high ranges of Hashimoto's thyroiditis.
- Nonspecific markers of inflammation are generally normal in contrast to granulomatous thyroiditis. ESR increased in 50% of patients to 20–40 mm/hr. WBC and serum proteins are normal.

## Recovery Phase

Complete in about 50%

- Serum $T_4$ and $T_3$ fall into normal range, but RAIU and TSH responses to TRH remain suppressed.

## Hypothyroid Phase

**(occurs in 20–30% of patients; few develop permanent hypothyroidism; recurs in >10%)**

- Antithyroid antibody titers are highest during this phase (especially in post-partum patients). Gradually decrease with time; 50% become negative within 6 months.
- Serum TSH, $T_4$, and $T_3$ gradually return to normal.
- RAIU, TRH test begin to normalize toward the end of this phase.

### Subacute Granulomatous (de Quervain's) Thyroiditis
*(probably viral origin)*

Biopsy of thyroid confirms diagnosis.

Antithyroglobulin antibodies may be present but the titer is never as high as in Hashimoto's thyroiditis. The level falls with recovery.

ESR is increased.

WBC is normal or decreased.

Four sequential phases may be identified: hyperthyroid, euthyroid, hypothyroid, recovery.

### Suppurative Thyroiditis, Acute

WBC and PMNs are increased in 75% of cases; absence may indicate anaerobic infection.

ESR is increased.

The 24-hr RAIU is decreased in <50% of cases.

Thyroid function tests normal in 80% of cases.

*Staphylococcus* causes one-third of cases.

### Riedel's Chronic Thyroiditis

Biopsy of thyroid confirms diagnosis.

Hypothyroidism when complete thyroid involvement occurs; otherwise, normal laboratory findings

# Tests of Parathyroid Function and Calcium/Phosphate Metabolism

## Calcium and Phosphorus, Serum

See Chapter 3.

## Calcitriol, Serum

### Interpretation

Suppressed during hypercalcemia unless there is autonomous source of PTH as in HPT. (Normal range <42 pg/mL in hypercalcemic and <76 pg/mL in normocalcemic patients.) Failure to suppress indicates extrarenal production, as it is normally secreted only by kidney.

### Increased in

Sarcoidosis (synthesized by macrophages within granulomas)
Non-Hodgkin's lymphoma (~15% of cases). Returns to normal after therapy.

### Not Increased in

HPT
Humoral hypercalcemia of malignancy (HHM)

## Parathyroid Hormone (PTH), Serum

See Fig. 13-6.

### Use

Differential diagnosis of HPT and hypoparathyroidism
Very sensitive in detecting PTH suppression by 1,25-dihydroxyvitamin D; therefore, used for monitoring that treatment of chronic renal failure.

### Interpretation

Serum calcium should always be measured at same time as PTH.
Assay of choice detects intact PTH and active N-terminal PTH. PTH is suppressed (<1 pmol/L) in 95% of cases of HHM unless there is coexisting parathyroid adenoma. Normal in chronic renal failure, in which almost all patients have increased C-terminal PTH (inactive) values.
PTH >25% above ULN occurs only in HPT (primary or tertiary), post–acute tubular necrosis, or post-transplant hypercalcemia. Some laboratories may assay different parts of PTH molecule.
PTH shows diurnal variation with low in morning and peak around midnight.

|  | PTH Increased | PTH Not Increased |
|---|---|---|
| **Serum calcium decreased**[a] | Secondary hyperparathyroidism (chronic renal disease) | Hypoparathyroidism (surgical, autoimmunity, hormone resistance, magnesium deficiency) |
| **Serum calcium increased**[b] | Primary HPT Familial hypocalciuric hypercalcemia Lithium-induced hypercalcemia Some neoplasms (HHM) | Hypercalcemia not due to HHM, milk-alkali syndrome, thiazide diuretics, vitamin intoxication, sarcoidosis, hyperthyroidism, immobilization) |
| **Serum calcium normal** | Pregnancy Nephrolithiasis Secondary hyperparathyroidism (chronic renal disease) | Normal |

[a]PTH may be normal or increased in hypocalcemic patients due to renal failure, acute pancreatitis, vitamin D deficiency.
[b]PTH may be normal or increased in hypercalcemic patients due to acromegaly, vitamin A intoxication, MEN type IIA, renal tubular acidosis, chronic renal failure.

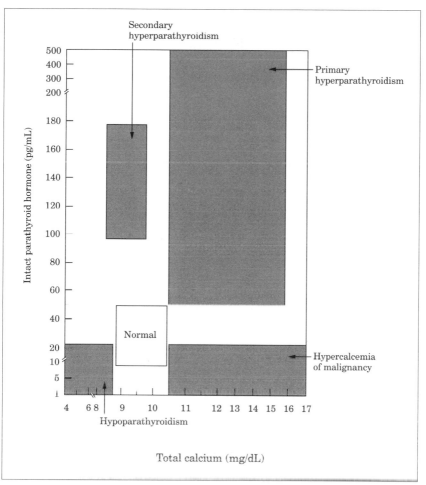

**Fig. 13-6.** Distribution of patients according to serum calcium and serum parathyroid hormone. The values of some patients may lie outside the exact boundaries indicated, and some conditions may overlap.

## Parathyroid Hormone–Related Protein (PTHRP), Serum

A PTH-related protein (PTHRP) can be measured in serum (>1.5 pmol/L) in >90% of cases of HHM. Increased in ~10% of cancers without hypercalcemia. Becomes normal when hypercalcemia is corrected by treatment of cancer. ~20% of cancers with hypercalcemia have only local osteolytic changes but not increased PTHRP. Not increased in other causes of hypercalcemia (e.g., sarcoidosis, vitamin D intoxication). C-terminal PTHRP is increased in renal insufficiency; may be increased in nonmalignant pheochromocytoma.

## Phosphate Deprivation Test

Low phosphate diet causes low serum phosphate and increased serum calcium in persons with HPT but not in normal persons.

## Vitamin D, Serum

### *1,25-Dihydroxyvitamin D*

Formed from 25-hydroxyvitamin D by kidney, placenta, granulomas
**Use**
Differential diagnosis of hypocalcemic disorders
Monitor patients with renal osteodystrophy
**Increased in**
HPT
Chronic granulomatous disorders
Hypercalcemia associated with lymphoma
**Decreased in**
Severe vitamin D deficiency
Hypercalcemia of malignancy (except lymphoma)
Tumor-induced osteomalacia
Hypoparathyroidism
Pseudohypoparathyroidism
Renal osteodystrophy
Type I vitamin D–resistant rickets

### *25-Hydroxyvitamin D*

**Use**
Evaluation of vitamin D intoxication or deficiency
**Increased in**
Vitamin D intoxication (distinguishes this from other causes of hypercalcemia)
**Decreased in**
Rickets
Osteomalacia
Secondary HPT
Malabsorption of vitamin D (e.g., severe liver disease, cholestasis)
Diseases that increase vitamin D metabolism (e.g., TB, sarcoidosis, primary
   HPT)

# Diseases of Parathyroid Glands and Calcium, Phosphorus, Alkaline Phosphatase Metabolism

See Table 13-3.

## Humoral Hypercalcemia of Malignancy

Hypercalcemia occurs in patients with cancer (typically squamous, transitional
   cell, renal, ovarian), 5–20% of whom have no bone metastases compared to
   patients with widespread bone metastases (myeloma, lymphoma, breast cancer). Both groups have large tumor burden and poor prognosis.
   • Rarely occurs in association with benign tumors (e.g., pheochromocytoma,
     dermoid cyst of ovary).
   • Very high serum calcium (e.g., >14.5 mg/dL) is much more suggestive of
     HHM than primary HPT; less marked increase with renal tumors.
Serum PTH is decreased or low-normal inappropriate for high serum calcium.
Serum PTHRP is increased (>1.5 pmol/L) in >90% of cases by some assay meth-
   ods (e.g., RIA) but not by others (e.g., IRMA).
Serum 1,25-dihydroxyvitamin D is usually decreased or low normal but increased
   in T-cell or B-cell lymphoma or Hodgkin's disease.
Urinary cyclic adenosine monophosphate (cAMP) is increased in 90% of cases
   HHM and of primary HPT.
Hypercalciuria is much greater than in HPT at any serum calcium level.
Decreased serum chloride

Decreased serum albumin

Alkalosis is present.

Decreased serum phosphorus in >50% of patients

Serum ALP is frequently increased.

Blood 1,25-dihydroxyvitamin D (calcitriol) is not increased in HHM but is increased in HPT.

Serum proteins are not consistently abnormal.

Occult cancer should be ruled out as the cause of hypercalcemia in presence of

- Hypercalcemia without increased serum PTH level together with increased urinary cAMP.
- Serum ALP >2 times ULN.
- Increased serum phosphorus.
- Serum chloride:phosphorus ratio <30.
- Serum calcium >14.5 mg/dL without florid HPT.
- Urine calcium >500 mg/24 hrs; urine calcium and phosphorus and renal tubular reabsorption of phosphate are not useful in differential diagnosis.
- Anemia, increased ESR.
- Positive cortisone suppression test in absence of osteitis fibrosa.

*Multiple and repeat tests may be necessary in differential diagnosis of some cases of hypercalcemia. Primary HPT occurs in up to 10% of patients with HHM as well as in those receiving thiazides, or with other causes of hypercalcemia.*

## Hyperparathyroidism, Primary (HPT)

Due to parathyroid adenoma (80%), hyperplasia (15%), carcinoma (<5%); no laboratory test can differentiate these. See Table 13-4 and Fig. 13-7.

Increased serum calcium is hallmark of HPT and first step in diagnosis. Drug-induced hypercalcemia should be reevaluated after discontinuation of drug therapy for 1–2 months; cessation of thiazides may unmask primary HPT. ≤5% of hypercalcemia patients have simultaneous HPT and HHM. Any increased serum calcium must be confirmed by repeat test in fasting state and discontinuance for several days of drugs that may increase serum calcium (e.g., thiazide diuretics). *Serum TP and albumin must always be measured simultaneously, as marked decrease may cause a decrease in calcium.*

Normal calcium level may occur with coexistence of conditions that decrease serum calcium level (e.g., malabsorption, acute pancreatitis, nephrosis, infarction of parathyroid adenoma). High-phosphate intake can abolish increased serum and urine calcium and decreased serum phosphorus; low-phosphate diet unmasks these changes.

Serum PTH concentration is increased; a few patients have only high-normal values. There is considerable overlap of serum PTH levels in normal and HPT patients. Serum calcium must always be measured concurrently, because PTH in the upper-normal range may be inappropriately high in relation to a distinctly increased calcium level, which is consistent with HPT. Blood should always be drawn after 10 AM because of circadian rhythm. PTH >2 times ULN is almost always due to primary HPT. Failure to detect PTH in the presence of simultaneous hypercalcemia militates against the diagnosis of primary HPT and surgical exploration of the parathyroid glands. In general, nonparathyroid disease causing hypercalcemia (e.g., sarcoidosis, vitamin D intoxication, hyperthyroidism, milk-alkali syndrome, most malignancies) will have a normal or low (suppressed) PTH value. Selective catheterization of veins draining the thyroid-parathyroid region for determination of PTH may confirm the diagnosis of HPT due to tumor by showing a significant elevation at one site compared to at least one other site. *A low PTH rules out HPT.*

Serum chloride is increased (>102 mEq/L; <99 mEq/L in other types of hypercalcemia). HPT patients tend toward hyperchloremic (nonanion gap) acidosis, whereas other hypercalcemic patients tend toward alkalosis.

Chloride:phosphorus ratio >33 supports the diagnosis of HPT and <30 contradicts this diagnosis.

**Table 13-3.** Laboratory Findings in Various Diseases of Calcium and Phosphorus Metabolism

| Disease | Serum Calcium[a] | Serum Phosphorus | Serum ALP | Urine Calcium[b] | Urine Phosphorus | Serum PTH | Serum 1,25-Di-hydroxyvitamin D |
|---|---|---|---|---|---|---|---|
| Primary hyper-parathyroidism | I | D (<3 mg/dL in 50%) | I slightly in 50% (N if no bone disease) | I in two-thirds | I | I | I |
| Humoral hypercalcemia of malignancy | I; frequently marked | D in 50% | Frequent | I | I | D | D |
| Familial hypocalciuric hypercalcemia | Mild I | D or slightly I | N | D or low N | | I or inappropri-ately N | Proportional to PTH |
| Hypoparathyroidism | D | I | N | D | D[c] | D | D |
| Pseudohypopara-thyroidism | D | I | N; occasionally D | D | D[c] | N or I | D |
| Pseudopseudohypo-parathyroidism | N | N | N | N | N | N | |
| Secondary hyperpara-thyroidism (renal rickets) | V | I | I or N | D or I | D | I | D |
| Vitamin D excess | I | N | D | I | I | D | I |
| Rickets and osteomalacia | D or N | D or N | I | D | D | D | D |

| | | | | | | |
|---|---|---|---|---|---|---|
| Osteoporosis | N | N | N | N | N or I | N |
| Polyostotic fibrous dysplasia | N | N | N or I | N or I | N | N |
| Paget's disease | N | N or I | I | I | N or I | I |
| Metastatic neoplasm to bone | N or I | V | N or I | N or I | V | I |
| Multiple myeloma | N or I | V | N or I | N or I | N or I | N or I |
| Sarcoidosis | N or I | N or I | N or I | I | I | N | I |
| Fanconi's syndrome or renal loss of fixed base | D or N | D | N or I | N or I | I | I |
| Histiocytosis X (Letterer-Siwe, Hand-Schüller-Christian, eosinophilic granuloma) | N | N | N or I | N or I | N or I | N |
| Hypercalcemia and excess intake of alkali (Burnett's syndrome) | I | I or N | N | N | N | N |
| Solitary bone cyst | N | N | N | N | N | N |

[a]Serum calcium. Repeated determinations may be required to demonstrate abnormalities. Serum TP level should always be known.
[b]Urine calcium. Patient should be on a low-calcium diet (e.g., Bauer-Aub).
[c]See Ellsworth-Howard test under Hypoparathyroidism.

**Table 13-4.** Comparison of Primary Hyperparathyroidism (HPT) and Humoral Hypercalcemia of Malignancy (HHM)

|  | HHM | HPT |
|---|---|---|
| Etiology | Squamous or large-cell carcinoma of bronchus, hypernephroma of kidney, cancer of ovary, colon, others | Primary hyperplasia, adenoma, carcinoma of parathyroids |
| Serum calcium | Very high: >14 mg/dL in 75% of patients<br>Suppressed by cortisone in 25–50% of patients | Moderately high: >14 mg/dL in 25% of patients<br>Suppressed by cortisone in 50% of cases with and 23% of cases without osteitis fibrosa |
| Serum PTH | D | I |
| Serum PTHRP | I | Not I |
| Serum chloride | Low: <99 mEq/L | High: >102 mEq/L |
| Serum chloride-phosphorus ratio | <30 | >33 |
| Serum bicarbonate | I or normal | Normal or low |
| pH | Alkalosis | Acidosis |
| Serum ALP | Increased in 50% of patients, even without bone disease | Seldom increased unless bone disease is present |
| Serum phosphorus | I, normal, or low | Normal or low |
| Urine calcium | Often >400 mg/24 hrs | Usually <400 mg/24 hrs |
| Serum 1,25-dihydroxy-vitamin D | D | I |
| Urine cyclic adenosine monophosphate | Increased in HHM but not due to bone metastases only | Increased in 90% of cases |
| ESR | Usually I | Normal |
| Anemia | May be present | Absent |
| Serum albumin | Often D | Usually normal |
| Renal stones | Absent | Common |
| Pancreatitis | Rare | Occurs |
| X-ray changes in hand bones | Absent | May be present |

PTHRP = parathyroid hormone–related protein.

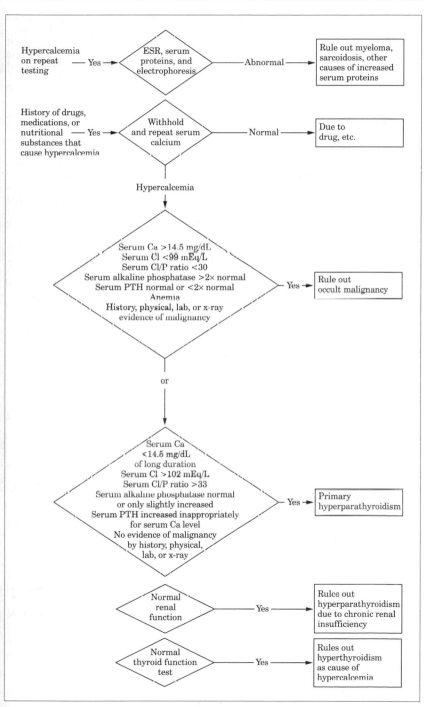

**Fig. 13-7.** Algorithm for diagnosis of hypercalcemia.

Serum phosphorus is decreased (<3 mg/dL) in ~50% of cases. It may be normal in the presence of high phosphorus intake or renal damage with secondary phosphate retention. It may be normal in one-half of patients, even without uremia. Low serum phosphorus supports the diagnosis of primary HPT, an increased level supports the diagnosis of nonparathyroid hypercalcemia, but a normal level is not useful.

Serum ALP is of limited value. Increase >2 times ULN and increased serum LD favors HHM rather than HPT.

Urine calcium is increased (>400 mg on a normal diet; 180 mg on a low-calcium diet); found in 70% of patients with HPT. Urine calcium excretion is often >500 mg/24 hrs in malignancy, sarcoidosis, hyperthyroidism. Is <200 mg/24 hrs in benign familial hypocalciuric hypercalcemia. Lithium-induced hypercalcemia resembles that of familial hypocalciuric hypercalcemia in that both show increased PTH levels and low urine calcium concentrations.

Urine phosphorus is increased unless there is renal insufficiency or phosphate depletion (e.g., antacids containing aluminum). Phosphate loading unmasks the increased urine phosphorus of HPT.

*Serum protein electrophoresis should be performed in HPT to rule out multiple myeloma and sarcoidosis.*

Serum 1,25-dihydroxyvitamin D may be elevated in primary HPT and in sarcoidosis (and other granulomatous diseases) but not in HMM; serum 25-hydroxyvitamin D may be useful to establish vitamin D intoxication.

Urinary cAMP may be high (>4.0 mmol/L) in >90% of cases of primary HPT and of HHM (not increased in hypercalcemia due to osteolytic metastases) but low in vitamin D intoxication and sarcoidosis. Not usually increased in multiple myeloma or other hematologic malignancies. Not widely used.

Uric acid is increased in >15% of patients. Increased uric acid favors hypercalcemia due to thiazides, neoplasm, or renal failure rather than HPT.

Increased ESR is infrequent in HPT.

*HPT must always be ruled out in the presence of*
- Renal colic and stones or calcification (2–3% have HPT)
- Peptic ulcer (occurs in 15% of patients with HPT)
- Calcific keratitis
- Bone changes (present in 20% of patients with HPT)
- Jaw tumors
- Multiple endocrine neoplasia
- Relatives of patients with HPT or "asymptomatic" hypercalcemia

## Hyperparathyroidism, Secondary

Diffuse hyperplasia of parathyroid glands usually secondary to chronic, advanced renal disease

Serum PTH should be monitored to identify autonomous (tertiary) HPT.

Classic findings in renal osteodystrophy are
- Serum calcium is low or normal.
- Serum phosphorus is increased.
- Serum ALP is increased.
- These levels can also be used to monitor response to treatment with calcitriol or alpha-calcidiol.
- Increased serum PTH level is suppressed by 1,25-dihydroxyvitamin D, which can be used to monitor this treatment of chronic renal failure.

## Hypervitaminosis D

Serum calcium may be increased; preceded by hypercalciuria.
Serum phosphorus is normal.
Serum ALP is decreased.
Serum PTH is low or normal.
Urine calcium excretion is increased.

Renal calcinosis may lead to renal insufficiency and uremia.
Serum 25-hydroxyvitamin D is increased.

## Hypoparathyroidism

Serum calcium is decreased (as low as 5 mg/dL) in presence of low or inappro-
priately low PTH and normal serum magnesium, which affects PTH secretion
and action. Hypocalcemia stimulates PTH secretion in pseudohypoparathy-
roidism but not in hypoparathyroidism.
Serum phosphorus is increased (usually 5–6 mg).
Serum ALP may be slightly decreased.
Urine calcium is decreased.
Serum PTH is decreased.
Renal resistance to PTH is shown by Ellsworth-Howard test
   • PTH challenge (IV administration of PTH) causes increased urine phosphate
      (>10 times) and cAMP in normal persons and in primary hypoparathy-
      roidism but little or no increase in urine phosphorus.
   • <2 times increase in urine phosphorus and cAMP in classical type I pseudo-
      hypoparathyroidism or pseudopseudohypoparathyroidism.
   • In type II pseudohypoparathyroidism cAMP increases without phosphaturia.
   • Decreased response may occur in basal cell nevus syndrome.
Alkalosis is present.
Serum uric acid is increased.
CSF is normal.
Hypoparathyroidism should be ruled out in presence of mental and emotional
changes, cataracts, faulty dentition in children, associated changes in skin and
nails (e.g., moniliasis is frequent). One-third of these patients may present as
"epileptics."
Congenital absence may be associated with thymic aplasia (DiGeorge syndrome).

# Tests for Diagnosis of Diabetes Mellitus (DM) and Hypoglycemia

## C-Peptide, Serum

C-peptide is formed during conversion of proinsulin to insulin; C peptide serum
levels correlate with insulin levels in blood, except in islet cell tumors and possibly in obese patients.

### Use

For estimating insulin levels in the presence of antibodies to exogenous insulin
In factitious hypoglycemia due to surreptitious administration of insulin in which
high serum insulin levels will occur with low C-peptide levels

### Increased in

Insulinoma
Type II DM

### Decreased in

Exogenous insulin administration (e.g., factitious hypoglycemia)
Type I DM

## Fructosamine, Serum

Measures concentration of nonlabile glycated serum proteins giving a reliable
estimate of mean blood glucose levels during preceding 1–3 wks

Should primarily be compared with previous values in same patient rather than reference range

Reference range in non-diabetic persons: fructosamine = 2.4–3.4 mmol/L; fructosamine:albumin ratio = 54–86 $\mu$mol/gm)

### Use

To monitor treatment of diabetic patients

### Interpretation

Correlates with Hb A1c but is not affected by abnormal hemoglobins or Hb F or increased RBC turnover and shows changed glucose levels earlier; is cheaper, faster, less subjective than Hb A1c.

### Interferences

Increased serum bilirubin may interfere.

Changes in fructosamine values correlate with significant changes in serum albumin or protein concentrations. Abnormal values also occur during abnormal protein turnover (e.g., thyroid disease) even though patients are normoglycemic. Obviated by using fructose:albumin ratio.

## Glycohemoglobin (Glycated Hemoglobin), Serum

May be reported as Hb A1c or as A1b, A1a, or A1c.

Different methodologies and different laboratories may not be comparable.

Glycosylated Hb will be proportional to mean plasma glucose level during previous 6–12 wks.

Glycosylated albumin has been used for monitoring degree of hyperglycemia during previous 1–2 wks.

### Use

*Monitor diabetic patients' compliance and long-term blood glucose level control.*
In known diabetics
- 7% indicates good diabetic control
- 10% indicates fair diabetic control
- 13–20% indicates poor diabetic control

### Interpretation

Does not require dietary preparation or fasting. Has low sensitivity but high specificity. Increase almost certainly means DM if other factors are absent (>3 standard deviations [SD] above the mean has 99% specificity and ~48% sensitivity), but a normal level does not rule out impaired glucose tolerance. Values less than normal mean are not seen in untreated diabetes. May rise within 1 wk after rise in blood glucose due to stopping therapy but may not fall for 2–4 wks after blood glucose falls when therapy is resumed.

### Normal ($A_{1a}$, $A_{1b}$, $A_{1c}$) = 4–8%

For level of 4–20%, this formula may estimate daily average plasma glucose:
Mean daily plasma glucose (mg/dL) = 10 × (glycohemoglobin level + 4)

### Increased in

Hb F > normal or 0.5%
Chronic renal failure with or without hemodialysis
Iron deficiency anemia
Splenectomy
Increased serum triglycerides
Alcohol
Lead toxicity

### Decreased in

(shortened RBC life span)
Hemolytic anemias
Presence of Hb S, Hb C, Hb D
Congenital spherocytosis
Acute or chronic blood loss
Pregnancy

## Insulin, Serum

### Use

Diagnosis of insulinoma

### Increased in

Insulinoma. Fasting blood insulin level >50 U/mL in presence of low or normal blood
glucose level. IV tolbutamide or administration of leucine causes rapid rise of
blood insulin to very high levels within a few mins with rapid return to normal.
Factitious hypoglycemia
Insulin autoimmune syndrome
Untreated obese mild diabetics. The fasting level is often increased.
Acromegaly (especially with active disease) after ingestion of glucose.
Reactive hypoglycemia after glucose ingestion, particularly when diabetic type
of glucose tolerance curve is present
Not useful for diagnosis of DM

### Absent in

Severe DM with ketosis and weight loss. In less severe cases, insulin is frequently
present but only at lower glucose concentrations.

### Normal in

Hypoglycemia associated with nonpancreatic tumors
Idiopathic hypoglycemia of childhood, except after administration of leucine

## Insulin:C-Peptide Ratio, Serum

### Use

To differentiate insulinoma from factitious hypoglycemia due to insulin

### Interpretation

<1.0 in molarity units (or <47.17 $\mu$g/ng in conventional units)
  • Increased endogenous insulin secretion (e.g., insulinoma, sulfonylurea
    administration)
  • Renal failure
>1.0 in molarity units
  • Exogenous insulin administration
  • Cirrhosis

## Proinsulin, Serum

Proinsulin level is normally ≤ 20% of total insulin. Proinsulin is included in the
immunoassay of total insulin and separation requires special technique.

### Increased in

Insulinoma. Proinsulin >30% of serum insulin after overnight fast suggests
insulinoma.

Factitious hypoglycemia due to sulfonylurea
Familial hyperproinsulinemia—heterozygous mutation affecting cleavage of proinsulin leading to secretion of excess amounts of proinsulin

### Interferences

May also be increased in renal disease.

## Tolerance Test, Glucose, Oral (OGTT)

Standards for OGTT: Prior diet of >150 gm of carbohydrate daily, no alcohol, and unrestricted activity for 3 days before test. Test in morning after 10–16 hrs of fasting. No medication, smoking, or exercise (remain seated) during test. Not to be done during recovery from acute illness, emotional stress, surgery, trauma, pregnancy, inactivity due to chronic illness; therefore, is of limited or no value in hospitalized patients. Certain drugs should be stopped several weeks before the test (e.g., oral diuretics, oral contraceptives, phenytoin).

### Use

OGTT should be reserved principally for patients with "borderline" fasting plasma glucose levels (i.e., fasting range 110–140 mg/dL).
Pregnant women should be tested for gestational diabetes with a 50-gm dose at 24–28 wks of pregnancy; if that is abnormal, OGTT should be performed after pregnancy.
OGTT is not indicated in
- Persistent fasting blood glucose >140 mg/dL or <110 mg/dL.
- Patients with typical clinical findings of DM and random plasma glucose >200 mg/dL.
- Suspected gestational diabetes.
- Secondary diabetes (e.g., genetic hyperglycemic syndromes, after administration of certain hormones).
- Should never be done to evaluate reactive hypoglycemia.
- Limited value in children and is rarely indicated for that purpose.

### Interpretation

For diagnosis of DM in nonpregnant adults, at least two values of OGTT should be increased (or fasting serum glucose ≥ 140 mg/dL on more than one occasion) and other causes of transient glucose intolerance must be ruled out.

### Decreased Tolerance in

Excessive peak
- Increased absorption
- Mechanical (e.g., gastrectomy, gastroenterostomy)
- Hyperthyroidism
- Excess intake of glucose
Decreased utilization with slow fall to fasting level
- DM
- Hyperlipidemia, types III, IV, V
- Hemochromatosis
- Steroid effect (Cushing's disease, administration of ACTH or steroids)
- CNS lesions
Decreased formation of glycogen with low fasting levels and subsequent hypoglycemia
- von Gierke's disease
- Severe liver damage
- Hyperthyroidism (normal return to fasting level)
- Increased epinephrine (stress, pheochromocytoma) (normal return to fasting level)
- Pregnancy (normal return to fasting level)

### Increased Tolerance in

Flat peak
- Pancreatic islet cell hyperplasia or tumor
- Poor absorption from GI tract (normal IV GTT curve)
- Intestinal diseases (e.g., steatorrhea, sprue, celiac disease, Whipple's disease)
- Hypothyroidism
- Addison's disease
- Hypoparathyroidism

Late hypoglycemia
- Pancreatic islet cell hyperplasia or tumor
- Hypopituitarism
- Liver disease

## Tolerance Test, Insulin

Administer insulin IV. *Use smaller dose if hypopituitarism is suspected. Always keep IV glucose available to prevent severe reaction.*

### Normal

Blood glucose falls to 50% of fasting level within 20–30 mins; returns to fasting level within 90–120 mins.

### Increased Tolerance

Blood glucose falls <25% and returns rapidly to fasting level.
Hypothyroidism
Acromegaly
Cushing's syndrome
DM (some patients)

### Decreased Tolerance

Increased sensitivity to insulin (excessive fall of blood glucose)
Hypoglycemic unresponsiveness (lack of response by glycogenolysis)
- Pancreatic islet cell tumor
- Adrenocortical insufficiency
- Adrenocortical insufficiency secondary to hypopituitarism
- Hypothyroidism
- von Gierke's disease (some patients)
- Starvation (depletion of liver glycogen)

## Tolerance Test, Tolbutamide

Administer sodium tolbutamide IV within 2 mins. *Always keep IV glucose available to prevent severe reaction.*

### Use

Diagnosis of insulinoma and to rule out functional hyperinsulinism

### Interpretation

In normal persons, glucose is a more potent stimulus for insulin release than tolbutamide, but the opposite is true in insulinoma, which shows an exaggerated early insulin peak (3–5 mins after injection), with a sustained elevation of insulin and depression of glucose at 150 mins.

In insulinoma, the fall in blood sugar is usually more marked than in functional hypoglycemia; more important, the blood sugar fails to recover even after 2–3 hrs. A mean serum glucose at 120, 150, 180 mins after tolbutamide ≤ 55 mg/dL in lean patients and 62 mg/dL in obese patients has 95% specificity and sensitivity for insulinoma; this is the most useful test.

In functional hypoglycemia, return of blood sugar to normal is usually complete by 90 mins.
Adrenal insufficiency—normal or low curve
Severe liver disease—low curve

# Diabetes Mellitus and Other Hyperglycemic and Hypoglycemic Disorders

## Diabetes Mellitus and Other Hyperglycemic Disorders, Classification

I. Type 1: Immune-mediated beta-cell destruction DM (formerly called *insulin-dependent* [IDDM], *juvenile-onset, ketosis-prone* or *brittle DM*): represents 10–20% of diabetic patients. Autoantibodies are present in 85–90% of cases. Insulin secretion is virtually absent. Plasma C-peptide low or undetectable. Other autoimmune disorders may be present (e.g., Graves' disease, Hashimoto's thyroiditis, Addison's disease, pernicious anemia). Idiopathic diabetes: 10–15% of cases; not due to autoimmunity; no autoantibodies; strongly inherited.

II. Type 2: (formerly called *non-insulin–dependent type* [NIDDM] or *adult-onset DM*: represents 80–90% of diabetic patients. Varies from predominantly insulin resistance with relative deficiency to predominantly insulin secretory defect with insulin resistance. Relative rather than absolute insulin deficiency. Not due to autoimmunity or other disorders in following list. Plasma insulin may be normal or increased but expected to be higher relative to blood glucose concentration. Ketosis occurs with stress (e.g., infection) but seldom spontaneously. Associated with dyslipidemia, obesity, increasing age, hypertension, and family history.

III. Other Specific Types
   A. Genetic defects of beta cell function (e.g., chromosome 7, 12, 20). Formerly referred to as *maturity-onset diabetes of the young*. Onset of mild hyperglycemia usually before age 25 yrs, impaired insulin secretion, autosomal dominant inheritance
   B. Genetic defects in insulin resistance (e.g., leprechaunism, type A insulin resistance, Rabson-Mendenhall syndrome, lipoatrophic diabetes)
   C. Diseases of exocrine pancreas (e.g., pancreatitis, pancreatectomy, neoplasia, cystic fibrosis, hemochromatosis)
   D. Endocrine disorders (e.g., Cushing's syndrome, acromegaly, pheochromocytoma, aldosteronoma, hyperthyroidism, glucagonoma)
   E. Drug/chemical induced (e.g., glucocorticoids, phenytoin [Dilantin], beta-adrenergic agonists, pentamidine, thiazides, alpha-interferon)
   F. Infections (e.g., cytomegalovirus, congenital rubella)
   G. Uncommon forms of immune-mediated diabetes (e.g., anti-insulin receptor antibodies, "stiff-man" syndrome)
   H. Other genetic syndromes that may be associated with DM (e.g., Down syndrome, Klinefelter's syndrome, Turner's syndrome, Friedreich's ataxia, Huntington's chorea, Laurence-Moon-Biedl syndrome, porphyria, Prader-Willi syndrome)
   I. Gestational DM (see Diabetes Mellitus, Gestational)

### Criteria for Diagnosis

**DM**
   • Random glucose >200 mg/dL when there are classical symptoms.
or
   • Fasting (>8 hrs) serum glucose >126 mg/dL.
or
   • 2-hr glucose >200 mg/dL after 75-gm glucose load (OGTT). OGTT not recommended for routine use.
   • Must be confirmed on another day by any of the above.

- Fasting blood glucose ≥ 126 mg/dL gives provisional diagnosis of DM; must be confirmed as noted under Tolerance Test, Glucose, Oral (OGTT).

### Impaired Glucose Tolerance (IGT)

- Fasting glucose ≥ 110 mg/dL but < 126 mg/dL in nonpregnant adult.
- With OGTT 2-hr value ≥ 140 and < 200 mg/dL. Replaces terms "latent" or "chemical" diabetes.

### Impaired Fasting Glucose (IFG)

- Fasting glucose ≥ 110 mg/dL but < 126 mg/dL, or
- With OGTT 2-hr value ≥ 140 but < 200 mg/dL.

In absence of pregnancy, IGT and IFG are risk factors for future DM and cardiovascular disease; not clinical entities.

*Other causes of transient glucose intolerance must be ruled out before an unequivocal diagnosis of DM is made.*

Test asymptomatic undiagnosed individuals older than age 45 every 3 yrs.

Test at younger age if
- HDL cholesterol ≤ 35 mg/dL or triglyceride ≥ 250 mg/dL
- Previous IGT or IFG
- Obese
- First-degree relative with DM
- High risk ethnic population (e.g., African-American, Native-American, Hispanic)
- Delivered baby weighing >9 pounds

See Table 13-5 (diabetic nephrosclerosis), and Chapters 12 (serum lipoproteins) and 16 (papillary necrosis and GU tract infection).

## Diabetes Mellitus, Gestational

Hyperglycemia that develops for the first time during pregnancy; affects ~4% of pregnant women; most will return to normal glucose tolerance after delivery. 60% become diabetic in next 16 yrs.

Diagnosis is necessary for short-term identification of increased risk of fetal morbidity (stillbirth, macrosomia, birth trauma, hypoglycemia, hyperbilirubinemia, hypocalcemia, polycythemia).

Screening of all pregnant women should include
- Random venous blood glucose 1 hr after ingestion of 50 gm of glucose at 24–28 wks' gestation. Values >140 mg/dL are indication for 3-hr 100-gm glucose GTT. 1 hr, 50-gm test is abnormal in ~15% of pregnant women, ~14% of whom have abnormal 3-hr OTT. Sensitivity ~79%, specificity ~87%.

Diagnosis is made if at least two of the following glucose plasma levels are found on OGTT with 100-gm glucose loading dose (see Tolerance Test, Glucose, Oral [OGTT]):

| | |
|---|---|
| Fasting | ≥ 105 mg/dL |
| 1 hr | ≥ 190 mg/dL |
| 2 hrs | ≥ 165 mg/dL |
| 3 hrs | ≥ 145 mg/dL |

If abnormal results during pregnancy, repeat GTT at first postpartum visit; if GTT is normal, diagnose as DM only during pregnancy, but blood glucose should be tested at every subsequent visit because of increased risk of developing DM. If postpartum GTT is abnormal, classify as IGT, IFG, or DM using the preceding criteria.

Glycosylated Hb and fructosamine are not recommended tests for detection of gestational diabetes.

For management of DM during pregnancy, goal is fasting plasma glucose of 60–110 mg/dL and postprandial levels < 150 mg/dL. Measure serum or 24-hr urine estriol for fetal surveillance. Amniotic fluid lecithin:spingomyelin ratio,

**Table 13-5.** Evolution of Renal Disease in Insulin-Dependent Diabetes Mellitus

| Stage | Time of Onset | Laboratory Findings* | Morphologic Findings | % of Cases That Progress |
|---|---|---|---|---|
| Early | At time of diagnosis | I GFR | Kidney size I | 100 |
| Renal lesions; no clinical signs | 2–3 yrs after diagnosis | I GFR; albuminuria cannot be detected | I thickness of glomerular and tubular capillary basement membrane; glomerulosclerosis | 35–40 |
| Incipient nephropathy | 7–15 yrs after diagnosis | Albuminuria 0.03–0.3 gm/day; or N or sl I GFR; beginning to decline | Glomerulosclerosis progressing | 80–100 |
| Clinical diabetic nephropathy | 10–30 yrs after diagnosis | Albuminuria >0.3 gm/day. N or sl D GFR; steady fall | Glomerulosclerosis widespread | >75 |
| End-stage renal disease | 20–40 yrs after diagnosis | GFR <10 mL/min. Serum creatinine ≥ 10 mg/dL | | |

sl = slightly.
*When albuminuria is 0.075–0.100 gm/day in insulin-dependent diabetes mellitus, there is significant renal disease and albuminuria will progress to clinical nephropathy. GFR declines ~10 mL/min/yr after nephropathy is established.

phosphatidylglycerol, shake test, or fluorescence polarization to evaluate fetal pulmonary maturity.

During labor, keep maternal glucose at 80–100 mg/dL; beware of markedly increased insulin sensitivity in immediate postpartum period.

## Diabetic Ketoacidosis (DKA)

See Table 13-6.

Blood glucose is increased (usually >300 mg/dL); range from slightly increased to very high. Very elevated glucose (>500–800 mg/dL) suggests nonketotic hyperosmolar hyperglycemia (because glucose levels become very high only when extracellular fluid volume is markedly decreased). Glucose <200 mg/dL may occur, especially in alcoholics or pregnant insulin-dependent diabetics. Glucose concentration is not related to severity of DKA.

Plasma acetone is increased (4+ reaction when plasma is diluted 1:1 with water). (Acetone is usually 3–4 times the concentration of acetoacetate but does not contribute to acidosis.) Nitroprusside reagent tests (e.g., Acetest [Miles, Inc., Elkhart, IN], Chemstrip [Boehringer Mannheim Corp., Indianapolis, IN]) react with acetoacetate, not with beta-hydroxybutyrate, and weakly with acetone; therefore, weak positive reaction with ketone does not rule out ketoacidosis. Beta-hydroxybutyrate:acetoacetate ratio varies from 3:1 in mild up to 15:1 in severe DKA. With correction of DKA, conversion of beta-hydroxybutyrate to acetoacetate gives a stronger nitroprusside test reaction; *do not mistake this for worsening of DKA.*

Metabolic acidosis (pH <7.3 and/or bicarbonate <15 mEq/L) is mainly due to beta-hydroxybutyrate and acetoacetate. Some lactic acidosis may exist, especially if shock, sepsis, or tissue necrosis is present; suspect this if pH and anion gap do not respond to insulin therapy. Whole spectrum of patterns from pure hyperchloremic acidosis to wide anion gap acidosis. May be obscured by complicating metabolic alkalosis.

Volume and electrolyte depletion (due to glucose-induced osmotic diuresis)

- Absence of volume depletion should arouse suspicion of other possibilities (e.g., hypoglycemic coma, other causes of coma).
- Very low sodium (120 mEq/L) is usually due to hypertriglyceridemia and hyperosmolality, although occasionally may be dilutional due to vomiting and water intake.
- Serum potassium is normal or increased due to potassium exit from cells secondary to acidosis; initial low potassium indicates severe depletion.
- Serum phosphate is usually increased, falls with onset of therapy. Excessive replacement may cause hypocalcemia and hypomagnesemia.
- Serum magnesium is usually increased.

Azotemia is present (BUN is usually 25–30 mg/dL); creatinine may be proportionally increased >BUN due to methodologic interference by acetoacetate.

Serum osmolality is slightly increased (≤ 340 mOsm/L).

WBC is increased (often >20,000/cu mm) even without infection; associated with decreased lymphocytes and eosinophils.

Hb, Hct, and TP may be increased due to intravascular volume depletion.

Serum amylase may be increased.

Serum AST, ALT, LD, and CK may be increased.

Precipitating medical problem should be sought.

Follow up lab tests every 2–4 hrs initially and less often with clinical improvement. Bedside fingerstick glucose can be determined initially every 30–60 mins to determine rate of fall of glucose and when to add glucose to IV fluids.

ESR may be increased in diabetic patients even in absence of infection.

## Hyperosmolar Hyperglycemic Nonketotic Coma
**(due to combination of severe dehydration caused by inadequate fluid intake and insulin deficiency; occurs predominantly in type II DM)**

See Tables 13-6 and 13-7.

**Table 13-6.** Differential Diagnosis of Diabetic Coma

| Condition | Serum Glucose (mg/dL) | Serum Ketones (undiluted) | Blood pH | Serum Osmolality (mOsm/kg) | Serum Lactate (mmol/L) | Plasma Insulin |
|---|---|---|---|---|---|---|
| Diabetic ketoacidosis | 300–1000 | + + + + | D | 300–350 | 2–3 | 0–L |
| Lactic acidosis | 100–200 | 0 | D | N–300 | ≥ 7 | L |
| Alcoholic ketoacidosis | 40–200 | + + + + | D | 290–310 | 2–6 | L |
| Hyperosmolar coma | 500–2000 | 0/+ | N | 320–400 | 1–2 | Some |
| Hypoglycemia | 10–40 | 0 | N | 285 ± 6 | Low | I |

L = low; 0 = none; + = small amount; + + + + = large amount. Normal serum lactate = 0.6–1.1 mmol/L.
*Lactic acidosis occurs in one-third of patients with diabetic ketoacidosis.*
*Hyperosmolar coma and alcoholic ketoacidosis may occur in diabetic ketoacidosis.*

**Table 13-7.** Comparison of Diabetic Ketoacidosis and Hyperosmolar Hyperglycemic Nonketotic Coma

|  | Diabetic Ketoacidosis | Hyperosmolar Hyperglycemic Nonketotic Coma |
|---|---|---|
| **Laboratory findings** | | |
| Serum glucose | Usually <800 mg/dL | >800 mg/dL |
| Plasma acetone | Positive in diluted plasma | Less positive in undiluted plasma |
| Serum sodium | Usually low | Normal, I, or low |
| Serum potassium | Normal, I, or low | Normal or I |
| Serum $HCO_3^-$ | <10 mEq/L | >16 mEq/L |
| Anion gap | >12 mEq/L | 10–12 mEq/L |
| Blood pH | <7.35 | Normal |
| Serum osmolality | <330 mOsm/L | >350 mOsm/L |
| Serum BUN | Not as high | Higher |
| Blood free fatty acids | >1500 mEq/L | <1000 mEq/L |
| **Clinical findings** | | |
| Dehydration | Less | More |
| Acidosis | More | Less |
| Coma | Rare | Frequent |
| Hyperventilation | Yes | No |
| Age | Younger | Usually elderly |
| Diabetes type | I—insulin dependent | II—non-insulin dependent |
| Previous history of diabetes | Almost always | 50% of cases |
| Prodrome | <1 day | Several days |
| Neurologic findings | Rare | Very common |
| Cardiovascular or renal disease | 15% | 85% |
| Thrombosis | Very rare | Frequent |
| Mortality | <10% | 20–50% |

Blood glucose is very high, often 600–2000 mg/dL, but contrary to expectation in diabetic coma, acidosis and ketosis are minimal and plasma acetone is not found.

Serum osmolality is very high (normal = 280–300 mOsm/L).

Serum sodium may be increased, normal, or decreased but is disproportionately decreased for degree of dehydration due to marked hyperglycemia (artifactual decrease 1.6 mEq/L for every 100 mg/dL increase of serum glucose). Increased sodium with marked hyperglycemia indicates severe dehydration.

Serum potassium may be increased (due to hyperosmolality), low (due to osmotic diuresis with urinary loss), or normal depending on balance of factors.

BUN is increased (70–90 mg/dL) more than diabetic ketoacidosis.

Laboratory findings due to complications or precipitating factors
* Renal insufficiency in 90% of cases
* Infection (e.g., pneumonia)
* Drugs (e.g., steroids, phenytoin, potassium-wasting diuretics such as thiazides and furosemide, others [propranolol, diazoxide, azathioprine])
* Other medical conditions (e.g., cerebrovascular or cardiovascular accident, subdural hematoma, severe burns, acute pancreatitis, thyrotoxicosis, Cushing's syndrome)

## Hypoglycemia, Classification

Diagnosis requires triad of low blood glucose at the time of spontaneous hypoglycemic symptoms and alleviation by administration of glucose that corrects hypoglycemia. *(Glucose concentration is 15% lower in whole blood than in serum or plasma.)*

Reactive (i.e., after eating)
* Alimentary (rapid gastric emptying [e.g., after subtotal gastrectomy, vagotomy])
* Impaired glucose tolerance as in DM (mild maturity-onset)
* Functional (idiopathic)
* Rare conditions (e.g., hereditary fructose intolerance, galactosemia)

Fasting (spontaneous)—almost always indicates organic disease
* Liver—severe parenchymal disease (including sepsis, congestive heart failure, Reye's syndrome) or enzyme defect (e.g., glycogen storage diseases, galactosemia)
* Chronic renal insufficiency
* Pancreatic
    Insulinoma (pancreatic islet cell tumor)
    MEN I
    Pancreatic hyperplasia
* Deficiency of hormones that oppose insulin (e.g., decreased function of thyroid, anterior pituitary, or adrenal cortex)
* Postoperative removal of pheochromocytoma
* Large extrapancreatic tumors (e.g., intra- or retroperitoneal)
* Certain epithelial tumors (e.g., hepatoma, carcinoid, Wilms' tumor)
* Drugs (including factitious)
    Insulin
    Sulfonylureas
    Alcohol
    Salicylates
    Pentamidine
    Quinine
    Propranolol (rare)
    Others may potentiate effect of sulfonylurea (e.g., sulfonamides, butazones, coumarins, clofibrate)
* Artifactual (high WBC or RBC count, e.g., leukemia or polycythemia)
* Starvation, anorexia nervosa, lactic acidosis, intense exercise
* Insulin antibodies or insulin receptor antibodies

Combined reactive and fasting types
- Insulinoma
- Adrenal insufficiency
- Insulin antibodies or insulin receptor antibodies

### *Infants*

### Transient
### (<14 days' duration)
- Maternal (e.g., diabetes, toxemia, complicated labor or delivery)
- Infant
  Prematurity, small size for gestational age
  Intrauterine malnutrition
  Erythroblastosis
  Secondary (e.g., sepsis, asphyxia, anoxia, cerebral or subdural hemorrhage)
  Congenital anomalies
  Iatrogenic (e.g., postoperative complications, abrupt cessation of glucose infusion, after exchange transfusion, cold injury)

### Persistent
Hyperinsulinism
- Beta-cell hyperplasia
- Nesidioblastosis
- Beckwith-Wiedemann syndrome
- Beta-cell tumor
- Teratoma

Endocrine disorder
- Hypothyroidism
- Congenital adrenal hyperplasia
- Anterior pituitary hypofunction
- Decreased glucagon

Hepatic enzyme deficiencies
- Glycogen storage diseases I, III, VI, 0
- Congenital fructose intolerance
- Galactose-1-phosphate deficiency
- Maple syrup urine disease
- Galactosemia
- Hereditary tyrosinemia
- Methylmalonic acidemia
- Propionicacidemia

## Endocrine-Secreting Tumors of Pancreas

| Cell Type | Hormone Secreted | Tumor |
| --- | --- | --- |
| B cell | Insulin | Insulinoma |
| D cell | Gastrin | Gastrinoma |
| A cell | Glucagon | Glucagonoma |
| H cell | VIP | Vipoma |
| D cell | Somatostatin | Somatostatinoma |
| Human pancreatic polypeptide (HPP) cell | HPP | HPP-secreting tumor (very rare) |

Other rare endocrine-secreting tumors have been identified as causing ectopic ACTH syndrome, atypical carcinoid syndrome, SIADH, ectopic hypercalcemia syndrome.

### *Islet Cell Tumors of Pancreas*

Insulin-secreting beta-cell tumor (benign or malignant, primary or metastatic) produces hyperinsulinism with hypoglycemia.

Non–insulin-secreting non–beta-cell tumor (benign or malignant, primary or metastatic) may produce several types of syndromes.
- Z-E syndrome.
- Profuse diarrhea with hypokalemia and dehydration.
- Profuse diarrhea with hypokalemia may occur as a separate syndrome without peptic ulceration. *(Some patients have histamine-fast achlorhydria.)* May be associated with MEN.
- Nonspecific diarrhea.
- Steatorrhea (due to inactivation of pancreatic enzymes by acid pH).

### Insulinoma
*(tumor of pancreatic islet beta-cell origin; ~5% are malignant; 5–10% may have MEN I)*

See Fig. 13-8.
*In patients with fasting hypoglycemia, insulinoma should be considered the cause until another diagnosis can be proved.* No single test is certain to be diagnostic.
Fasting 24–36 hrs will provoke hypoglycemia in ≤ 90% of these patients; 72 hrs of fasting will provoke hypoglycemia in >95% of these patients, especially if punctuated with exercise. Absence of ketonuria implies surreptitious food intake or excess insulin effect (differentiate by blood glucose level). Low serum glucose and high serum insulin establishes the diagnosis, i.e., insulin level is inappropriately elevated for the degree of hypoglycemia (in normal persons, insulin level becomes <5 $\mu$U/mL or undetectable). *Serum insulin rarely reaches these high levels in patients with reactive hypoglycemia.* Serum C-peptide is similarly inappropriately elevated in contrast to factitious hypoglycemia. In women, serum glucose during fasting can fall to 20–30 mg/dL and return to normal without treatment; in men, a fall in serum glucose to <50 mg/dL is considered abnormal.
Serum insulin:C-peptide ratio <1.0 in molarity units
Proinsulin level is normally ≤ 20% of total insulin; increased in insulinoma.
Proinsulin >30% of serum insulin after overnight fast suggests insulinoma. (May also be increased in renal disease.) *(Proinsulin is included in the immunoassay of total insulin and separation requires special technique.)*
Serum insulin values are not useful in reactive hypoglycemia but should always be performed in cases of fasting hypoglycemia.
Occasional patients with insulinoma have very low serum insulin levels; their serum shows very high proinsulin level that interferes with the insulin immunoassay, giving falsely low values.
Serum insulin:glucose ratio >0.3 when serum glucose >50 mg/dL indicates inappropriate hyperinsulinism, and this usually indicates insulinoma if factitious hypoglycemia is ruled out. Has no diagnostic value in insulinoma.
Stimulation tests are usually not necessary and may be dangerous if serum glucose <50 mg/dL. Too many false-positive and false-negative results make these tests unreliable.
- Tolbutamide tolerance test.
- Glucagon stimulation test: After glucagon IV serum insulin is measured at intervals. Patients with insulinoma show an exaggerated response of serum immunoreactive insulin. Serum insulin >100 $\mu$/mL after glucagon stimulation in a patient with fasting hypoglycemia and inappropriate insulin secretion strongly suggests insulinoma.
- Infusion of exogenous insulin to reduce serum glucose level will also suppress the secretion of insulin and of C-peptide in normal persons but not in patients with insulinoma. C-peptide level usually remains elevated if insulinoma is present (C-peptide is also not suppressed in islet cell hyperplasia and nesidioblastosis) but falls to very low level if beta-cell function is normal.
- Oral glucose tolerance test is useless for diagnosis.

### Zollinger-Ellison (Z-E) Syndrome (Gastrinoma)

Increased basal serum gastrin. >500 pg/mL (normal <100 pg/mL) is highly suggestive for gastrinoma in absence of achlorhydria or renal failure. <100 pg/mL

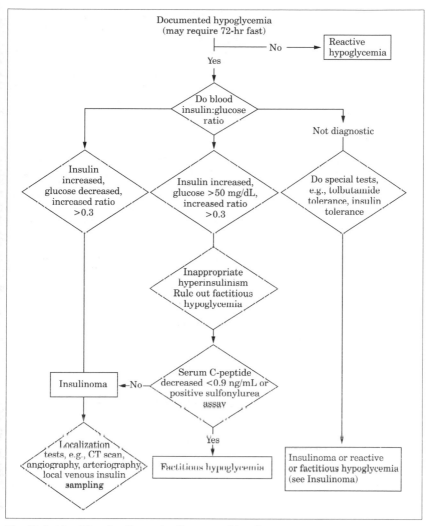

**Fig. 13-8.** Algorithm for diagnosis of suspected insulinoma.

is unlikely to be gastrinoma. 100–500 pg/mL occurs in ~40% of gastrinoma patients and ~10% of ulcer patients without gastrinoma. If fasting serum gastrin is increased but <1000 pg/mL, secretin-provocative test and acid secretory rate should be performed.

IV injection of secretin is the most sensitive and accurate provocative test. This will provoke an increase of serum gastrin ≥ 110 pg/mL within 10 mins. Some ulcer patients may increase serum gastrin ≤ 200 pg/mL. Serum gastrin decreases in most nongastrinoma patients. Postoperative fasting serum gastrin and secretin are both necessary to determine cure.

Other provocative tests, such as IV injection of calcium gluconate or a standard test meal, are not as sensitive or specific as secretin test. Response after calcium infusion is positive if serum gastrin ≥ 395 pg/mL.

There is a large volume of highly acid gastric juice in the absence of pyloric obstruction. (12-Hr nocturnal secretion shows acid of >100 mEq/L and volume of >1500 mL; baseline secretion is >60% of the secretion caused by histamine or betazole stimulation.) It is refractory to vagotomy and subtotal gastrectomy. Hypochlorhydria or achlorhydria excludes diagnosis of Z-E syndrome.

Basal acid output >15 mEq/hr (normal <10 mEq/hr) occurs in 90% of cases if no previous gastric surgery was performed or >5 mEq/hr if previous vagotomy or gastric resection was performed. pH >3 excludes Z-E syndrome if patient is not on antisecretory drugs. Fasting serum gastrin >1000 pg/mL and gastric pH <2.5 almost certainly indicates Z-E syndrome; both should be measured because there may be a poor correlation between them in individual patients.

Hypokalemia is frequently associated with chronic severe diarrhea that may be a clue to this diagnosis.

Serum albumin may be decreased.

*Clues to Z-E syndrome are ulcers in unusual locations or giant or multiple ulcerations, rapid or severe recurrence of ulcer after adequate therapy or surgery, prominent gastric folds, gastric acid hypersecretion with hypergastrinemia, family history of peptic ulcer or ulcers with other endocrine disorders, duodenal ulcers without* Helicobacter pylori.

Gastrinomas (non–beta-cell tumors often arising in pancreas) *are malignant* in 62% of patients.

*Diffuse hyperplasia occurs in 10% of patients.*

*MEN I should be ruled out in all patients with Z-E syndrome, which may be the initial manifestation of MEN I. 25% of cases of this syndrome are associated with MEN I. 40–60% of patients with MEN-I have Z-E syndrome.*

# Laboratory Tests for Evaluation of Adrenal-Pituitary Function

See Fig. 13-9.

Increased function is tested by suppression tests, and decreased function is tested by stimulatory tests.

Cortisol measurements have largely replaced other steroid determinations in diagnosis of Cushing's syndrome.

## Adrenocorticotropic Hormone (ACTH), Plasma

### Decreased in

Cushing's syndrome due to adrenal tumor (usually <5 pg/mL)
Factitious Cushing's syndrome
Secondary adrenal insufficiency

### Increased in

Pituitary Cushing's disease (usually >10 pg/mL)
Cushing's syndrome due to ectopic ACTH syndrome (e.g., carcinoma of lung)
Primary adrenal insufficiency

## Adrenocorticotropic Hormone Stimulation (Cosyntropin) Test

### Use

Differential diagnosis of adrenal insufficiency
Not helpful in diagnosis of Cushing's syndrome

### Rapid Screening Test

Administer synthetic ACTH (cosyntropin) and measure plasma cortisol levels baseline and at intervals. If response is abnormal, perform long test.

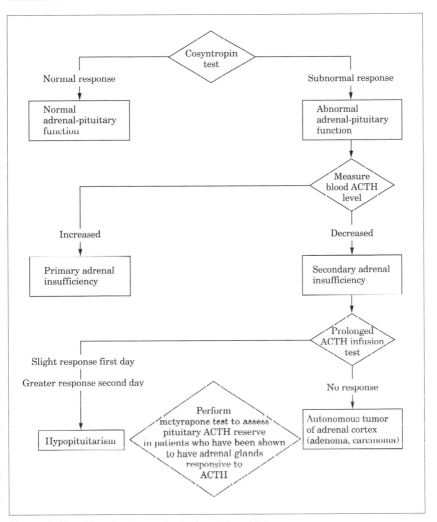

**Fig. 13-9.** Algorithm for diagnosis of adrenal insufficiency.

## Interpretation

Normal—baseline plasma cortisol >5.0 $\mu$g/dL with increase to 2 times baseline level $\geq$ 20 $\mu$g/dL is sufficient criterion of normal adrenal function to preclude need for further work-up.

Addison's disease—is ruled out by a positive response.

Hypopituitarism—a slight increase is shown the first day and a greater increase the next day.

Adrenal carcinoma—little or no response

Adrenal hyperplasia increases 3–5 times baseline level.

### *Long Test*

Daily infusion of ACTH for 5 days, with before and after measurement of serum cortisol, 24-hr urine for cortisol. (Protect possible Addison's disease patient against adrenal crisis with dexamethasone.)

### Interpretation

Normal—at least 3 times increase with maximum > upper reference value
Complete primary adrenal insufficiency (Addison's disease)—increase of <2 mg/day
Incomplete primary adrenal insufficiency—less than normal increases on all 5 days or slight increase on first 3 days that may be followed by decrease on days 4 and 5
Secondary adrenal insufficiency (due to pituitary hypofunction)—"staircase" response of progressively higher values each day (delayed but normal response)
Adrenal insufficiency due to chronic steroid therapy—may require prolonged ACTH testing to elicit the staircase response.
Congenital adrenal hyperplasia.

## Aldosterone, Plasma

### Use

Diagnosis of primary hyperaldosteronism
Differential diagnosis of fluid and electrolyte disorders
Assessment of adrenal aldosterone production

### Increased in

Primary aldosteronism
Secondary aldosteronism
Bartter's syndrome
Pregnancy
Very-low-sodium diet
Urine aldosterone is also increased in nephrosis.

### Decreased in

Hyporeninemic hypoaldosteronism
Congenital adrenal hyperplasia
Congenital deficiency of aldosterone synthetase
Addison's disease
Very-high-sodium diet

## Androstenedione, Serum
**(also produced by testes and ovaries)**

### Use

Diagnosis of virilism and hirsutism

### Increased in

Congenital adrenal hyperplasia due to 21-hydroxylase deficiency; marked increase is suppressed to normal levels by adequate glucocorticoid therapy. Suppressed level reflects adequacy of therapeutic control.
Adrenal tumors
Cushing's disease
Polycystic ovarian disease

### Decreased in

Addison's disease

## Corticotropin-Releasing Hormone (CRH) Stimulation Test

CRH is given IV; blood is drawn at intervals for ACTH and cortisol. Comparison of ACTH concentration from both inferior petrosal sinuses and peripheral vein after CRH stimulation. Use of only peripheral plasma ACTH and cortisol has little value.

## Use

Differentiates pituitary and nonpituitary causes of Cushing's syndrome, especially ectopic ACTH production; sensitivity, specificity, accuracy approach 100%. Different values between right and left petrosal sinuses suggests on which side tumor is located. Especially useful when the high-dose dexamethasone suppression test is equivocal or when biochemical data indicate a pituitary source but radiographic examination is normal.

### Interpretation

Cushing's syndrome due to pituitary adenoma: Positive response is exaggerated increase above baseline of >50% in plasma ACTH and >20% in cortisol concentrations.

Hypercorticalism of adrenal origin: Plasma ACTH is low or undetectable before and after CRH without any cortisol response.

Ectopic ACTH syndrome: No ACTH or cortisol response

Psychiatric states associated with hypercortisolism (e.g., depression, anorexia nervosa, bulimia): In uni- or bipolar depression, obsessive-compulsive disorders, and alcoholism both peak and total ACTH response is decreased; only a small decrease in cortisol occurs (normal); after recovery response is not distinguishable from normal persons.

# Dehydroepiandrosterone Sulfate (DHEA-S), Serum

## Use

Indicator of adrenal cortical function, especially for differential diagnosis of virilization

Replaces 17-ketosteroids (17-KS) urine excretion

### Increased in

Congenital adrenal hyperplasia—markedly increased values can be suppressed by dexamethasone.

Adrenal carcinoma—markedly increased levels cannot be suppressed by dexamethasone.

Cushing's syndrome due to bilateral adrenal hyperplasia shows higher values than Cushing's syndrome due to benign cortical adenoma in which values may be normal or low.

Cushing's disease (pituitary etiology)—moderate increase

In hypogonadotropic hypogonadism, DHEA-S is usually normal for chronologic age and high for bone age in contrast to idiopathic delayed puberty in which DHEA-S is low relative to chronologic age and normal relative to bone age.

First few days of life, especially in sick or premature infants

### Decreased in

Addison's disease
Adrenal hypoplasia

# Dexamethasone Suppression of Pituitary ACTH Secretion

## Low-Dose Test

0.5 mg of dexamethasone (synthetic glucocorticoid) is given orally every 6 hrs for eight doses. A rapid overnight variation for screening uses a single 1-mg dose at 11 PM with plasma cortisol collection the following 8 AM.

## Use

Good screening test to rule out Cushing's syndrome and to identify cases for further testing because there are few false-negative results. Should be reserved primarily for cases with mildly increased urine cortisol or pseudo–Cushing's syndrome.

### Interference

False-positive results may occur in acute and chronic illness, alcoholism, depression, and due to certain drugs (e.g., phenytoin, phenobarbital, primidone); estrogens may cause a false-positive overnight dexamethasone test.

Noncompliance (check by measuring plasma dexamethasone)

### Interpretation

Normal response is a fall in urine free cortisol to <25 μg/24 hrs plasma, cortisol to <5 μg/dL, or urine 17-hydroxyketosteroid (OHKS) to <4 mg/24 hrs. Fall in urine free cortisol >90% (i.e., normal result) excludes hypercortisolism.

Patients with Cushing's of any cause almost always have abnormal lack of suppressibility.

#### High-Dose Test

Dexamethasone is given orally every 6 hrs for eight doses and plasma cortisol is measured 6 hrs after last dose and urine free cortisol is measured on day 2; baseline specimens for 2 days before test.

### Use

The high-dose test is the basic test to differentiate Cushing's disease (in which there is only relative resistance to glucocorticoid negative feedback) from adrenal tumors or ectopic ACTH production (usually complete resistance).

### Interpretation

Cushing's disease (pituitary tumor)
- Suppression of urine free cortisol to <90% of baseline strongly differentiates Cushing's disease from ectopic ACTH production, but not all pituitary tumor patients show such marked suppression. Some patients with large ACTH-producing pituitary adenomas have marked resistance to high-dose dexamethasone suppression. In long-standing cases, nodular adrenal hyperplasia may develop, causing autonomous cortisol production and resistance to dexamethasone test.

Ectopic ACTH syndrome or nodular adrenal hyperplasia
- No suppression in 80% of cases.

Adrenal adenoma or carcinoma or ectopic ACTH syndrome
- Urinary 17-OHKS and urine and plasma cortisol are not decreased after high or low doses of dexamethasone. Adrenal tumors do not reproducibly suppress.

Patients with psychiatric illness may be resistant.

### Interferences

Atypical or false-positive responses may occur due to drugs (e.g., alcohol, estrogens and birth control pills, phenytoin, barbiturates, spironolactone), pregnancy, obesity, acute illness and stress, severe depression.

## 11-Deoxycortisol (Compound S), Serum

### Use

In metyrapone test, in which blood level parallels changes in urine 17-OHKS,
- Functioning pituitary-adrenal system shows increase from <200 ng/dL baseline to >7000 ng/dL 8 hrs after large dose of metyrapone, whereas in nonfunctioning system there is very little increase in blood level.

### Increased in

Congenital adrenal hyperplasia
After metyrapone administration in normal persons

### Decreased in

Adrenal insufficiency

## Metyrapone Test

Adrenal suppression of pituitary secretion of ACTH is inhibited by metyrapone (which blocks cortisol production leading to increased ACTH secretion and therefore of 11-deoxycortisol).

Do not perform metyrapone test until ACTH test proves that adrenals are sensitive to ACTH.

### Use

Distinguish Cushing's disease from ectopic ACTH production.
To assess if adrenal insufficiency is secondary to pituitary disease. Some increase in 11-deoxycortisol indicates some pituitary reserve exists; in primary adrenal insufficiency, no rise occurs.

### Interpretation

ACTH deficiency (secondary Addison's disease)
Normal persons and pituitary Cushing's disease: Basal plasma 11-deoxycortisol increases $\geq$ 400 times or $>10\ \mu g/dL$ if cortisol falls to $<7\ \mu g/dL$ and rise in plasma ACTH to $>100$ ng/dL.
Adrenal tumor with excess cortisol production: No increase or fall in urinary 17-OHKS and 17-KS. Test is positive in 100% of adrenal hyperplasias without tumor, 50% of adrenal adenomas, and 25% of adrenal carcinomas.
Ectopic ACTH syndrome: May not be accurate in this condition.

## Renin Activity, Plasma (PRA)

See Renovascular Hypertension.

## 17-Hydrocorticosteroids in Urine
(derived from cortisol and cortisone)

### Use

Evaluation of adrenocortical function

### Increased in

Cushing's syndrome
Adrenal tumors
Marked stress (e.g., burns, surgery, infections)

### Decreased in

Addison's disease
ACTH deficiency

# Diseases of the Adrenal Glands

## Adrenal Feminization

Adult males with adrenal tumor (usually unilateral carcinoma, occasionally adenoma) that secretes estrogens
Urinary estrogens are markedly increased.
17-KS is normal or moderately increased and cannot be suppressed by low doses of dexamethasone when due to adrenal tumor.

## Adrenal Insufficiency, Acute (Waterhouse-Friderichsen Syndrome)

Dehydration
Azotemia is due to dehydration and shock affecting renal function.
Serum sodium and chloride are decreased and potassium is increased in some patients.

Hypoglycemia occurs regularly.
Direct eosinophil count is >50/cu mm (<50/cu mm in other kinds of shock).
Blood cortisol is markedly decreased (<5 μg/dL).

## Addison's Disease
### (chronic adrenocortical insufficiency)

Low serum cortisol and increased ACTH are diagnostic of adrenal failure. In primary deficiency, both cortisol and aldosterone are deficient with salt loss; in secondary, aldosterone production is maintained but other secondary endocrine deficiencies may appear (e.g., hypothyroidism, hypogonadism).

Serum potassium is increased; may be low in secondary adrenal insufficiency.

Increased blood ACTH (200–1600 pg/mL) with wide variation between morning and evening levels in primary adrenal hypofunction but decreased or absent ACTH in pituitary (secondary) hypoadrenalism. Increased ACTH level is quickly suppressed by replacement therapy.

Decreased ACTH with low cortisol indicates ACTH deficiency.

Decreased blood cortisol (<5 μg/dL in 8–10 AM specimen) is useful screening test. High or high-normal result excludes both primary and secondary adrenocortical insufficiency. Low or borderline result is indication for ACTH stimulation test.

Long ACTH stimulation test is necessary for diagnosis of secondary adrenal insufficiency.

Metyrapone inhibition test is performed if ACTH test causes some increase in blood cortisol.

Cortisol treatment will interfere with all of the previous tests and must be discontinued for prior 24–48 hrs. Dexamethasone will interfere with metyrapone test and plasma ACTH levels.

Urine 17-OHKS is absent or markedly decreased.

Urine 17-KS and 17-KGS are markedly decreased.

Antiadrenal autoantibodies are found in most cases of idiopathic Addison's disease and rule out adrenal TB and adrenoleukodystrophy.

Serum sodium and chloride are decreased.

BUN and creatinine may be moderately increased; may be decreased in secondary adrenal insufficiency.

Fasting hypoglycemia is present, with insulin hypersensitivity.

Neutropenia and relative lymphocytosis are common.

Eosinophilia is present (300/cu mm). *(A total eosinophil count of <50 is evidence against severe adrenocortical hypofunction.)*

Normocytic anemia is slight or moderate but difficult to estimate because of decreased blood volume.

## Adrenocortical Insufficiency

Acute
- Primary (e.g., Waterhouse-Friderichsen syndrome)
- Secondary to pituitary or hypothalamic disorders
- Following cessation of prolonged steroid therapy

Chronic
- Primary
    Granulomas (e.g., TB)
    Metastatic carcinoma
    Amyloid
    Autoimmune adrenalitis
    Adrenal hypoplasia (neonates)
    Adrenoleukodystrophy
- Secondary
    Simmonds' disease
    Destruction of pituitary by granulomas, tumor, etc.

**Table 13-8.** Differentiation of Primary Aldosteronism Due to Adenoma and Hyperplasia

| Test | Adenoma | Idiopathic Hyperplasia |
|---|---|---|
| During normal sodium intake<br>  Plasma renin activity | | Tend to higher values<br>  than adenoma patients |
| After salt depletion | | |
| Plasma renin activity | | Significantly higher values<br>  than adenoma patients |
| Urinary aldosterone | Relatively unaffected | Higher than adenoma<br>  patients |
| After saline infusion | | |
| Plasma aldosterone-cortisol<br>  ratio | I | Unchanged or D (<2.2) |
| Plasma 18-hydroxycortico-<br>  sterone-cortisol ratio | I | Unchanged or D (<3.0) |
| Plasma 18-hydroxycortico-<br>  sterone | >100 ng/dL | <50 ng/dL |
| | $\vdash$————— 50–100 ng/dL less helpful————— $\dashv$ | |
| Plasma aldosterone circadian<br>  rhythm correlates with<br>  plasma ACTH and cortisol | Yes | No |
| Effect of posture on plasma<br>  aldosterone | Slight/none | I ≥ 33% over baseline |
| Adrenal vein measurements | See Aldosteronism<br>  (Primary) | |

## Aldosteronism (Primary)

See Table 13-8 and Figs. 13-10 and 13-11.

### Due to

Solitary adrenal cortical adenoma
Idiopathic bilateral hyperplasia
Adrenal carcinoma
Ectopic production of aldosterone by adrenal embryologic rest within kidney or ovary (rare)
Ectopic production of ACTH or aldosterone by nonadrenal neoplasm (rare)
Glucocorticoid suppressible hyperaldosteronism

Excessive mineralocorticoid hormone secretion causes renal tubules to retain sodium and excrete potassium. Classic biochemical abnormalities are increased aldosterone production, suppressed PRA, and decreased serum potassium.

Hypokalemia (usually <3.0 mEq/L) not related to use of diuretics or laxatives in a hypertensive patient is the first indication. Present in 80–90% of cases; is often mild (3.0–3.5 mEq/L). Aldosteronism should be *suspected* in any hypertensive patient with spontaneous or easily provoked hypokalemia. May be normal in cases of shorter duration. Hypokalemia is usually less in hyperplasia than adenoma, but

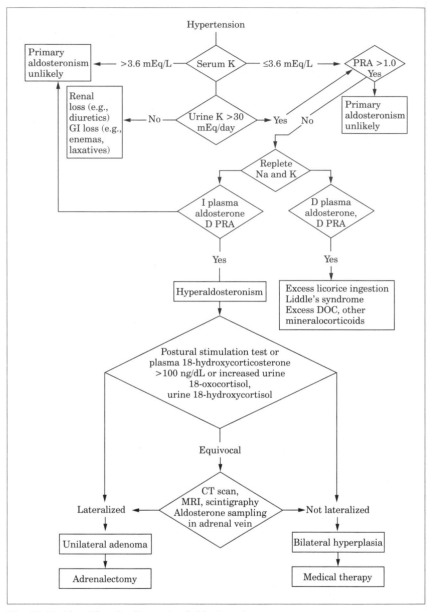

**Fig. 13-10.** Algorithm for diagnosis of aldosteronism.

considerable overlap occurs. Hypokalemia ≤ 2.7 mEq/L in a hypertensive patient is usually due to primary aldosteronism, especially adenoma. Normokalemic aldosteronism should be considered when urine potassium is >30 mEq/24 hrs when serum potassium is <3.5 mEq/L. Intermittent hypokalemia or normokalemia may occur, especially in adrenal hyperplasia etiologies. In essential hypertensive patients on diuretic therapy, urine potassium decreases to <30 mEq/L in 2–3 days after cessation of diuretics but continues in primary aldosteronism patients.

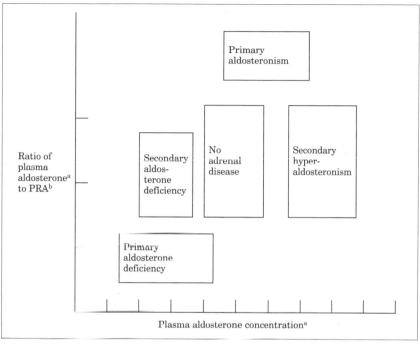

**Fig. 13-11.** Relationship between plasma aldosterone concentration and ratio of plasma aldosterone to PRA in disorders of mineralocorticoid deficiency or excess. [a]pmol/L, [b]ng/mL/hr.

Hypokalemia is alleviated by administration of spironolactone and by sodium restriction but not by potassium therapy. Administration of spironolactone for 3 days increases serum potassium >1.2 mEq/L. It also increases urine sodium and decreases urine potassium. Negative potassium balance recurs in 5 days. It increases urinary aldosterone (this is variable in hypertensive and normal people).

Saline infusion causes significant fall in serum potassium and in corrected potassium clearance. This hypokalemia is a reliable screening test.

There is hyperkaluria even with low potassium intake; <30 mEq/24 hrs essentially rules out primary aldosteronism. Sodium output is reduced.

Hypernatremia (>140 mEq/L), hypochloremia, and metabolic alkalosis (carbon dioxide content >25 mEq/L; blood pH tends to increase >7.42); correlates with severity of potassium depletion. Are clues in all etiologies of primary aldosteronism.

*Suggestive screening* tests are appropriate kaliuresis, low PRA (<3.0 ng/mL/hr), high plasma aldosterone:PRA ratio (>20).

*Diagnosis is confirmed* by nonsuppressible aldosterone excretion with normal cortisol excretion. Discontinue interfering drugs (for at least 2 wks) and assess plasma volume before beginning testing.

Increased plasma and/or urinary aldosterone that is relatively nonsuppressible by salt loading or volume expansion. May be normal in 30% of cases; therefore, must replete potassium before measurement if serum <3.0 mEq/L. Plasma aldosterone is normal in recumbent hypertensive and nonhypertensive persons without aldosteronism and increases 2–4 times after 4 hrs of upright posture; increases ≥ 33% in aldosteronism due to adrenal hyperplasia, but no increase occurs if due to adrenal adenoma.

Increased urinary aldosterone is best initial screening procedure (normal salt intake, no drugs; not detectable on all days). Cannot be reduced by high sodium intake or DOC administration. Therefore, high NaCl intake (10–12 gm/day) will cause 24-hr urine aldosterone >14 $\mu$g/24 hrs and sodium >250 mEq/24 hrs.

Volume expansion (by high salt intake, infusion of 2 L of NaCl in 4 hrs, or DOC) suppresses aldosterone level to >50–80% of baseline level in hypertensive patients without primary aldosteronism but not in patients with primary aldosteronism. Since plasma aldosterone levels vary from moment to moment, a single specimen may not properly reflect adrenal secretion.

PRA fails to rise to ≥ 4 ng/mL 90 mins after stimulus of low sodium diet, furosemide-induced volume contraction and upright posture.

Plasma aldosterone:PRA ratio ≥ 50 at 8 AM or in random blood sample after ambulating 2 hrs in patient not on medication is said to indicate primary aldosteronism except in chronic renal insufficiency. Does not distinguish adenoma from hyperplasia.

Captopril (angiotensin-converting enzyme [ACE] inhibitor that blocks angiotensin II production) administered at 8 AM decreases aldosterone in plasma 2 hrs later in normal persons and essential hypertension but remains increased in primary aldosteronism.

Urine is neutral or alkaline (pH >7.0) and not normally responsive to ammonium chloride load. Its large volume and low specific gravity are not responsive to vasopressin or water restriction (decreased tubular function, especially reabsorption of water).

Glucose tolerance is decreased in ≤ 50% of patients.

Plasma cortisol and ACTH are normal.

Urine 17-KS and 17-OHKS are normal.

It is important to distinguish cases due to adenoma (treated surgically) from idiopathic hyperplasia (treated medically). Aldosterone concentration in adrenal vein plasma is higher on side of adenoma. Patients with adenomas have higher plasma 18-oxocortisol (>15 $\mu$g/day) and 18-hydroxycorticosterone (>60 $\mu$g/day) concentrations, which decrease on standing; plasma aldosterone also decreases or fails to increase >30% on standing. In patients with bilateral adrenal hyperplasia and normal persons, plasma aldosterone increases with upright position. Hypokalemia is more severe with adenoma than with hyperplasia (normal in ~20% of latter). A small subset of hyperplasia mimics adenoma because it is associated with angiotensin-independent aldosterone overproduction and is cured by unilateral adrenalectomy.

## Aldosteronism (Secondary)

See Figs. 13-12 and 13-13.

### *Due to*

Decreased effective blood volume
- Congestive heart failure
- Cirrhosis with ascites
- Nephrosis
- Sodium depletion

Hyperactivity of renin-angiotensin system
- Renin-producing renal tumor
- Bartter's syndrome
- Toxemia of pregnancy
- Malignant hypertension
- Renovascular hypertension
- Oral contraceptive drugs

## Aldosteronism, Normotensive, Secondary (Bartter's Syndrome)
**(renal concentrating defect resistant to antidiuretic hormone [ADH])**

Hypokalemia with renal potassium wasting associated with juxtaglomerular hyperplasia; not due to laxatives, diuretics, or GI loss of potassium and chlo-

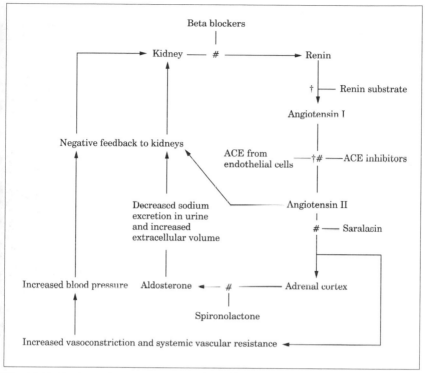

**Fig. 13-12.** Renin-angiotensin system and blocking sites. (ACE = angiotensin-converting enzyme; # = sites of action of blocking agents; † = sites where other substances form reaction.)

ride. It is almost impossible to maintain normal plasma potassium levels despite therapy.

Chloride-resistant metabolic alkalosis

Increased PRA is characteristic feature.

Frequently, there is decreased serum magnesium and increased uric acid; often the hypokalemia cannot be corrected without adequate magnesium replacement.

Increased plasma and urine aldosterone in the absence of edema, hypertension, or hypovolemia

Excrete large quantities of Na and Cl in urine

## Congenital Adrenal Hyperplasia

**(errors of metabolism due to specific deficiencies of enzymes needed for normal steroid synthesis of three main hormone classes; mineralocorticoids [17- deoxy pathway], glucocorticoids [17-hydroxy pathway], and sex steroids; all forms have decreased cortisol production that stimulates compensatory secretion of pituitary ACTH that causes the adrenal hyperplasia and hypersecretion of other pathways)**

See Table 13-9 and Fig. 13-13.

Establish diagnosis by increase in specific precursor steroids in blood or urine, which can be suppressed by administration of glucocorticoids.

Finding of increased 17-hydroxyprogesterone or androstenedione in amniotic fluid permits prenatal diagnosis.

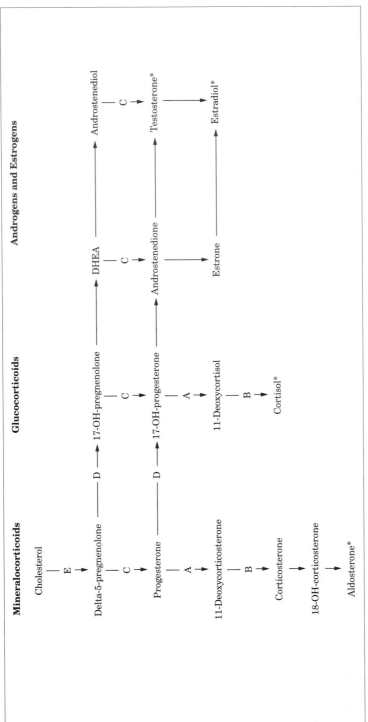

**Fig. 13-13.** Pathway of adrenal hormone synthesis. Hormones above the level of the deficient enzyme are present in increased amount; those below this level are decreased in amount. Shunting to other pathways may occur. Findings depend on completeness of enzyme deficiency, degree of hormone deficiency, or excessive accumulation. *Hormone produced in excess causing clinical manifestations. (A = 21-hydroxylase; B = 11-hydroxylase; C = 3-beta-hydroxysteroid dehydrogenase; D = 17-hydroxylase; E = 20,22-desmolase; DHEA = dehydroepiandrosterone.)

**Table 13-9.** Comparison of Different Forms of Congenital Adrenal Hyperplasia

| Enzyme Deficiency | Sexual Ambiguity in Newborn Female | Sexual Ambiguity in Newborn Male | Postnatal Virilization | Hypertension | Salt-Wasting | Urine Hormone Concentrations | | | | Blood Hormone Concentrations | | | | |
|---|---|---|---|---|---|---|---|---|---|---|---|---|---|---|
| | | | | | | 17-KS | 17-OH | Pregnanetriol | Aldosterone | 17-OHP | Delta-4 | DHEA | Testosterone | Renin |
| **21-Hydroxylase** | | | | | | | | | | | | | | |
| Salt-wasting | + | 0 | + | 0 | + | II | D | II | D | II | II | N/I | I | II |
| Simple virilizing | + | 0 | + | 0 | 0 | II | N/D | II | N/I | II | II | N/I | I | N/I |
| Late-onset | 0 | 0 | + | 0 | 0 | I | N | I | N/I | I | I | N/I | N/I | N |
| 11-Beta-hydroxylase[a] | + | 0 | + | + | 0 | II | II | I | D | I | II | I | I | DD |
| **3-Beta-HSD** | | | | | | | | | | | | | | |
| Salt-wasting | + | + | + | 0 | + | I | DD | N/D | D | N/I | N/I | III | [b] | I |
| Non-salt-wasting | + | + | + | 0 | 0 | I | DD | N/D | N | N/I | N/I | III | [b] | N |
| Late-onset | 0 | ? | + | 0 | 0 | N/I | N | N | N | N/I | N/I | I | N/I | N |
| 17-Alpha-hydroxylase[a] | 0 | + | 0 | + | 0 | DD | DD | DD | D | D | D | D | D | D |
| Cholesterol desmolase | 0 | + | 0 | 0 | + | DD | DD | DD | DD | D | D | D | D | I |

17-OH = 17-hydroxylase; 17-OHP = 17-hydroxyprogesterone; DHEA = dehydroepiandrosterone; I, II = degrees of increased; D, DD = degrees of decreased; 0 = none; + = present.
[a] Increased 17-deoxycortisol (corticosterone) and 11-deoxycortisol (compound B).
[b] N/D in males; N/I in females.

## Cushing's Syndrome

See Fig. 13-14 and Table 13-10.

### Due to

Pituitary (Cushing's *disease*) 50–80% in adults
- Pituitary tumor (may be part of MEN I)
- Hyperplasia of pituitary adrenocorticotropic cells
- Ectopic CRH syndrome

Adrenal (adrenal cause is predominant in children)
- Adenoma
- Carcinoma
- Micronodular hyperplasia
- Macronodular hyperplasia

Ectopic ACTH production
- Neoplasms

Iatrogenic
- Therapeutic (glucocorticoids or ACTH)
- Illicit use by athletes
- Factitious

Pseudo–Cushing's syndrome
- Major depressive disorder
- Chronic alcoholism

Definitive diagnosis or exclusion is made only by laboratory tests in two parts:
1. Establish autonomous hypercortisolism and loss of diurnal rhythm,
2. Determine etiology

Diagnosis of excessive cortisol production may include increased plasma cortisol ($>30 \mu g/dL$ at 8 AM and $>15 \mu g/dL$ at 4 PM), 24-hr urine free cortisol, 17-OHKS, 17-KS, dexamethasone suppression test.

### Interferences

More than one test may be needed because these are misleading in one-third or more cases
- Baseline measurements are increased by stress.
- Baseline measurements may vary daily and make dexamethasone suppression test difficult to interpret.
- Some drugs alter ACTH production or interfere with assays.
- Impaired renal function.
- Cortisol production is somewhat proportional to obesity or large muscle mass.
- Cortisol production is pulsatile rather than uniform even in ectopic ACTH production or Cushing's disease.
- Cortisol secretion may not be very increased on every determination.

### 24-Hr Urinary Free Cortisol

#### Use

Screening for
- Cushing's syndrome (increased)
- Adrenal insufficiency (decreased)

#### Interpretation

Increase is most useful screening test (best expressed per gm creatinine), which should vary by <10% daily. Should be measured in three consecutive 24-hr specimens. Found in 95% of Cushing's syndrome. $<100 \mu g/24$ hrs excludes and $>300 \mu g/24$ hrs establishes the diagnosis of Cushing's syndrome. If values are intermediate, low-dose dexamethasone suppression test is indicated.

#### Interferences

False positives or false negatives are very rare and test is more reliable than blood levels, which vary with time of day, require standardized collection, and are secreted in pulsatile fashion, making 24-hr urine cortisol preferred test.

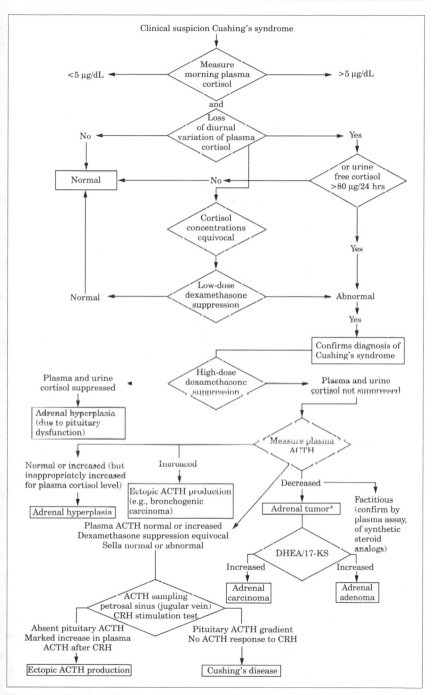

**Fig. 13-14.** Algorithm for diagnosis of Cushing's syndrome. (More than 90% of patients with Cushing's syndrome are found to follow this scheme.) *Adrenal computed tomography, magnetic resonance imaging, scintigraphy, and adrenal vein sampling to detect and localize adrenal tumor. (DHEA = dehydroepiandrosterone.)

**Table 13-10.** Comparison of Different Causes of Cushing's Syndrome

| | Normal | Pituitary Cushing's | Adrenal Adenoma | Adrenal Carcinoma | Adrenal Hyperplasia | Ectopic ACTH Production | Other Illness |
|---|---|---|---|---|---|---|---|
| Frequency | | 70% | 9% | 8% | ? | 15% | |
| Free cortisol Urine (µg/24 hr) | <100 | >300 establishes diagnosis of Cushing's syndrome if increased | | | | | False positive may occur in alcoholism, depression, drugs, etc. |
| Plasma (µg/dL) | 7–25 at 8 AM 2–14 at 4 PM | >30 at 8 AM and >15 at 4 PM | | | | | |
| Low-dose dexamethasone suppression Urine free cortisol | Falls to <25 µg/24 hr | Does not fall to <25 µg/24 hr in Cushing's syndrome due to any cause | | | | | |
| Plasma cortisol | Falls to <5 µg/dL | Not suppressed | | | | | |
| High-dose dexamethasone suppression | | Suppressed in >90% of cases | Not suppressed but not reproducible | | Not suppressed in 80% of cases | | |
| Plasma ACTH (pg/mL) | 60 | I or high-normal range Not >200 | Decreased or not detectable | | | >200 in % cases; 100–200 in % cases | |
| CRH stimulation | | ACTH increases | Flat plasma ACTH response to CRH | | | | |
| ACTH ratio inferior petrosal sinus:peripheral blood | | High; enhanced by CRF | Ratio = 1 | | | | |

CRH = corticotropin-releasing hormone.

Increased values may occur in depression or alcoholism but do not exceed 300 µg/24 hrs.
Alcoholism
Various drugs (e.g., phenytoin, phenobarbital, primidone)
Acute and chronic illnesses
Depression
Not affected by body weight

## *Plasma Free Cortisol*

### Use

Loss of normal diurnal variation for screening for Cushing's syndrome (normal persons have highest concentration at 8 AM and lowest between 8 PM and midnight); this diurnal variation disappears early and may be absent or reversed in 70% of Cushing's syndrome and 18% of patients without Cushing's (due to depression, alcoholism, stress, etc.). Midnight cortisol >7.5 µg/dL indicates Cushing's syndrome whereas <5 µg/dL virtually rules it out.
Normal urine free cortisol and normal diurnal variation in plasma cortisol virtually exclude Cushing's syndrome.

### Interferences

False negatives are frequent if blood is drawn before 8 PM (PM blood is commonly drawn at 4 PM to coincide with hospital employee working hours).
Because episodic rise and fall occurs in Cushing's disease, ectopic ACTH production, as well as in normal persons, should be measured on at least 2 separate days.
To determine the etiology of Cushing's syndrome after hypercortisolism has been established, the most useful tests are
• High-dose dexamethasone suppression
• CRH stimulation test
• Metyrapone test
• ACTH stimulation test
• DHEA-S concentration
• Plasma ACTH concentration

## *Basal Plasma ACTH Concentration*

### Interpretation

Cushing's syndrome due to autonomous cortisol production (e.g., adrenal tumor or exogenous steroids): Low or undetectable
Pituitary Cushing's disease: High or high-normal range but rarely >200 pg/mL.
Inferior petrosal sinus sampling
Ectopic ACTH syndrome (e.g., carcinoma of lung): Very high concentrations with no diurnal variation. Two-thirds of patients have high concentrations (>200 pg/mL); the other one-third usually have moderately elevated values (100–200 pg/mL). In these cases, difference in ACTH concentrations is measured in blood obtained simultaneously from both inferior petrosal sinuses and a peripheral vein in basal state and after CRH stimulation; ratio of inferior petrosal sinus:peripheral vein ≥ 2 indicates pituitary rather than ectopic source of ACTH. Ratio ≥ 3.0 is sensitive and specific for pituitary tumor.

### Interferences

ACTH has diurnal variation, episodic secretion, short plasma half-life.

### Urinary Steroid Findings in Different Etiologies of Cushing's Syndrome

Urinary 17-OHKS is increased (>10 mg/24 hrs) in virtually all patients with Cushing's syndrome but less useful for screening because increased in 20% of persons without Cushing's (e.g., obesity, hyperthyroidism).
• Night collection sample > day sample (reverse is true in normal persons).
• ACTH stimulation test produces lowest 17-OHKS in Cushing's syndrome due to adrenal carcinoma and the highest 17-OHKS due to adrenal adenoma.
• Increased urinary 17-KS.
• Cushing's syndrome: may be normal in 35% of patients and increased (>25 mg/24 hrs) in 20% of obese persons without Cushing's. Not useful except if virilism or marked hirsutism is present.

- Normal or low in 70% of adrenal adenomas (<20 mg/24 hrs) but increased in 90% of adrenal carcinomas; averages 50–60 mg/24 hrs in carcinoma (always >15 mg/hrs); >4 times normal in 50% of adrenal carcinomas; higher values increase likelihood of diagnosis of adrenal carcinoma and >100 mg/24 hrs is virtually diagnostic.
- Adrenal carcinoma: most of the increase is usually due to DHEA-S which is markedly increased; DHEA-S is slightly increased in Cushing's disease and often very low in adrenocortical adenoma (<0.4 mg/dL).
- Adrenal hyperplasia: Increased total 17-KS (in 50% of cases) is due to elevation of all of the 17-KS.
- Ectopic ACTH syndrome: Increased in 15% of cases.

*Isolated urine measurements of 17-KS or 17-OHKS are not recommended as screening tests for Cushing's syndrome. In general, free cortisol is best for screening, 17-OHKS with free cortisol in dexamethasone suppression tests, 17-KS to screen for possible adrenal carcinoma or to help differentiate adrenal adenoma from pituitary or ectopic ACTH syndrome causes.*

- Increased urinary 17-KGS (>20 mg/24 hrs)

Plasma renin activity is increased; suppressed activity suggests ectopic ACTH syndrome or adrenal adenoma or carcinoma (causing increased secretion of DOC or aldosterone).

Hypokalemic acidosis due to renal tubular loss of potassium chloride is characteristic but compensatory metabolic alkalosis occurs in ~10% of patients due to attempt to conserve potassium with $H^+$ exchange. Hypokalemic alkalosis may indicate ectopic ACTH production (e.g., bronchogenic carcinoma). Increased serum sodium and bicarbonate and decreased potassium and chloride is due to increased aldosterone production.

Glucose tolerance is diminished in 75% of cases.

Hematologic changes

- WBC is normal or increased.
- Relative lymphopenia is frequent (differential is usually <15% of cells).
- Eosinopenia is frequent (usually <100 cu mm).
- Hct is usually normal; if increased, it indicates an androgenic component.

Changes due to osteoporosis in long-standing cases. Serum and urine calcium may be increased. Kidney stones occur in 15% of cases.

Serum uric acid may be decreased due to uricosuric effect of adrenal steroids.

## Cushing's Syndrome Due to Adrenal Disease

### Is Suggested by

- Failure of high-dose dexamethasone test to cause suppression
- Very low plasma ACTH
- Positive metyrapone test

Adenoma is indicated by low or normal 17-KS with increased 17-OHKS, low DHEA-S.

Adrenal carcinoma is suggested by very high 17-KS. Carcinoma cases show hypercortisolism (50%), virilism (20%), or both (10–15%); nonfunctioning (10–15%). *Virilism favors diagnosis of carcinoma rather than adenoma.*

Nodular adrenal hyperplasia: ACTH levels are variable, unpredictable response to dexamethasone suppression making it difficult to distinguish from other adrenal causes.

## Cushing's Syndrome Due to Ectopic ACTH Production

**(by neoplasm, e.g., small cell carcinoma of lung, thymoma, islet cell tumor of pancreas, medullary carcinoma of thyroid, bronchial carcinoid, pheochromocytoma)**

Plasma ACTH is markedly increased (500–1000 pg/mL) compared to pituitary Cushing's disease (≤ 200 pg/mL) but overlap in 20% of ectopic ACTH cases. Morning basal level in normal persons is 20–100 pg/mL.

Increased plasma and urine free cortisol, which may show marked spontaneous variation; lack of diurnal variation

Increased ACTH in plasma from inferior petrosal sinus identifies ACTH-producing pituitary adenomas; combining with CRH stimulation improves the differentiation of pituitary from ectopic ACTH production.

High-dose dexamethasone suppression does not occur in ectopic ACTH production but does occur in Cushing's disease.

Use of both dexamethasone suppression and CRH stimulation has diagnostic accuracy of 98% in distinguishing Cushing's disease from ectopic ACTH production.

Metyrapone test may not be accurate in distinguishing from Cushing's disease.

Increased urinary 17-OHKS and 17-KS

Marked hypokalemic alkalosis (occurs in ≤ 60% of such patients) rather than metabolic acidosis may suggest this diagnosis.

## Cushing's Syndrome Due to Ectopic Corticotropin-Releasing Hormone Production
(usually due to bronchial carcinoids; clinically indistinguishable from ectopic ACTH production because most of these tumors also secrete ACTH)

Plasma CRH increased and CRH-stimulated secretion of ACTH suppressed by high doses of dexamethasone may not be present in many cases.

## Neuroblastoma, Ganglioneuroma, Ganglioblastoma

Urinary concentrations of catecholamines (norepinephrine, normetanephrine, dopamine, VMA, and HVA are increased. Excretion of epinephrine is not increased. If only one of these substances is measured, only ~75% of cases are diagnosed. If VMA and HVA, or VMA and total catecholamines are measured, 95–100% of cases are diagnosed.

These tests are also useful to show response to therapy, which should bring return to normal in 1–4 months. Continued increase indicates need for further treatment.

Cystathionine in urine suggests active disease but absence is not significant because is not normally present.

Serum neuron-specific enolase may be increased in neuroblastoma.

## Pheochromocytoma
(tumor of chromaffin cells of sympathetic nervous system; may secrete epinephrine, norepinephrine, dopamine)

See Figs. 13-15 and 13-16.

Secretory patterns
- Normally: Epinephrine is secreted primarily by adrenal medulla and norepinephrine secreted primarily at sympathetic nerve endings.
- Epinephrine is secreted by tumors usually of adrenal medulla.
- Norepinephrine is secreted by almost all extra-adrenal tumors and many adrenal tumors.
- Dopamine secretion is not associated with hypertension.
- Malignancy: Increased dopamine and almost as much norepinephrine with very low epinephrine.
- Part of familial syndrome: More likely to secrete both dopamine and epinephrine.
- Most common: Norepinephrine predominant with much less epinephrine and dopamine.
- Less common: Equal norepinephrine and epinephrine and some dopamine.

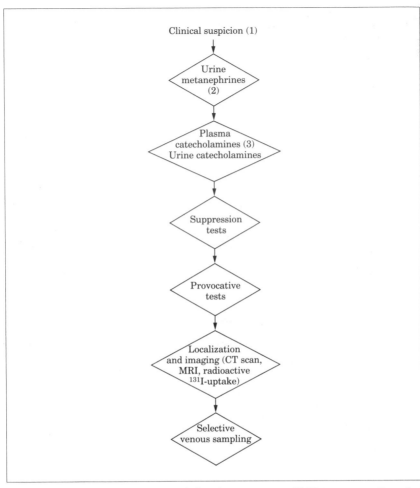

**Fig. 13-15.** Algorithm for diagnosis of pheochromocytoma. (1) History suggestive of MEA II. <30-year-old hypertensive patient. Any hypertensive patient with unusual symptoms. Only 20% of patients with pheochromocytoma have intermittent hypertension. Pheochromocytoma is more likely in younger patients. (2) Because of high sensitivity, normal metanephrines in urine virtually rule out pheochromocytoma if MEA II is not suspected. Because of low prevalence of pheochromocytoma, even <10%. Urine metanephrines may be decreased by various drugs (e.g., L-dopa, x-ray contrast media) and may be increased by stress (e.g., MI, CNS trauma) and certain drugs (e.g., MAO inhibitors, hydrazines and prochlorperazine, chlorpromazine, imipramine, methyldopa, oxytetracycline, phenacetin, phenothiazines). If urine metanephrines are increased, urine VMA should be performed next because of high specificity. Combination of increased metanephrines and VMA in urine is presumptive evidence of pheochromocytoma and should be followed by localizing tests. (3) Measurement of catecholamines (especially in plasma) should be performed along with localizing tests when MEA II is suspected. Although urinary catecholamine determinations commonly show false-negative and false-positive results, it may be particularly useful in possible MEA II but must beware of interfering factors (e.g., increased by exercise, stress, emotion, hypoglycemia, certain drugs).

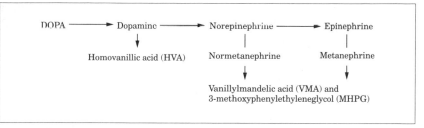

**Fig. 13-16.** Synthesis and breakdown of catecholamines. Since the hormones are broken down before release, metabolites are present in much larger amounts. When excretion of free catecholamines is greater compared to metabolites, it is said that the tumor is likely to be very small and difficult to locate. (DOPA = dihydroxyphenylalanine.)

- Rare: Epinephrine very high with small amounts of norepinephrine and dopamine. Usually indicates adrenal rather than extra-adrenal tumor.

Biochemical diagnosis is based on increased blood or urine concentrations of catecholamines (norepinephrine and, to a lesser extent, epinephrine) and their metabolites (normetanephrine and metanephrine), which are usually increased even when patient is asymptomatic and normotensive; rarely are increases found only following a paroxysm. The diagnosis is never ruled out by a normal concentration, and repeated testing may be necessary. Increase of either epinephrine or norepinephrine should be considered positive. Concentrations are usually 5–100 times normal although there is considerable overlap and wide range of normals. Plasma concentrations are often >2000 pg/dL, which is rarely seen in other conditions and is considered diagnostic; plasma concentrations <500 pg/dL essentially rule it out; concentrations >500 pg/dL indicate need for further testing. Plasma concentrations are particularly useful to compare paroxysm and basal concentrations and to localize tumors by selective venous sampling. Blood should be drawn in the unstressed supine patient without interfering conditions or drugs. 24-Hr urine free norepinephrine has also been reported.

### Plasma and Urine Catecholamines May Also Be Increased in

Neural crest tumors (neuroblastoma, ganglioneuroma, ganglioblastoma)
Adrenal medullary hyperplasia
Diabetic ketoacidosis (markedly elevated)
AMI (markedly elevated)
Acute CNS disturbance (e.g., infarct, hemorrhage, encephalopathy, tumor)
Heavy exercise before urine collection (≤ 7 times)
After surgery
Hypothyroidism
Thyrotoxicosis
Volume depletion induced by diuretics
Renal disease
Heavy alcohol intake
Hypoglycemia
Stress (emotional, physical)
Various drugs

*Plasma concentrations may not be increased when secretion is intermittent rather than continuous; for these cases, 24-hr urines are more accurate. Plasma concentrations are useful if 24-hr urine cannot be collected.*

Urine VMA excretion is increased; is urinary metabolite of both epinephrine and norepinephrine. Because this analysis is simpler than for catecholamines, it has been more commonly used but is less sensitive than other tests. Beware of false increase due to foods (e.g., vanilla; fruits, especially bananas; coffee; tea) and drugs (e.g., vasopressor agents).

Urinary metanephrines (are reliable screening tests with fewer interferences by drugs and diet than VMA or catecholamines) confirmed by urine catecholamine fraction determinations are an excellent routine to identify pheochromocytoma patients.

Urinary catecholamines are less reliable than VMA or metanephrines in screening for pheochromocytoma due to technical problems.

Fractionation that shows predominance of epinephrine suggests tumor in adrenal or organ of Zuckerkandl. Presence of HVA suggests malignancy.

Increased catecholamine concentrations after surgery may indicate recurrence of tumor.

Plasma chromogranin A as a marker for pheochromocytoma has sensitivity ~50%.

Suppression tests
- Pheochromocytomas (which secrete autonomously): High plasma catecholamine concentrations are not suppressed by pentolinium (pre-ganglionic blocking agent) or by clonidine.
- Patients without tumor: High basal concentration is decreased to normal.

Provocative tests: IV injection of glucagon or histamine causes marked rise in plasma catecholamines but false results may occur. A 3 times increase or an absolute concentration >2000 pg/mL within 3 mins is considered positive.

PRA is increased.

Other hormones may be secreted (e.g., serotonin, PTH, calcitonin, ACTH, gastrin, VIP, FSH, insulin).

*All patients with pheochromocytoma should be screened for other components of MEN IIa and IIb present in ~4% of cases.*

### Renovascular Hypertension

Sudden increase in serum creatinine and BUN, especially after onset of ACE inhibitor therapy

Hypokalemia (<3.4 mEq/L) in ~15% of patients

Proteinuria

Peripheral PRA (indexed against sodium excretion): *Low PRA in untreated patients virtually rules out renovascular hypertension.*

Captopril test causes
- Stimulated peripheral PRA 12 $\mu$g/L (ng/mL)/hr
- Increases peripheral PRA ≥ 10 $\mu$g/L/hr
- Increases peripheral PRA ≥ 150%, or 400% if baseline value <3 $\mu$g/L/hr
- Does not differentiate unilateral and bilateral disease

PRA is assayed in blood from each renal vein, inferior vena cava, aorta, or renal arteries. The test is considered diagnostic when the concentration from the ischemic kidney is at least 1.5 times greater than the concentration from the normal kidney (which is equal to or less than the concentration in the vena cava that serves as the standard) or as increment of PRA between each renal artery and vein. Increased accuracy by repeating test after captopril administration. This is due to high PRA in the peripheral blood, increase in PRA in the renal vein compared to the renal artery of the affected kidney, and suppression of PRA in the other kidney. Maximum renin stimulation accentuates the difference between the two kidneys and should always be obtained at pretest conditions. This is the most useful diagnostic test in renovascular hypertension as judged by surgical results but is not a sufficiently reliable guide to nephrectomy in patients with hypertension due to parenchymal renal disease. Little value in patients with bilateral disease.

Split renal function tests may show disparity between kidneys.

## Plasma Renin Activity

### Use

PRA is particularly useful to diagnose curable hypertension (e.g., primary aldosteronism, unilateral renal artery stenosis).

PRA measurement may be useful for preliminary screening to differentiate patients with volume excess (e.g., primary aldosteronism) with low PRA from those with medium to high PRA; if latter group shows marked rise in PRA during captopril test, should be worked up for renovascular hypertension, but patients with little or no rise are not likely to have curable renovascular hypertension.

Captopril test criteria for renovascular hypertension: Stimulated PRA ≥ 12 μg/L/hr, absolute increase PRA ≥ 10 μg/L/hr, increase PRA ≥ 150% (or ≥ 400% if baseline PRA <3 μg/L/hr).

### PRA Is Decreased (<1.5 ng/mL/3 hrs) in

98% of cases of primary aldosteronism. Usually absent or low and can be increased less or not at all by sodium depletion and ambulation in contrast to secondary aldosteronism. PRA may not always be suppressed in primary aldosteronism; repeated testing may be necessary. Normal PRA does not preclude this diagnosis; not a reliable screening test.

Hypertension due to unilateral renal artery stenosis or unilateral renal parenchymal disease

Increased plasma volume due to high-sodium diet, administration of salt-retaining steroids.

18–25% of essential hypertensives (low-renin essential hypertension), and 6% of normal controls.

Advancing age in both normal and hypertensive patients (decrease of 35% from the third to the eighth decade)

May also be decreased in congenital adrenal hyperplasia secondary to 11-hydroxylase or 17-hydroxylase deficiency with oversecretion of other mineralocorticoids.

Various drugs (propranolol, clonidine, reserpine; slightly with methyldopa)

Usually cannot be stimulated by salt restriction, diuretics, and upright posture that deplete plasma volume; therefore, measure before and after furosemide and 3–4 hrs of ambulation. *Drugs should be discontinued before measurement of PRA. Renin level should be indexed against 24 hr level of sodium in urine.*

### PRA May Be Increased in

15% of patients with essential hypertension (high-renin hypertension)

50–80% of patients with renovascular hypertension. Normal or high PRA is of limited value to diagnose or rule out renal vascular hypertension. Very high PRA is highly predictive but has poor sensitivity. Low PRA using renin-sodium nomogram in untreated patient with normal serum creatinine is strongly against this diagnosis.

Renin-producing tumors of the kidney

Reduced plasma volume due to low-sodium diet, diuretics, hemorrhage, Addison's disease

Secondary aldosteronism (usually very high levels), especially malignant or severe hypertension

Some edematous normotensive states (e.g., cirrhosis, nephrosis, congestive heart failure)

Sodium or potassium loss due to GI disease or in 10% of patients with uremia

Normal pregnancy

Pheochromocytoma

Last half of menstrual cycle

Erect posture for 4 hrs

Ambulatory patients compared to bed patients

Bartter's syndrome

Various drugs (diuretics, ACE inhibitors, vasodilators; sometimes by calcium antagonists and alpha blockers)

*In children with salt-losing form of congenital adrenal hyperplasia due to 21-hydroxylase deficiency, severity of disease is related to degree of increase.*

# Tests of Gonadal Function

## Estrogens (Total), Serum/Urine
**(includes estradiol produced by ovaries, placenta, and smaller amounts by testes and adrenals; estrone and estriol)**

### Increased in

Granulosa cell tumor of ovary

Theca cell tumor of ovary

Luteoma of ovary

Pregnancy

Secondary to stimulation by hCG-producing tumors (e.g., teratoma)

Gynecomastia

### Decreased in

Primary hypofunction of ovary
- Autoimmune oophoritis is the most common cause: Usually associated with other autoimmune endocrinopathies (e.g., Hashimoto's thyroiditis, Addison's disease, insulin-dependent DM). May cause premature menopause.
- Resistant ovary syndrome.
- Toxic (e.g., irradiation, chemotherapy).
- Infection (e.g., mumps).
- Tumor (primary or secondary).
- Mechanical (e.g., trauma, torsion, surgical excision).
- Genetic (e.g., Turner's syndrome).
- Menopause.

Secondary hypofunction of ovary
- Disorders of hypothalamus-pituitary axis

## Cytologic Examination of Vaginal Smear (Papanicolaou's [Pap] Smear) for Evaluation of Ovarian Function

Maturation index (MI) is the proportion of parabasal, intermediate, and superficial cells in each 100 cells counted.
- Lack of estrogen effect shows predominance of parabasal cells (e.g., MI = 100/0/0).
- Low estrogen effect shows predominance of intermediate cells (e.g., MI = 10/90/0).
- Increased estrogen effect shows predominance of superficial cells (e.g., MI = 0/0/100), as in hormone-producing tumors of ovary, persistent follicular cysts.

Karyopyknotic index (KI) is the percent of cells with pyknotic nuclei. Increased estrogen effect (e.g., KI $\geq$ 85%) is seen, as in cystic glandular hyperplasia of the endometrium.

Eosinophilic index is the percent of cells showing eosinophilic cytoplasm; it may also be used as a measure of estrogen effect.

## Chromosome Analysis

Turner's syndrome (gonadal dysgenesis)—usually negative for Barr bodies

Klinefelter's syndrome—positive for Barr bodies

Pseudohermaphroditism—chromosomal gender corresponding to gonadal gender

## Follicle-Stimulating Hormone and Luteinizing Hormone (LH), (Pituitary Gonadotropins), Serum

### Use

Differential diagnosis of gonadal disorders
Diagnosis and management of infertility

### Increased in

Primary hypogonadism (anorchia, testicular failure, menopause)
Gonadotropin-secreting pituitary tumors
Precocious puberty (secondary to a CNS lesion or idiopathic)
Complete testicular feminization syndrome
Luteal phase of menstrual cycle

### Decreased in

Secondary hypogonadism
  • Kallmann's syndrome (inherited autosomal isolated deficiency of hypothalamic gonadotropin releasing hormone)
  • Pituitary LH or FSH deficiency
  • Gonadotropin deficiency

## Progesterone, Serum

### Increased in

Luteal phase of menstrual cycle
Luteal cysts of ovary
Ovarian tumors (e.g., arrhenoblastoma)
Adrenal tumors

### Decreased in

Amenorrhea
Threatened abortion
Fetal death
Toxemia of pregnancy
Gonadal agenesis

## Testosterone, Free, Plasma

### Use

Evaluation of gonadal hormonal function

### Decreased in (Men)

Primary hypogonadism (e.g., orchiectomy)
Secondary hypogonadism (e.g., hypopituitarism)
Testicular feminization
Klinefelter's syndrome levels lower than in normal male but higher than in normal female and orchiectomized male
Estrogen therapy
Total testosterone decreased due to decreased sex hormone binding globulin (e.g., cirrhosis, chronic renal disease)

### Increased in

Adrenal virilizing tumor causing premature puberty in boys or masculinization in women

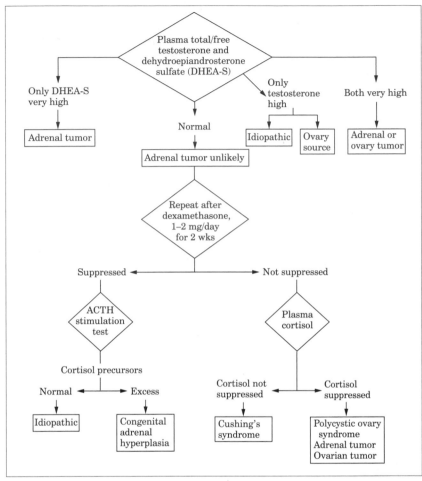

**Fig. 13-17.** Algorithm for work-up of hirsutism.

Congenital adrenal hyperplasia
Idiopathic hirsutism—inconclusive
Stein-Leventhal syndrome—variable; increased when virilization is present
Ovarian stromal hyperthecosis
Drugs that alter $T_4$-binding globulins may also affect testosterone-binding globulins; however the free testosterone level will not be affected.

# Gonadal Disorders

See Fig. 13-17.

## Amenorrhea, Hormone Profiles in

Normal LH, FSH, prolactin, estradiol, testosterone, $T_4$, and TSH (eugonadal)
- Drugs

- Diet, anorexia
- Exercise
- Stress, illness
- Structural genital tract disorders (see previous section)

Increased LH and normal FSH
- Early pregnancy
- Polycystic ovarian disease (Stein-Leventhal syndrome)
- Ectopic gonadotropin production by neoplasm (e.g., lung, GI tract)

Increased LH and FSH (>30 mIU/mL), decreased estrogen (<50 pg/mL)
- Primary ovarian hypofunction

Normal or low LH and FSH, decreased estrogen
- Hyperprolactinemia
- Isolated gonadotropin deficiency due to pituitary or hypothalamic impairment.
  Clomiphene citrate should be administered for 5–10 days; if gonadotropin
  level rises or menses return, cause is probably hypothalamic.
  Administer hypothalamic luteinizing hormone-releasing factor; normal or
  exaggerated response in hypothalamic amenorrhea (cause in 80% of
  patients); smaller or no response in pituitary tumor or dysfunction.

Increased androgen
- Polycystic ovarian disease (testosterone level usually <200 ng/dL)
- Tumor of adrenal or ovary (testosterone level may be >200 ng/dL)
- Testicular feminization
- Use of anabolic steroids (e.g., in athletes)

## Klinefelter's Syndrome
### (patients have two or more X chromosomes)

Plasma LH and FSH are increased; high FSH is best demarcator between nor-
mal men and men with Klinefelter's syndrome.
Urinary gonadotropin level is elevated.
Plasma testosterone levels are decreased to normal.
Azoospermia
Buccal smears are helpful if positive for Barr bodies but a negative smear does
not rule out mosaicism. If negative, chromosome analysis should be performed,
but in 70% of patients, mosaic pattern may only occur in testes, requiring chromosomal analysis of testicular cells for definite diagnosis.
Abnormal chromosomal pattern. XY males have an extra X; 47,XXY is the classic type; 10% of patients have the mosaic form (46,XY/47,XXY); may have additional X (e.g., XXXY, XXXXY).
Biopsy of testicle shows atrophy, with hyalinized tubules lined only by Sertoli's
cells, clumped Leydig's cells, and absent spermatogenesis.

## Polycystic Ovarian Disease (Stein-Leventhal Syndrome)

Serum LH is increased ~3 times normal (>35 mIU/mL) in ~60% of patients with
normal or slightly low FSH. Abnormally high LH:FSH ratio (>2) is more consistently evidence of an abnormality than are abnormal levels of either measurement alone. Ratio ≥ 2 is considered highly suggestive; ratio ≥ 3 is considered
diagnostic.
Plasma free testosterone is increased ≤ 200 $\mu$g/dL in 40–60% of cases; (>200 $\mu$g/dL
usually indicates an androgen-producing tumor); not suppressed by dexamethasone.
Plasma androstenedione (DHEA) is increased in ≤ 50% of cases.
Serum 3-alpha-androstanediol glucuronide (metabolite of dihydrotestosterone)
is markedly increased in this and in idiopathic hirsutism.
Synthetic estrogens and progestins (as in oral contraceptives) for 21 days with
before and after measurement of free testosterone and androstenedione
- Free testosterone and androstenedione decrease by 50% or become normal
  in LH-dependent hyperandrogenism (e.g., polycystic ovaries).

- No suppression occurs in patients with ovarian tumors or adrenal disorders.
- Change in free testosterone accounts for estrogen-caused increase in sex hormone–finding globulin that could result in unchanged or increased total testosterone level.

~85% of these patients have one or more abnormalities of serum LH:FSH ratio, testosterone, or androstenedione. Hyperandrogenism does not differentiate condition from congenital adrenal hyperplasia (CAH) but CAH is more likely if LH:FSH ratio is <2:1 and ovaries are normal in size.

Urinary 17-KS is somewhat increased (higher values occur in congenital virilizing adrenal hyperplasia and hyperadrenalism due to Cushing's syndrome). Dexamethasone administration (0.5 mg qid for 5–7 days) causes partial suppression in cases of ovarian origin, but complete suppression suggests adrenal origin (e.g., late-onset congenital adrenal hyperplasia). Administration of gonadotropin increases urinary 17-KS.

Plasma cortisol, urinary 17-OHKS, and 17-KGS are normal.

Plasma prolactin is increased in ~30% of patients.

Hyperinsulinemia occurs for unknown reason; correlates with degree of increased androgens.

Some patients have partial 21-hydroxylase defects.

Increased serum LH (>35 mIU/mL), LH/FSH >2, and mild increase of ovarian androgen level are sufficient for diagnosis in the presence of the symptoms and clinical signs. *Because of erratic daily fluctuations of LH and androgens, daily plasma specimens for 3–5 days may be necessary.*

If testosterone is >2 ng/mL or DHEA >7,000 ng/mL, ovarian or adrenal tumor should be ruled out.

Biopsy of ovary is not specific.

*Increased serum LH with normal or decreased FSH may occur in simple obesity, hyperthyroidism, liver disease.*

## Testicular Cancer

Increased serum hCG (>1–2 ng/mL or >5–10 mIU/mL) is found in 40–60% of patients with nonseminomatous tumors and in some patients with apparently pure seminoma. In the latter case, immunochemical staining of paraffin-embedded tumor should be performed, because isolated syncytiotrophoblastic cells may show the hormone but are not by themselves evidence of choriocarcinoma.

Increased serum AFP (>20 ng/mL) is found in ≤ 70% of patients with teratocarcinoma or embryonal carcinoma. Not increased in pure seminoma without teratomatous component.

Both markers should always be measured simultaneously. 40% of patients with nonseminomatous tumors have elevation of only one marker. 90% of patients with testicular tumors are positive for AFP or hCG or both; these are valuable for gauging efficacy of chemotherapy. AFP levels may remain elevated although lower than pretreatment levels.

20–30% of patients have false-negative results preoperatively despite tumor in the retroperitoneal lymph nodes. Lymphadenectomy should not be omitted simply because of normal marker levels.

Serum markers for AFP and beta-hCG may be elevated in conditions other than testicular cancer.

- The most important use is for follow-up after surgery or chemotherapy. Failure of increased preoperative levels to fall after surgery suggests metastatic disease and the need for chemotherapy. Rise of levels that had previously declined to normal suggests recurrent tumor even with no other evidence of disease.

Negative markers are not useful for differential diagnosis of scrotal mass, but elevated levels indicate testicular cancer.

Serum LD is a third marker; not specific for testicular cancer.

## Tumors, Germ Cell of Ovary and Testicle

| Tumor | AFP* | beta-HCG* |
|---|---|---|
| Seminoma | — | + |
| Seminoma with syncytiotrophoblastic giant cells (STGCs) | — | + |
| Embryonal carcinoma | + | — |
| Embryonal carcinoma with STGCs | + | + |
| Yolk sac tumor | + | — |
| Yolk sac tumor with STGCs | + | + |
| Choriocarcinoma | — | + |
| Mature teratoma | — | — |

*See Chapter 16.

When both markers are positive, both should be assayed after therapy as recurrence or metastases may be reflected by increase of only one marker.

## Tumors, Ovarian

### Feminizing Ovarian Tumors
*(e.g., granulosa cell tumor, thecoma, luteoma)*

Pap smear of vagina and endometrial biopsy show high estrogen effect and no progestational activity; no signs of ovulation during reproductive phase.
Urinary FSH is decreased (inhibited by increased estrogen).
Urine 17-KS and 17-OHKS are normal.
Pregnanediol is absent.

### Masculinizing Ovarian Tumors
*(e.g., arrhenoblastoma, hilar cell tumors, adrenal rest tumors)*

Androgen-secreting tumor of ovary or adrenal is highly likely if serum total testosterone >200 ng/dL or DHEA-S >800 μg/dL. Localization may require androgen measurement in blood from adrenal and ovarian veins.
Pap smear of vagina shows decreased estrogen effect.
Endometrial biopsy shows moderate atrophy of endometrium.
Urine FSH (gonadotropins) is low.
Urine 17-KS is normal or may be slightly increased in arrhenoblastoma. May be markedly increased in adrenal tumors of ovary ("masculinovoblastoma"). The higher the urine 17-KS level, the greater the likelihood of adrenocortical carcinoma; >100 mg/24 hrs is virtually diagnostic. It may be moderately increased in Leydig cell tumors.
*In arrhenoblastoma, there may be an increase of androsterone, testosterone, etc., excreted in urine even though the 17-KS is not much increased. Urine 17-KS normal or slightly increased associated with plasma testosterone in male range is almost certainly due to ovarian tumor.*
*In adrenal cell tumors of ovary, laboratory findings may be the same as in hyperfunction of adrenal cortex with Cushing's syndrome, etc.*
*In some cases, there are no endocrine effects from these tumors.*
*Some cases of arrhenoblastoma with masculinization also show evidence of increased estrogen formation.*

### Struma Ovarii

About 5–10% of cases are hormone-producing. Classic findings of hyperthyroidism may occur; these tumors take up radioactive iodine.

### Primary Chorionepithelioma of Ovary

Urinary chorionic gonadotropins are markedly increased.
Estrogen and progesterone secretion may be much increased.

### Nonfunctioning Ovarian Tumors

Only effect may be hypogonadism due to replacement of functioning parenchyma.

### Tumor Markers

Serum CA-125
Beta-hCG
AFP
CEA

# Laboratory Tests for Diagnosis of Disorders of Pituitary and Hypothalamus

## Arginine Vasopressin (AVP) (Antidiuretic Hormone, ADH)

### Use

Diagnosis of central diabetes insipidus (DI) and of SIADH and differentiation
from nephrogenic DI
Differential diagnosis of hyponatremias

### Increased in Serum

SIADH (inappropriately increased for degree of plasma osmolality)
Ectopic ADH syndrome
Certain drugs (e.g., chlorpropamide, phenothiazine, carbamazepine [Tegretol])
Nephrogenic DI (normal for degree of plasma osmolality)

### Decreased in Serum

Central DI

### In Urine

Central DI—low AVP and osmolality
Nephrogenic DI—high AVP and low osmolality
SIADH—normal AVP relative to osmolality

## Growth Hormone (GH)

### Use

Differential diagnosis of short stature, slow growth
Evaluation of pituitary function

### Increased in

Acromegaly and gigantism due to certain pituitary adenomas
Laron dwarfism (GH resistance; growth hormone binding protein cannot be
detected)
Renal failure
Uncontrolled DM
Drugs (e.g., estrogens, oral contraceptives, tranquilizers, antidepressants)
Starvation
2 hrs after sleep

### Decreased in

Hypothalamic defect causes most cases (e.g., tumors, infection, diseases such as
hemochromatosis, perinatal insult such as birth trauma).

Hypopituitarism (e.g., familial isolated GH deficiency, tumors, infection, granulomas, trauma, irradiation)
Dwarfism
Corticosteroid therapy
Obesity

*Low levels must be measured after stimulation (e.g., insulin, arginine).*

## Growth Hormone–Releasing Hormone (GHRH)

### Increased in

1% of cases of acromegaly due to GHRH by hypothalamus or ectopic secretion by neoplasms (e.g., pancreatic islet, carcinoid of thymus or bronchus, neuroendocrine tumors)

### Normal in

Most cases of acromegaly due to pituitary tumors

## Prolactin

See Prolactinomas.

## Somatomedin-C
**(mediates most growth-promoting effects of growth hormone)**

### Use

Screening growth disorders (acromegaly, pituitary deficiency); preferable to hCG because it is constant after eating and during the day)
Assessing nutritional status
Monitor effectiveness of nutritional repletion.

### Increased in

Acromegaly and gigantism
Pregnancy (2–3 times nonpregnant values)

### Decreased in

Pituitary deficiency
Laron dwarfism
Anorexia or malnutrition
Acute illness
Hepatic failure
Hypothyroidism
Diabetes mellitus
Normal aging

# Diseases of the Pituitary and Hypothalamus

## Acromegaly and Gigantism

Serum somatomedin C is uniformly increased in untreated cases; is superior to serum GH because GH levels fluctuate and have short serum half-life.
Autonomous serum growth hormone (GH) is increased. Annual random blood GH levels, FTI, and ACTH are used for treatment follow-up.
* Fasting levels >5 ng/mL in men or >10 ng/mL in women are suggestive but not diagnostic of acromegaly.

- Most patients show a fall of <50% or even an increase 60–90 mins after glucose load, whereas normal subjects show almost complete suppression of GH (or to <5 ng/mL) by induced hyperglycemia. This is the most reliable test. Failure to suppress GH to <2 ng/mL after oral glucose load is essential to diagnosis.

If borderline response to hyperglycemia, perform TRH test. (TRH IV causes transient increase [>50% over basal levels] of GH in 15–30 mins in acromegaly patients but little effect in normal persons.)

GHRH excess secretion (e.g., ectopic source, such as pancreatic tumor or carcinoid causes, <1% of acromegaly cases)

All patients with acromegaly should have baseline serum prolactin measured because ≤ 40% of these adenomas may secrete both prolactin and GH.

IV ACTH administration may cause excessive increase in urine 17-KS but normal 17-OHKS excretion.

Adrenal virilism and increased urine 17-KS are common in women.

Hypogonadism develops in up to 50%.

In inactive cases, all secondary laboratory findings may be normal.

In late stage, panhypopituitarism may develop.

Biopsy of costochondral junction evidences active bone growth.

After successful surgery: Basal plasma GH <5 ng/mL should decrease to ≤ 2 ng/mL after glucose administration and IGF-I should become normal.

### *Due to*

Excess GH secretion
- Pituitary adenomas, hyperplasia, or carcinoma
- Ectopic pituitary tumor (sphenoid or parapharyngeal sinus)
- Ectopic hormone production (e.g., tumor of pancreas, lung, ovary, breast)

Excess GHRH secretion
- Hypothalamic tumor (e.g., hamartoma, ganglioneuroma)
- Ectopic hormone production (e.g., carcinoid of bronchus, GI tract, pancreas; pancreatic islet cell tumor, small cell carcinoma of lung, adrenal adenoma, pheochromocytoma)

## Carcinoid Syndrome
### (in malignant carcinoids [argentaffinomas])

Liver metastases are present in 95% of cases except in lung and ovary primary sites.

Urinary 5-hydroxyindoleacetic acid (5-HIAA) is increased but may be normal despite massive metastases. Only useful in diagnosis in ~45% of those with liver metastases. Disease extent and prognosis correlates generally with urine 5-HIAA excretion; becomes normal after successful surgery. May also be increased in Whipple's disease and nontropical sprue; small increases may occur in pregnancy, ovulation, after surgical stress. Increased by various foods (e.g., pineapples, kiwi, bananas, eggplant, plums, tomatoes, avocados, walnuts, pecans, coffee) and drugs. If urine 5-HIAA is normal, check blood level of serotonin or a precursor, 5-hydroxytryptophan. Urine 5-HIAA may be decreased in renal insufficiency. Normal = 2–9 mg/day; >40 mg/day in carcinoid syndrome, often 300–1000 mg/day.

Serum and urine serotonin may be increased (>0.4 μg/mL) but without increased urine 5-HIAA.

Platelet serotonin and urine serotonin is increased.

Some tumors produce histamine, ACTH, gastrin, and bradykinin.

VMA and catecholamines levels in urine are normal.

Laboratory findings due to other aspects of carcinoid syndrome (e.g., valvular stenosis or insufficiency, heart failure, liver metastases, electrolyte disturbances)

Nonfunctioning tumors can only be diagnosed by histologic examination.

# Diabetes Insipidus
## *Due to*

Central (pituitary)
Nephrogenic
Psychogenic
High-set osmoreceptor


# Diabetes Insipidus, Central
## *Due to*

Primary
  • Idiopathic
  • Heredity
Secondary
  • Supra- and intrasellar tumors
    Primary (e.g., craniopharyngioma, cyst)
    Metastatic
  • Histiocytosis (e.g., eosinophilic granuloma)
  • Granulomatous lesions (e.g., sarcoidosis, tuberculosis, syphilis)
  • Trauma, with or without basal skull fracture; neurosurgical procedures
  • Vascular lesions (e.g., aneurysms, thrombosis, sickle-cell disease, Sheehan's syndrome)
  • Infections (e.g., meningitis, encephalitis, Guillain-Barré syndrome)
  • Others (e.g., hypoxemic encephalopathy)

Urine is inappropriately dilute (low specific gravity [usually <1.005] and osmolality [50–200 mOsm/kg]) in presence of increased serum osmolality (295 mOsm/kg) and increased or normal serum sodium.
Large urine volume (4–15 L/24 hrs) is characteristic.
Plasma vasopressin level is decreased.
Dehydration test fails to increase urine specific gravity or osmolality, and serum osmolality remains elevated. After administration of vasopressin, urine osmolality will double.
Partial central DI shows intermediate values between complete central and normal.


# Diabetes Insipidus, Nephrogenic
## *Due to*

Chronic renal failure
Diuretic phase of acute tubular necrosis
After renal transplant or relief of urinary tract obstruction
Primary hyperaldosteronism
Sickle cell anemia
Hypergammaglobulinemia (e.g., multiple myeloma, amyloidosis)
Drugs (e.g., lithium, amphotericin)
Prolonged potassium depletion and hypokalemia (is reversed by restoring potassium level to normal)
Prolonged hypercalciuria, usually with hypercalcemia (is reversed by restoring the calcium level to normal)
Hereditary renal tubular unresponsiveness to vasopressin due to X-linked genetic defect; severe form occurs in males; family history of this condition is frequent.

Laboratory findings are the same as in hypophyseal (central) DI except that nephrogenic type shows
  • Normal or increased plasma vasopressin level.
  • Dehydration test does not cause urine osmolality to rise above plasma osmolality.
  • Dehydration test causes the plasma vasopressin level to increase.
  • Urine osmolality does not rise with subsequent injection of vasopressin.

## Hypopituitarism

### Due to

Pituitary disease
- Neoplasms
- Infiltrative diseases
    Granulomatous lesions (e.g., sarcoidosis, Hand-Schüller-Christian syndrome, histiocytosis X)
    Infection (e.g., TB, mycoses)
    Hemochromatosis
    Autoimmune inflammation
- Hemorrhage
    Pituitary necrosis secondary to postpartum hemorrhage
    Hemorrhage into pituitary tumor
- Miscellaneous
    Head trauma
    Internal carotid artery aneurysm
    Empty sella syndrome
- Iatrogenic (e.g., hypophysectomy, radiation, section of stalk)
- Familial pituitary deficiency (deficient hormone production or production of abnormal hormone)
- Partial growth hormone deficiency (some forms of "constitutional short stature" with delayed onset of adolescence)
Hypothalamic dysfunction
End-organ resistance to GH (normal or increased serum GH with low somatomedin level)

*Serum somatomedin-C levels are 5–15% of normal in most hypopituitary dwarfs and 4–12 times normal in all active acromegaly patients.*
Endocrinologic findings: Diagnosis is based on low serum level of target organ hormone and of the corresponding pituitary stimulating hormone
- Hypogonadism
- Hypothyroidism: Low serum $T_4$ and FTI, inappropriately low serum TSH
- Hypocortisolism: Low serum cortisol and ACTH
- Low serum GH unresponsive to provocative tests
- Low serum prolactin unresponsive to provocative tests
*Dynamic tests are usually needed to detect partial deficiencies.*

## Hypothalamus, Diseases of

### Due to

Neoplasms (most frequent cause)
Inflammation (e.g., tuberculosis, encephalitis)
Head trauma (e.g., basal skull fractures, gunshot wounds)
Granulomas (e.g., histiocytosis X, sarcoidosis)
Releasing hormone deficiency, genetic or idiopathic
Radiation for childhood cancer

### Manifestations

Sexual abnormalities are the most frequent manifestations
Precocious puberty
Hypogonadism (frequently as part of Frohlich's syndrome)
DI
Hypopituitarism

## Hyponatremias, Causes of

See Table 13-11 and Fig. 13-18.

**Table 13-11.** Comparison of Hyponatremia Due to Various Causes

| Cause | Urine Sodium | Urine Osmolarity | BUN |
|---|---|---|---|
| Hypervolemic (e.g., congestive heart failure, cirrhosis, nephrotic syndrome) | | | |
| Early | D (usually <10–15 mEq/L) | I (usually >350–400 mOsm/L) | N |
| Late | D with isotonic urine is ominous finding | (>200 mmol/kg) | I disproportionate to creatinine |
| Hypovolemic | | | |
| Extrarenal<br>Gastrointestinal<br>Skin (burns, sweat)<br>Third space | D (<10 mEq/L) | I (>400 mOsm/L) | N |
| Renal<br>Diuretic (most common)<br>Chronic renal disease (especially interstitial)<br>Mineralocorticoid deficiency | I (>20 mEq/L) | Isotonic to plasma<br>If severe volume contraction, 300–450 mOsm/kg | Usually I |
| Normovolemic<br>SIADH (almost always) (see Syndrome of Inappropriate Secretion of Antidiuretic Hormone [SIADH]) | I (>20 mmol/L) | I (>200 mmol/kg)<br>D in plasma | Often D (<8–10 mg/dL) |
| Reset osmostat | V | V | N or D |

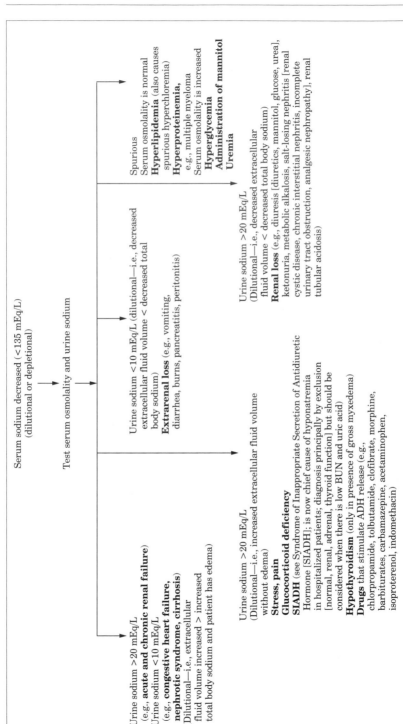

**Fig. 13-18.** Algorithm for hyponatremia.

Isotonic (artifactual—occurs with flame photometer but not with ion-selective electrode technology)
- Hyperlipidemia (plasma looks milky) "falsely" lowers serum sodium; measured serum osmolality exceeds calculated serum osmolality.

Calculated serum osmolality = $2 \times Na + (serum glucose/18) + (BUN/2.8)$

- Hyperproteinemia (e.g., myeloma, macroglobulinemia).

Hypertonic
- Hyperglycemia (each increase of blood sugar of 100 mg/dL decreases serum sodium by 1.7 mEq/L)
- Excess mannitol treatment

Hypotonic
- Hypervolemic, usually with clinical edema.
  With low urine sodium (<10 mEq/L) may be due to congestive heart failure, cirrhosis with ascites, nephrotic syndrome
  With high urine sodium (>20 mEq/L) may be due to acute tubular necrosis or end-stage chronic renal failure in which Na and $H_2O$ intake exceeds excretion. Serum uric acid and BUN tend to be increased.
- Hypovolemic.
  Urine sodium <10 mEq/L. Due to extrarenal loss of sodium (e.g., GI tract, fistulas, pancreatitis, exercise, sweating, burns).
  Urine sodium > 20mEq/L. Due to renal loss of sodium (e.g., diuretics, such as furosemide, or osmotic diuresis due to glucose or urea, diabetic ketoacidosis, renal tubular acidosis, salt-losing nephritis, adrenal insufficiency, hyporeninemia, hypoaldosteronism.)
- Normovolemic—usually no edema is present.
  Large amounts of sodium appear in urine (>20 mEq/L). May be due to SIADH, hypothyroidism, hypopituitarism, low reset osmostat syndrome, physical or emotional stress, potassium depletion, renal failure, water poisoning, certain drugs (e.g., ADH analogues, amitriptyline, diuretics, haloperidol, thioridazine, vincristine).

*Hyponatremic patients with BUN <10 mg/dL and uric acid <3.0 mg/dL should be considered to have SIADH or reset osmostat until proved otherwise.*

Pseudohyponatremia when sodium is measured with flame photometer rather than ion-selective electrode. May be secondary to hyperlipidemia, hyperproteinemia, increased concentration of osmotically active substances (e.g., glucose in absence of insulin, mannitol). Serum osmolality is normal.

## Hypernatremia, "Essential"
**(due to a hypothalamic lesion that causes impaired osmotic regulation but intact volume regulation of ADH secretion)**

See Fig. 13-19.

Serum sodium shows sustained but fluctuating elevations, corrected by administration of ADH but not corrected by fluid administration.

Serum osmolality is increased.

Serum creatinine, BUN, and creatinine clearance are normal.

There is spontaneous excretion of random specimens of urine that may be very concentrated or very dilute and opposite to plasma osmolality.

## Multiple Endocrine Neoplasia (MEN I; Werner's Syndrome)

HPT in >88% of patients is usual presenting feature.

Pancreatic endocrine tumors in >81% of patients; most are functional; usually multiple
- Gastrinomas with Z-E syndrome, occur in ~50% of cases. 50% of patients with Z-E syndrome have MEN I.
- Insulinomas (beta cells) in ~25% of MEN I patients.

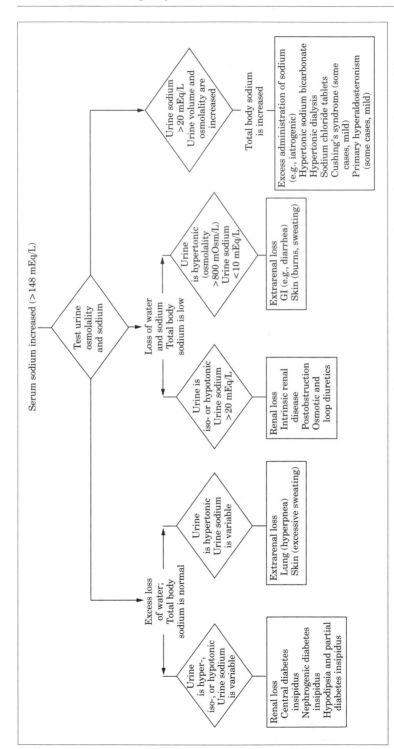

**Fig. 13-19.** Algorithm for hypernatremia. (Hypotonic urine = urine osmolality <800 mOsm/L; isotonic urine = urine osmolality between 800 mOsm/L and plasma osmolality; hypertonic urine = urine osmolality >800 mOsm/L.)

- Glucagonomas (alpha cells) syndrome of DM, anemia.
- Vipomas occur less often.

Pituitary adenomas in >21–65% of cases
- Nonfunctional chromophobe adenomas causing hypopituitarism due to space-occupying effect may be most common.
- ~15% are prolactinomas.
- ~15% are eosinophilic adenomas causing acromegaly.
- ~5% are basophilic adenomas causing Cushing's syndrome.

Adrenal cortical adenomas or hyperplasia in 27–36% of cases are nonfunctional. Adrenal medulla is not involved.

Thyroid disease in ~20% of cases include benign and malignant tumors, colloid goiter, thyrotoxicosis, Hashimoto's disease.

Uncommon lesions include carcinoids, schwannomas, multiple lipomas, gastric polyps, testicular tumors.

### MEN II (or IIa) (Sipple's Syndrome)

Medullary thyroid carcinoma in >90% of cases. Produce calcitonin and sometimes ACTH or serotonin.

Pheochromocytoma in 10–50% of cases. 10% of pheochromocytomas occur as part of MEN.

HPT in ~20% of cases; occurs late in disease; may occur without medullary thyroid carcinoma.

DNA analysis detected carriers of the gene before biochemical manifestations.

### MEN III (or IIb)
*(features in common with MEN II but is a separate genetic syndrome)*

Medullary thyroid carcinoma in 75% of cases
Pheochromocytoma in 33% of cases
HPT is rare.
Other lesions
- Multiple mucosal gangliomas in >95% of cases appear early in life.
- Marfan's syndrome habitus, hypertrophy of corneal nerves, ganglioneuromas of GI tract, characteristic retinal changes and facial appearance are frequent

## Nonendocrine Neoplasms Causing Endocrine Syndromes

**(Tumors secrete proteins, polypeptides, or glycoproteins that have hormonal activity. Diagnosed by arteriovenous gradient of hormone across tumor bed or between tumor and nontumor tissue; confirm by in vitro demonstration of hormone production by tumor cells and by resolution of endocrine syndrome after successful removal of tumor.)**

Cushing's syndrome*
- Bronchogenic oat cell carcinoma (causes ~50% of cases) and carcinoid
- Thymoma
- Hepatoma
- Carcinoma of ovary
- Also medullary carcinoma of thyroid, islet-cell tumor of pancreas, etc.

Hypercalcemia simulating HPT
- Renal carcinoma
- Squamous and large cell carcinoma of respiratory tract
- Carcinoma of breast (occurs in 15% of patients with bone metastases)

---

*Increased blood ACTH level (>200 pg/mL), inability to suppress with high dose dexamethasone test (except in bronchial carcinoids), loss of diurnal variation of cortisol levels (usually >40 $\mu$g/dL). Therefore cannot be distinguished from excessive pituitary secretion of ACTH by use of dexamethasone suppression test. Typically, malignant disease causing ectopic ACTH production has acute effects on adrenals manifested predominantly by excess mineralocorticoid production with hypokalemia and hypertension. May sometimes require selective venous catheterization for ACTH levels to establish the diagnosis. Patients with lung cancer may have elevated ACTH levels without Cushing's syndrome.

- Malignant lymphoma, myeloma, etc.
- Cancer of ovary, pancreas, etc.

SIADH
- Especially with oat cell carcinoma of lung

Hypoglycemia—serum insulin is low in presence of fasting hypoglycemia.
- Bronchogenic carcinoma
- Carcinoma of adrenal cortex (6% of patients)
- Hepatoma (23% of patients)
- Retroperitoneal fibrosarcoma (most frequently)

Thyrotoxicosis—signs and symptoms are rare, but laboratory findings are present.
- Tumors of GI tract, hematopoietic, pulmonary, etc.
- Trophoblastic tumors in women
- Choriocarcinoma of testis

Precocious puberty in boys
- Hepatoma

Acromegaly
- Pancreatic tumors producing GH or growth hormone releasing factor in presence of normal sella, elevated GH not suppressed by glucose
- Carcinoid

Erythrocytosis (due to erythropoietin production)
- Carcinoma of kidney, liver
- Fibromyoma of uterus
- Cerebellar hemangioblastoma

## Pituitary Growth Hormone Deficiency

There may be isolated deficiency with dwarfism or associated with TSH deficiency, with ACTH deficiency, or with TSH and ACTH deficiencies. GH deficiency is usually due to hypothalamic GHRH deficiency.

Serum GH basal levels are decreased ($<1.0$ ng/mL). Use pooled or average of three samples.

Stimulation tests have greater sensitivity. Increased basal or random serum level excludes this diagnosis but low levels do not distinguish normal persons from GH deficiency.

Stimulation (functional) tests
- Draw serum at intervals.
- Insulin should normally produce at least 2 times increase in serum GH level and 3 times increase in serum prolactin level at 60-min peak. This is the most reliable challenge for GH secretion.
- Levodopa (500 mg orally) should normally produce at least 2 times increase in serum GH level at 60-min peak.
- Arginine should normally produce at least 3 times increase in serum GH and at least 2 times increase in serum prolactin level at 30- to 60-min peak.
- Failure to produce these minimal responses indicates a lesion of pituitary or hypothalamus but does not differentiate between them.
- A normal response is at least 10 ng/mL peak value; 5–10 ng/mL is indeterminate, $\leq 5$ ng/mL is subnormal. A normal value rules out GH deficiency.

About one-fourth of patients with normal GH secretory capacity are unable to secrete GH in response to provocative tests indicated at any given time. Therefore, at least two of these tests should be used to confirm diagnosis of GH deficiency. Nonpituitary factors that impair GH response include obesity, primary hypothyroidism, thyrotoxicosis, primary hypogonadism, Kallmann's syndrome, Cushing's syndrome, use of various drugs. *Normal response may also occur in patients with partial deficiency.* GH response is normal or exaggerated in growth failure due to resistance to GH or resistance to somatomedins.

Serum prolactin baseline level is low and does not rise appropriately after TRH or other stimulation. In hypothalamic disease, basal prolactin level is increased and response may be normal or blunted.

Laboratory findings due to involvement of other endocrine organs
- TSH deficiency.
- ACTH deficiency.
- Gonadotropins are decreased or absent from urine in postpubertal patients (but increased levels occur in primary hypogonadism).

## Pituitary Tumors

Findings due to increased production of hormones or effect of growing mass.
Microadenomas (<10 mm in size) may be present in 10–20% of the population by autopsy and x-ray studies ("incidentaloma") but >10 mm in size are quite rare.

## Prolactinomas

### Serum Prolactin Reference Values

Normal <25 ng/mL in females; lower in males and children
Gradual increase from birth until adolescence
13- to 15-year-old boys: 2.5 times adult levels
13- to 15-year-old girls: 3 times adult levels
Serum samples should be collected under basal conditions by pooling three blood samples collected at 20-min intervals for one assay; all drugs should be discontinued for at least 2 wks before testing.

### Interpretation

40–85 ng/mL: seen in craniopharyngioma, hypothyroidism, effect of drugs
50 ng/mL: 25% chance of a pituitary tumor
100 ng/mL: 50% chance of a pituitary tumor
<200 ng/mL with a macroadenoma, particularly with extrasellar extension, is most likely due to compression of pituitary stalk rather than prolactinoma.
200–300 ng/mL: nearly 100% chance of a pituitary tumor
High levels may be seen with simultaneous multiple additive factors that usually cause lesser increases (e.g., chronic renal failure plus methyldopa).
Immediate postoperative level <7.0 ng/mL indicates long-term cure but higher levels are associated with recurrence.
Repeated serum levels in late morning or early afternoon increased 3–5 times normal in men or nonlactating women are usually considered diagnostic of pituitary adenoma or rarely of hypothalamic disease or pituitary stalk section or hypothyroidism. One elevated level is not adequate for diagnosis.

### Increased Serum Prolactin in

Amenorrhea/galactorrhea
- 10–25% of women with galactorrhea and normal menses
- 10–15% of women with amenorrhea without galactorrhea
- 75% of women with both galactorrhea and amenorrhea/oligomenorrhea
- Causes 15–30% of cases of amenorrhea in young women
Pituitary lesions (e.g., prolactinoma, section of pituitary stalk, empty-sella syndrome, acromegaly, chromophobe adenomas)
Hypothalamic lesions (e.g., sarcoidosis, eosinophilic granuloma, histiocytosis X, TB, glioma, craniopharyngioma)
Other endocrine diseases
- ~20% of cases of hypothyroidism (second most common cause of hyperprolactinemia). *Therefore, serum TSH and $T_4$ should always be measured.*
- Addison's disease.
- Polycystic ovaries.
- Glucocorticoid excess—normal or moderately elevated prolactin
Ectopic production of prolactin (e.g., bronchogenic carcinoma, renal cell carcinoma, ovarian teratomas, acute myeloid leukemia)

Children with sexual precocity—may be increased into pubertal range

Neurogenic causes (e.g., nursing and breast stimulation, spinal cord lesions, chest wall lesions such as herpes zoster)

Stress (e.g., surgery, hypoglycemia, vigorous exercise)

Pregnancy (increases to 8–20 times normal by delivery, returns to normal in 2–4 wks postpartum unless nursing occurs)

Lactation

Chronic renal failure

Liver failure (due to decreased prolactin clearance)

Idiopathic causes

### Interferences

Drugs—*most common cause*; usually subsides a few wks after cessation of using drug; these elevations are usually <100 ng/mL
- Neuroleptics (e.g., phenothiazines, thioxanthenes, butyrophenones)
- Antipsychotic drugs (e.g., prochlorperazine [Compazine, Thorazine], trifluoperazine [Stelazine], thioridazine [Mellaril])
- Dopamine antagonists (e.g., metoclopramide)
- Opiates (morphine, methadone)
- Reserpine
- Alpha-methyldopa (Aldomet)
- Estrogens and oral contraceptives
- TRH
- Amphetamines
- Isoniazid

### Serum Prolactin May Be Decreased in

Hypopituitarism
- Postpartum pituitary necrosis
- Idiopathic hypogonadotropic hypogonadism

Drugs
- Dopamine agonists
- Ergot derivatives (bromocriptine mesylate, lisuride hydrogen maleate)
- Levodopa, apomorphine, clonidine

### Interpretation

Normal value in child with growth retardation virtually rules out hypopituitarism but a low value is not diagnostic. Single blood value may be more reliable than multiple measurements of growth hormone in diagnosis of active acromegaly. Multiple basal prolactin levels have replaced stimulation tests.

Normal or decreased serum FSH, LH, and testosterone may occur in men.

Women may also present with hirsutism, infertility. Men may present with decreased libido, impotence, oligospermia, low serum testosterone levels, and sometimes galactorrhea.

Hypothyroidism

Acute fasting, and chronic protein-calorie deprivation (when growth hormone often rises)

## Syndrome of Inappropriate Secretion of Antidiuretic Hormone (SIADH)
**(syndrome of continuing release of vasopressin in presence of low plasma osmolality; kidney responds normally to AVP)**

### Due to

CNS disease of all types (e.g., neoplastic, degenerative, infective, trauma, vascular, psychogenic)

Advanced endocrinopathies (e.g., myxedema, ACTH deficiency, adrenal insufficiency)

Neoplasms (most commonly oat cell carcinoma of lung; adenocarcinoma of lung, carcinoma of pancreas, carcinoma of duodenum, lymphoma) some of which show ectopic production of ADH

Pulmonary infection (e.g., TB, pneumonia, chronic infections)

Miscellaneous (e.g., acute intermittent porphyria, postoperative state)

Idiopathic

Various drugs

- Oral hypoglycemic agents (chlorpropamide, tolbutamide, phenformin)
- Antineoplastic agents (vincristine, cyclophosphamide)
- Diuretics (chlorothiazide)
- Sedatives, analgesics (morphine, barbiturates, acetaminophen)
- Psychotropic drugs (amitriptyline, phenothiazines)
- Miscellaneous (clofibrate, isoproterenol, nicotine)

*Etiology should be established since some causes are curable with resolution of SIADH.*

*Cortisol deficiency and hypothyroidism should always be excluded.*

Dilutional hyponatremia with appropriately decreased osmolality (usually <280 mOsm/kg) when urine is not at maximum dilution; this is basis for diagnosis in patient with no evidence of cardiac, liver, kidney, adrenal, pituitary, thyroid disease, or hypovolemia and not on drug therapy.

Increased urine sodium (>20 mmol/L; >30 mmol/day) with inappropriately high urine osmolality (>500 mOsm/kg) is essential for diagnosis since it excludes hypovolemia as the cause of hyponatremia (in absence of abnormal renal function or causative drugs).

Increased urine osmolality > serum osmolality

Normal serum potassium, $CO_2$, BUN, and creatinine

Decreased serum chloride

Decreased anion gap

Decreased uric acid (due to dilution)

Increased plasma vasopressin that is inappropriately elevated for the degree of plasma osmolality is not helpful in diagnosis because most causes of true hyponatremia are associated with detectable or increased vasopressin.

Clinical and biochemical response to fluid restriction but not to administration of isotonic or hypertonic saline

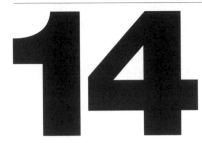

## Genitourinary Diseases

# Renal Function Tests

## Biopsy, Renal

Examination should include histology (stained by hematoxylin and eosin stain, trichrome, PAS, silver; other stains [e.g., for amyloid] when indicated), immunofluorescence (with antisera specific for IgG, IgA, IgM, C1q, C3, C4, fibrinogen, albumin, kappa and lambda light chains), and electron microscopy (e.g., necessary for diagnosis of Alport's syndrome, thin basement membrane nephritis).

### Indicated in

Acute renal allograft dysfunction
- Primary nonfunction for >10–14 days
- Unexplained deterioration of graft function
- Unexplained proteinuria
- Before beginning antilymphocyte therapy to prove diagnosis of rejection

Nephritic syndrome for differential diagnosis or to assess disease severity
Nephrotic syndrome—biopsy only if no response to corticosteroids
Non-nephrotic proteinuria with progressive disease

## Concentration Test, Urine

### Interpretation

Normal: Urine specific gravity is ≥ 1.025.
With decreased renal function, specific gravity is <1.020.
As renal impairment becomes more severe, specific gravity approaches 1.010.
The test is sensitive for early loss of renal function, but a normal finding does not rule out active kidney disease.

### Interferences

The test is unreliable in the presence of any severe water and electrolyte imbalance, low-protein or low-salt diet, chronic liver disease, pregnancy.

## Dilution Test, Urine

*Water loading may be contraindicated in kidney and heart disease.*

### Interpretation

Normal: Urine volume is >80% of ingested amount (1200 mL).
Specific gravity is 1.003 in at least one specimen.
With decreased renal function, there is a smaller volume of urine.

Specific gravity may not fall below 1.010.
Loss of dilution ability occurs later than loss of concentrating ability.

# Vasopressin (Pitressin) Concentration Test

The bladder is emptied, and urine is collected after injection of vasopressin.

## Interpretation

Same as in the urine concentration test
Normal: The specific gravity should reach ≥ 1.020.
In diabetes insipidus, urine specific gravity becomes normal after vasopressin
administration but not after fluid restriction.

# Osmolality, Urine

Measurement of urine osmolality during water restriction is an accurate, sensitive test of decreased renal function.

## Interpretation

Normal: Concentration of >800 mOsm/kg
Minimal impairment of renal concentrating ability: 600–800 mOsm/kg
Moderate impairment: 400–600 mOsm/kg
Severe impairment: <400 mOsm/kg
Urine osmolality may be impaired when other tests are normal. May be especially
useful in diabetes mellitus, essential hypertension, silent pyelonephritis.
Also should measure serum osmolality and calculate urine:serum ratio (nor-
mal >3)

# Glomerular Filtration Rate (GFR)

GFR is measured with urea clearance, creatinine clearance, or inulin clearance.

## Use

The creatinine clearance test, particularly serial measurements, is the most reliable test of renal function; is best measurement of GFR.

## Interpretation

Elderly patients with a normal serum creatinine and diminished muscle mass
may have a 30% decrease in GFR.
*Usually, there is good correlation between urine concentrating function and GFR.
A normal GFR in association with impaired concentrating ability may be found
in sickle cell anemia, diabetes insipidus, nephronophthisis, and various
acquired disorders (e.g., pyelonephritis, potassium deficiency, hypercalciuria).*
Impairment may be more severe than indicated by laboratory studies if signs and
symptoms are more disabling.
Estimate of creatinine clearance from single serum creatinine clearance may be
required for prompt therapy of nephrotoxic drug reaction or because of difficulty of accurate 24-hr urine collection. This estimate may be calculated by
the following formulas or by a nomogram.
To *estimate* GFR from serum creatinine, this equation may be used but may only
be accurate in patients in chronic renal failure with stable renal function who
are not massively obese or edematous:

$$GFR = \frac{(140 - age\ in\ years)\ (weight\ in\ kg)}{72 \times serum\ creatinine}$$

(Values for women are 85% of predicted.)

$$\text{Creatinine clearance (mL/min/1.73 sq m)} = \frac{(98 - 0.8) \times (\text{age} - 20)}{\text{Serum creatinine}}$$

(Values for women are 90% of predicted.)

## Other Renal Function Tests

### *Measurement of Effective Plasma Flow (RPF) and Tubular Function*

Para-aminohippurate (PAH)
Diodrast
Filtration fraction (FF) = GFR/RPF
Maximal Diodrast excretory capacity, TmD

### *Interpretation*

Urea clearance is normal until >50% of renal parenchyma is inactivated. With renal insufficiency, the clearance test parallels the parenchymal destruction.

Urinary acidification is impaired in chronic renal disease with azotemia. It is decreased without parallel impairment of GFR in renal tubular acidosis, some cases of Fanconi's syndrome, and some cases of nephrocalcinosis.

Proximal tubular malfunction is indicated by urinary excretion of substances normally reabsorbed by tubules: in renal glycosuria (blood glucose <180 mg/dL as in Fanconi's syndrome, heavy metal poisoning), aminoaciduria, phosphaturia. Serum creatinine and BUN are not useful in discovering early renal insufficiency because they do not become abnormal until 50% of renal function has been lost.

Serum creatinine increase occurs in 10–20% of patients taking aminoglycosides and up to 20% of patients taking penicillins.

## Phenolsulfonphthalein (PSP) Excretion Test

Rarely used now

## Split Renal Function Tests

### *Interpretation*

Affected kidney shows decreased urine volume and sodium excretion and decreased urine concentration of creatinine, inulin, or PAH.

### *Use*

Aid in diagnosis of renal artery stenosis
*Not useful in presence of GU tract obstruction (e.g., in men older than age 50)*

# Kidney Diseases

See Table 14-1.

## Allergic (Schönlein-Henoch) Purpura, Renal Disease in

Urine is abnormal in 50% of patients, but renal biopsy is abnormal in most.

Varies from minimal urinary abnormalities to severe, rapidly progressive nephritis that is indistinguishable from glomerulonephritis. Nephrotic syndrome may occur. Chronic course, with remissions and exacerbations and permanent renal damage, may occur.

Platelet count is normal.

**Table 14-1.** Urinary Findings in Various Diseases

| Disease | Volume | Specific Gravity | Protein[a] | RBCs[b] | WBCs and Epithelial Cells[b] | Casts[c, d] | Comment |
|---|---|---|---|---|---|---|---|
| Normal | 600–2500 | 1.003–1.030 | 0 (0.05 gm) | 0–occ. (0–0.130) | 0–0.65 | 0–occ. (2000/24 hrs) | |
| Acute febrile states | D | I | Trace to + | | | Few | |
| Orthostatic proteinuria | N | N | 1 (≤ 1 gm) | N (0–0.130) | 0–3 | V; H & G | Normal when recumbent; abnormalities after upright posture |
| Glomerulonephritis | | | | | | | |
| Acute | D | I | 2–4+ (0.5–5.0) | 1–4 + (1–1000) | 1–400 | 2–4+; H & G; *RBC, epithelial, mixed PBC* & epithelial | Gross hematuria or "smoky" urine |
| Latent | | | (0.1–2.0) | (1–100) | 1–20 | *RBC,* H & G | |
| Nephrosis ("nephrotic stage") | D | I | 4 + (4–40) | 0–few (0.5–50.0) | 20–1000 | *Epithelial, fatty, waxy;* H & G | Fat-laden epithelial cells, anisotropic fat in epithelial cells and casts |
| Terminal | I or D | D; fixed | 1–2+ (2–7) | Trace–1+ (0.5–10.0) | 1–50 | 1–3+ *broad, waxy,* H & G, epithelial | |
| Pyelonephritis | | | | | | | |
| Acute | N | N | 0–2+ (0.5–2.0) | Few (0–1) | 20–2000 | *WBC,* H & G, *bacteria* | Bacteria, many WBCs in clumps |

**Table 14-1.** (continued)

| Disease | Volume | Specific Gravity | Protein[a] | RBCs[b] | WBCs and Epithelial Cells[b] | Casts[c, d] | Comment |
|---|---|---|---|---|---|---|---|
| Chronic | N or D | N or D | 2–4+ (0–5) | Few (0–1) | 0.5–50.0 | Same as acute; often few or none | Same as acute; findings may be intermittent |
| Renal TB | | | (0.1–3.0) | (1–20) | 1–50 | WBC, H & G | Tubercle bacilli |
| Disseminated lupus erythematosus | V | N or D | 1–4+ (0.5–20.0) | 1–4+ (1–100) | 1–100 | 1–4+ RBC, *fatty*, *waxy*; H & G | |
| Toxemia of pregnancy | D | I | 3–4+ (0.5–10.0) | 0–1+ (0–1) | 1–5 | 3–4+ H & G | |
| Malignant hypertension | V | D; fixed | 1–2+ (1–10) | Trace–1+ (1–100) | 1–200 | 1–2+ H & G, RBC, fatty | Increasing uremia with minimal or marked proteinuria and hematuria |
| Benign hypertension | N or I | N or D | 0–1+ | 0–trace (1–5) | | 0–1+ H & G | |
| Congestive heart failure | D | I | 1–2+ | 0–1+ | | 1+ H & G | |
| Intercapillary glomerulosclerosis (Kimmelstiel-Wilson syndrome) | | | 1–4+ (2–20) | (0–1) | 1–30 | Epithelial, fatty, H & G | Frequently associated: pyelonephritis and nephrosclerosis |

Lower nephron
nephrosis

| | D | I | | | 1-4+ | 1-4- | REC; H & G, epithelial |
|---|---|---|---|---|---|---|---|
| Acute | | | | | | | |
| Diuretic | | I | | 0.5–10.0 | (0–1) | 1–100 | Broad, waxy, epithelial, H & G |

occ. = occasionally; H & G = hyaline and granular casts.
[a]Protein = quantitative values in ( ) given as gm/24 hrs.
[b]Quantitative values given in ( ) as cells × $10^6$ 24 hrs.
[c]Casts require examination of fresh or preserved urine and acid pE.
[d]Italics denote most important or diagnostic finding.

### Berger's Disease (IgA Nephropathy)
**(a focal, proliferative glomerulonephritis; immunologic mediation; probably the most common form of glomerulonephritis)**

Persistent or intermittent microscopic hematuria with episodes of painless gross hematuria and minimal proteinuria, often associated with (rather than following by 4–10 days) infection of any type.

Progression to renal failure in 10–20 yrs is not uncommon.

Diagnosis is based on renal biopsy with immunofluorescence showing predominant mesangial IgA, IgG, and C3.

### Glomerulonephritis, Acute Poststreptococcal in Children

See Table 14-2.

Evidence of infection with Group A beta-hemolytic *Streptococcus* by
- Culture of throat
- Serologic findings of recent beta-hemolytic streptococcal infection

Urine
- Hematuria—gross or only microscopic. Microscopic hematuria may occur during the initial febrile URI and then reappear with nephritis in 1–2 wks. It lasts 2–12 months.
- RBC casts show glomerular origin of hematuria.
- WBC casts and WBCs show inflammatory nature of lesion.
- Granular and epithelial cell casts are present.
- Fatty casts and lipid droplets occur several weeks later.
- Proteinuria is usually <2 gm/day (but may be ≤ 6–8 gm/day).
- Oliguria is frequent.

Blood
- Azotemia is found in ~50% of patients.
- ESR is increased.
- Leukocytosis with increased PMNs.
- Mild anemia, especially when edema is present.
- Serum proteins are normal or show nonspecific changes.

Renal biopsy shows characteristic findings with EM and immunofluorescence.

*Azotemia with high urine specific gravity and normal PSP excretion usually means acute glomerulonephritis.*

### Glomerulonephritis, Rapidly Progressive Nonstreptococcal

Preceded by associated systemic diseases in many patients

Infections
- Poststreptococcal glomerulonephritis
- Infective endocarditis
- Sepsis
- Hepatitis B, C

Multisystem diseases
- SLE
- Goodpasture's syndrome
- Necrotizing vasculitis
- Polyarteritis nodosa
- Wegener's granulomatosis
- Henoch-Schonlein purpura
- Cryoglobulinemia

No cultural or serologic evidence of recent streptococcus infection

Oliguria with urine volume often <400 mL/day

Hematuria is often gross.

RBCs, WBCs, and casts are present in urine.

Proteinuria is usually >3 gm/day.

Azotemia is usually marked, with BUN >80 mg/dL and serum creatinine >10 mg/dL (in poststreptococcal type, BUN is usually 30–100 mg/dL and serum creatinine 1.5–4.0 mg/dL).
Serum complement levels are normal.
Renal biopsy and immunofluorescent antibody findings

## Glomerulonephritis, Focal Proliferative

Attacks of hematuria usually occur at height of upper respiratory infection (bacterial or viral).
Serum IgA is often increased.
Azotemia is usually absent.
Proteinuria is slight or absent.
Progressive nephritis causing renal failure may occur, especially in adults.

## Glomerulonephritis, Membranoproliferative

Marked proteinuria and nephrotic type of syndrome is found in 70% of patients.
Normal serum C4 but prolonged or permanent depression of C3 is found in 60–80% of patients.
Renal biopsy and immunofluorescent antibody findings
GFR <80 mL/min/1.73/sq m in two-thirds of patients

## Glomerulonephritis, Chronic

### Various Clinical Courses

Early death after marked proteinuria, hematuria, oliguria, progressive increasing uremia, anemia
Intermittent or continuous proteinuria, hematuria with slight or absent azotemia, and normal renal function tests (may develop into late renal failure or may subside)
Exacerbation of chronic nephritis (with accentuation of proteinuria, hematuria, and decreased renal function) shortly after streptococcal upper respiratory infection
Nephrotic syndrome
*Compared to pyelonephritis, chronic glomerulonephritis shows lipid droplets and epithelial and RBC casts in urine, more marked proteinuria (>2–3 gm/day), poorer prognosis for equivalent amount of azotemia.*

## Hemolytic-Uremic Syndrome

(See Thrombotic Thrombocytopenic Purpura in Chapter 11.)
Urine indices resemble those of prerenal azotemia and contrast with acute tubular necrosis in which urine has low fixed specific gravity and high sodium content and a characteristic sediment may be found.
Usually appears in patients with decompensated cirrhosis with ascites. Hyponatremia, hyperkalemia, hepatic encephalopathy, and coma may be present.

## Hypercalciuria, Idiopathic

See Table 14-3.
Increased excretion of urinary calcium >350 mg/24 hrs on diet containing 600–800 mg/day
  • >4 mg/kg
  • >140 mg/gm of urinary creatinine
Normal blood calcium levels
Serum 1,25-dihydroxyvitamin $D_3$ levels are usually high.

Table 14-2. Classification of Glomerulonephritis

| Glomerular Disorder | Situations in Which May Be Found | Hematuria (% of cases) | | Proteinuria (% of cases) | | Renal Function Decreased | Comment |
|---|---|---|---|---|---|---|---|
| | | Micro RBCs Present | RBC Casts Present | 1–3 gm Present | >3 gm Present | | |
| IgA nephropathy (Berger's disease) | Focal proliferative GN | 100 | 50 | 75 | 25 | 25% or NS; N in 75% | |
| IgM mesangial nephropathy | | 50 | Rare | 50 | 50 | >75% or NS | |
| Acute GN secondary to infection (focal GN) | SBE, bacterial pneumonia, viral infections, infection of implanted devices | 100 | 50 | 75 | 25 | 100% | |
| Crescentic (rapidly progressive) GN | | | | | | | |
| Anti-GBM | Goodpasture's syndrome in ⅔ of patients | 100 | 50 | 50 | 50 | 100% | 90% have HLA-DR2 antigen. |
| Immune complex | SLE, mixed cryoglobulinemia, Schönlein-Henoch purpura | 100 | 50 | 50 | 50 | 100% | |

| Classification | Associated conditions / synonyms | | | | | Serum complement | Comments |
|---|---|---|---|---|---|---|---|
| **Non-immune complex** | | | | | | | |
| GN and vasculitis | Wegener's granulomatosis, polyarteritis | 100 | 50 | 50 | 50 | 100% | |
| | Wegener's granulomatosis, Schönlein-Henoch purpura, mixed cryoglobulinemia; Goodpasture's syndrome may occur | 100 | 50 | 50 | 50 | 100% | See Chapter 16. |
| **SLE** | | | | | | | |
| Mesangial | | 15 | 10 | | | N | Most frequent type in SLE. |
| Focal proliferative | | 50 | 25 | | | N or D | |
| Membranous | | 50 | | 85 | | N or D | |
| Diffuse proliferative (<25% of SLE patients) | | 75 | | 75 | | Usually D; uremia develops in 50–75% | |
| Minimal change disease | Lipid nephrosis, nil disease | 20 | | 100 | | N | 85% respond to steroid therapy. Most common cause of NS in children. |
| Focal sclerosis | | 75 | 25 | 75 | | Usually D | Frequent cause of NS. |

**Table 14-2.** (continued)

| Glomerular Disorder | Situations in Which May Be Found | Hematuria (% of cases) | | Proteinuria (% of cases) | | Renal Function Decreased | Comment |
|---|---|---|---|---|---|---|---|
| | | Micro RBCs Present | RBC Casts Present | 1–3 gm Present | >3 gm Present | | |
| Membranous nephropathy | Usually idiopathic; occasionally due to heavy-metal toxicity (e.g., gold, mercury), persistent hepatitis B infection, other viruses (e.g., measles, varicella, Coxsackie), other infections (e.g., malaria, syphilis, leprosy, schistosomiasis), neoplasias (e.g., colon carcinoma, lymphoma, leukemia), sarcoidosis, SLE, others | 50 | | 25 | 75 | N early; D late | Frequent cause of NS. Strong association with HLA-DR3. Spontaneous remission in 25–50%. Persistent proteinuria without progression in 25%. Progressive glomerular sclerosis causing renal failure in 50%. Common in adults; uncommon in children. |

| Membranoproliferative GN | | 75 | 25 | 50 | 5C | Usually; D; NS at onset in 75% | Renal failure within 5 yrs common in adults but may be delayed 10–20 yrs. Persistent, marked proteinuria is poor prognostic sign. Renal vein thrombosis may occur. |
|---|---|---|---|---|---|---|---|
| Type I (idiopathic) | SBE, essential cryoglobulinemia, Schönlein-Henoch purpura, SLE, sickle cell disease, hepatitis and cirrhosis, C2 deficiency, alpha$_1$-antitrypsin deficiency, infected shunts (*Staphylococcus, Corynebacterium*) | | | | | | |
| Type II (idiopathic) | Infection with streptococci, pneumococci, *Candida*, lipodystrophy | | | | | | |

GN = glomerulonephritis; NS = nephrotic syndrome; SBE = subacute endocarditis. *Goodpasture's syndrome occurs in <5% of cases of GN.*

**Table 14-3.** Comparison of Types of Idiopathic Hypercalciuria

|  | Resorptive | Absorptive | Renal |
|---|---|---|---|
| Due to | Primary hyper-parathyroidism | Primary increase in intestinal absorption; autosomal dominant | Abnormal renal tubular reabsorption |
| Frequency | Least common | Most common | $\frac{1}{10}$ as common as absorptive type |
| 2-Hr urine after fasting |  |  |  |
| Calcium | 30 mg | <20 mg | Increased |
| Calcium: creatinine ratio | >0.15 | <0.15 | >0.15 |

Diagnosis requires exclusion of all other causes of hypercalciuria; may be familial. Occurs in ~40% of patients who form calcium renal stones.

## Hypernephroma of Kidney

Even in the absence of the classic loin pain, flank mass, and hematuria, hypernephroma should be ruled out in the presence of these *unexplained* laboratory findings.
- Abnormal liver function tests in absence of metastases to liver
- Hypercalcemia
- Polycythemia
- Leukemoid reaction
- Refractory anemia and increased ESR
- Amyloidosis
- Cushing's syndrome
- Salt-losing syndrome
- Increased serum ferritin (due to hemorrhage within tumor)

For laboratory assistance in diagnosis
- Exfoliative cytology of urine for tumor cells
- Test for increased urine LD concentration

*Needle biopsy is not recommended.*

## Hypertension, Renovascular

See Chapter 13 and Fig. 14-1.

## Interstitial Nephritis, Chronic

Due to infections
- Pyelonephritis

Not due to infections
- Analgesic abuse
- Diabetes mellitus

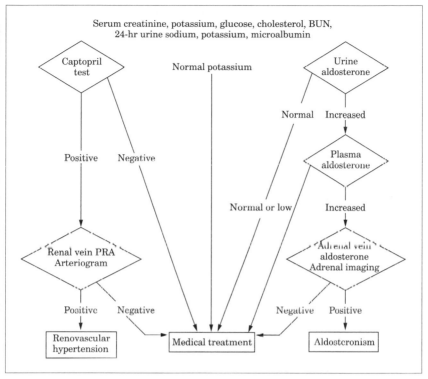

**Fig. 14-1.** Algorithm for diagnosis of suspected renovascular hypertension.

- Nephrocalcinosis
- Drugs
    Allergic (e.g., antibiotics, diuretics, phenytoin, cimetidine, NSAIDs)
    Toxic (e.g., cyclosporine, lithium, cisplatin, amphotericin B)
- Toxic substances
    Exogenous (e.g., lead, mercury, cadmium)
    Endogenous
        Uric acid
        Hypercalcemic nephropathy
        Oxalate
- Irradiation nephritis
- Sarcoidosis

Diagnosis is usually by exclusion. Renal biopsy may be helpful.
May be associated with metabolic acidosis and hyperkalemia out of proportion
    to degree of renal insufficiency, decreased urine concentrating capacity, and
    renal salt wasting

## Obstructive Uropathy

Partial obstruction of both kidneys may cause
- Increasing azotemia with normal or increased urinary output.
- Inexplicable wide variations in BUN and urine volume in patients with
  azotemia. PSP excretion is less in first 15-min period than in any later
  period; considerable PSP excretion after the 2-hr test period.

• In unilateral obstruction, BUN usually remains normal unless underlying renal disease is present.

## Papillary Necrosis of Kidney

Hematuria
Sudden diminution in renal function; occasionally oliguria or anuria with acute renal failure
Findings of associated diseases
• Diabetes mellitus
• Urinary tract infection
• Chronic overuse of phenacetin
• Sickle-cell disease

## Polycystic Kidneys

**(Autosomal dominant form [ADPKD] is usually slowly progressive. Autosomal recessive form is more severe, with few adult survivors. Acquired form is often seen in progressive renal failure due to diabetes mellitus, glomerulonephritis, especially after dialysis.)**

Polyuria is common.
Hematuria may be gross and episodic or an incidental microscopic finding.
Proteinuria occurs in ~one-third of patients and is mild (<1 gm/24 hrs).
Renal calculi may be associated.
Superimposed UTI is frequent.
Renal failure affects 45% of patients by age 60.
Hypertension
Anemia of renal failure is less severe than in other forms of kidney disease.
Prenatal diagnosis using DNA from amniocentesis or chorionic villus sampling

## Pyelonephritis

### Tests for Bacteriuria and Pyuria

Diagnosis of UTI and determination of antibiotic sensitivity of causative organism

### Interferences

Urine allowed to remain at room temperature.
False low colony counts may occur with a high rate of urinary flow, low urine specific gravity or pH, presence of antibacterial drugs, or inappropriate cultural techniques.
High doses of vitamin C may cause false-negative test for nitrite on dipstick.

### Interpretation

Dipstick test for neutrophils and bacteria. Combined positive esterase and nitrate strips is indication for colony count.
Direct microscopic examination of uncentrifuged urine unstained or gram-stained that shows 1 PMN or 1 organism/HPF for detection of bacteriuria; >10% false-positive results. Uncentrifuged urine showing 1 organism/oil-immersion field correlates with count ≥ 10,000 colonies/mL. Gram's stain of cytospin specimen has good sensitivity and specificity. With pyuria and bacteriuria, a Gram's stain to differentiate gram-positive cocci from gram-negative bacilli will indicate appropriate initial therapy. Patients with chronic UTI and asymptomatic bacteriuria may not show significant numbers of WBCs on urine microscopic examination. Bacteriuria and pyuria are often intermittent; often absent in the chronic atrophic stage of pyelonephritis. In acute pyelonephritis, marked pyuria and bacteriuria are almost always present;

hematuria and proteinuria may also be present during first few days. WBC casts are very suggestive of pyelonephritis.

A colony count >100,000 bacteria/cu mm indicates active infection under the following conditions: A midstream, clean-catch, first morning specimen is submitted in a sterilized container and refrigerated until the colony count is performed; periurethral area first thoroughly cleaned with soap. The presence of any organisms on culture from suprapubic sterile needle aspiration is diagnostic of UTI; it is the only acceptable method in infants. Colony counts <10,000/cu mL in the absence of therapy largely rule out bacteriuria. Colony counts 10,000–100,000/mL should be repeated and cultured. <100,000/mL with clinical findings of acute pyelonephritis with no obvious explanation, such as recent use of antibiotics, suggests urinary tract obstruction or perinephric abscess.

A culture should be performed for identification of the organism and determination of antibiotic sensitivity when these screening tests are positive. This is useful to subsequently identify the same organism in relapsing infections. If culture shows a common gram-positive saprophyte, it should be repeated because the second culture is often negative. Causative bacteria are usually enteric organisms; <10% are gram-positive cocci. Positive significant single culture or predominant organism should be considered positive in symptomatic patients and repeat is unnecessary. Three or more species with none being predominant (i.e., >80% of the growth) almost always represents specimen contamination and culture should be repeated; but true mixed infections may occur after instrumentation or with chronic infection. *If* Pseudomonas *or* Proteus *is found, the patient may have an anatomic abnormality. If organism other than* Escherichia coli *is found, patient probably has chronic pyelonephritis, even if this is the first clinical episode of infection.* In women, >80% of UTI are due to *E. coli* and smaller percent are due to *Staphylococcus saprophyticus,* and less often to other aerobic gram-negative bacilli. In men, gram-negative bacilli cause ~75% of UTI but *E. coli* causes only ~25% of infections in men and <50% of infections in boys. Other common gram-negative bacilli are *Proteus* and *Providencia* species. Gram-positive organisms (especially enterococci and coagulase-negative staphylococci) cause ~20% of infections in men and boys. If *Candida* are isolated, rule out contaminated specimen, diabetes mellitus, papillary necrosis, indwelling catheter, broad-spectrum antibiotic exposure, immunosuppressive chemotherapy, etc. "Sterile" (i.e., pyogenic infection is absent) pyuria (> 10 WBCs/HPF in centrifuged urine) and absence of bacilli (<1 bacillus in multiple oil-immersion fields or 20–40 bacteria/HPF in centrifuged sediments) should cast doubt on diagnosis of untreated bacterial UTI; may occur in renal TB, chemical inflammation, mechanical inflammation (e.g., calculi, instrumentation), early acute glomerulonephritis before appearance of hematuria or proteinuria, polycystic kidney disease, papillary necrosis, chronic prostatitis, interstitial cystitis, transplant rejection, sarcoidosis, GU tract neoplasm, uric acid and hypercalcemic nephropathy, lithium and heavy metal toxicity, extreme dehydration, hyperchloremic renal acidosis, genital herpes, nonbacterial gastroenteritis and respiratory tract infections, and after administration of oral polio vaccine; may persist for several months after transurethral prostatectomy. *When urine cultures are persistently negative in the presence of other evidence of pyelonephritis, specific search should be made for tubercle bacilli.*

With pyuria and bacteriuria, persistent alkaline pH may indicate infection with urea-splitting organism (e.g., *Proteus;* less often *Pseudomonas* or *Klebsiella*) suggesting a calculus.

Bacteria should be cleared from urine within 48 hrs of antibiotic therapy; persistence indicates need to change antibiotic treatment or search for another explanation.

In pregnancy, asymptomatic bacteriuria has ≤ 15% prevalence. Routine urinalysis is performed on first prenatal visit because 20–40% of untreated patients with positive culture develop acute pyelonephritis during pregnancy.

Persistent or recurrent infection may be due to stones or obstruction.

Acute pyelonephritis shows two consecutive colony counts ≥ 100,000 organisms/mL with or without upper GU tract symptoms.

Acute urethral syndrome and acute cystitis have colony count ≥ 100 organisms/mL and lower GU tract symptoms. Pyuria is rarely present unless bacterial count >10,000/cu mL.

Suprapubic aspiration, cystoscopy, nephrostomy, or renal transplant urines with bacteriuria plus positive dipstick test suggests infection but with a negative test suggests colonization.

Catheterization for <30 days or intermittent catheterization—criterion for bacteriuria is ≥ 100 organisms/mL; >95% of patients progress to >100,000 organisms/mL within days. Multiple organisms are common.

Catheterization for >30 days—mixed infections >100,000 organisms/mL in >75% of cases. Organisms constantly change with new ones every ~2 wks.

Dye tests do not detect 10–50% of infections. Urine should incubate in patient's bladder for ≥ 4 hrs.

Beta$_2$ microglobulin is increased in 24-hr urine in pyelonephritis (due to tubular damage) but not in cystitis.

## Nephrotic Syndrome

### Characterized by

Marked proteinuria—usually >4.5 gm/day

Hyperlipidemia: Increased serum cholesterol—usually >350 mg/dL. (Low or normal with poor nutrition)

Decreased serum albumin (usually <2.5 gm/dL) and TP

Serum alpha$_2$ and beta globulins are markedly increased; gamma globulin is decreased; alpha$_1$ globulin is normal or decreased.

Urine containing doubly refractive fat bodies as seen by polarizing microscopy; many granular and epithelial cell casts

Hematuria—may be present in 50% of patients but is usually minimal and not part of syndrome

Azotemia—may be present but not part of syndrome

Increased ESR

Increased susceptibility to infection (most frequently peritonitis) during periods of edema

Serum C3 complement is normal in idiopathic lipoid nephrosis but decreased when there is underlying glomerulonephritis.

Associated renal vein thrombosis in ~35% of patients (≤ 40% of these will have pulmonary emboli), especially when due to membranous nephropathy, membranoproliferative glomerulonephritis, rapidly progressive glomerulonephritis

Renal biopsy. Minimal change disease—fused epithelial podocytes by electron microscopy

### Etiology

Renal
- Glomerulonephritis (>50% of patients)
    Membranous nephropathy—50% of adults, <5% of children; ~65% have spontaneous complete or partial remission of proteinuria and ~15% develop end stage renal disease.
    Membranoproliferative—10% of children, 10% of adults
    Rapidly progressive
- Minimal change disease (formerly called *lipoid nephrosis* or *nil lesion*; 10% in adults; 80% in children; may be associated with Hodgkin's disease and non-Hodgkin's lymphoma)
Systemic
- Diabetic glomerulosclerosis (15% of patients)
- SLE (20% of patients)

- Amyloidosis
- Schönlein-Henoch purpura
- Multiple myeloma
- Goodpasture's syndrome (rare)
- Berger's disease
- Polyarteritis (rare)
- Takayasu's syndrome
- Sarcoidosis
- Sjögren's syndrome
- Wegener's granulomatosis (rare)
- Dermatitis herpetiformis
- Cryoglobulinemia

Venous obstruction
- Obstruction of inferior vena cava (thrombosis, tumor)
- Constrictive pericarditis
- Tricuspid stenosis
- Congestive heart failure

Infections
- Bacterial (poststreptococcal glomerulonephritis, bacterial endocarditis)
- Viral (hepatitis B; also HIV, CMV, infectious mononucleosis, varicella)
- Protozoal (malaria, toxoplasmosis)
- Parasitic (schistosomiasis, filariasis)

Allergic (e.g., serum sickness)

Neoplasm associated in 10% of adults and 15% >age 60 yrs (e.g., Hodgkin's disease; carcinoma of colon, lung, stomach, and others; lymphomas and leukemia); paraproteinemia (multiple myeloma, light chain nephropathy). *In adult with minimal-change nephrotic syndrome without evident cause, first rule out Hodgkin's disease. With membranous lesion, carcinoma may be more likely.*

Toxic (e.g., heavy metals, heroin, drugs)

Hereditary (e.g., sickle-cell disease)

Miscellaneous
- Preeclampsia
- Chronic allograft rejection

## Renal Calculi

See Fig. 14-2.

Calcium oxalate alone or with phosphate is the constituent of kidney stones in 75% of patients in the United States.
- 35% of patients have increased urinary calcium (i.e., >275 mg/24 hrs in females and >300 mg/24 hrs in males).
- 50–75% of hyperparathyroidism patients have renal calculi; ~5% of patients with nephrolithiasis have primary hyperparathyroidism.
- 20–30% of patients have
   Bone diseases—destructive or osteoporosis
   Milk-alkali syndrome
   Hypervitaminosis D
   Sarcoidosis
   Renal tubular acidosis, type I (hypercalciuria, highly alkaline urine)
   Hyperthyroidism
   Other.
- ~50% of patients have idiopathic hypercalciuria.

Oxalate is a constituent of renal calculi in 65% of all patients, but hyperoxaluria is a relatively rare cause of these calculi and may be due to primary or secondary hyperoxaluria.

Magnesium ammonium phosphate is the constituent of renal calculi in 15% of patients. It occurs almost exclusively in patients with recurrent UTIs by urea-splitting organisms, particularly *Proteus* species, and in patients with persistently alkaline urine.

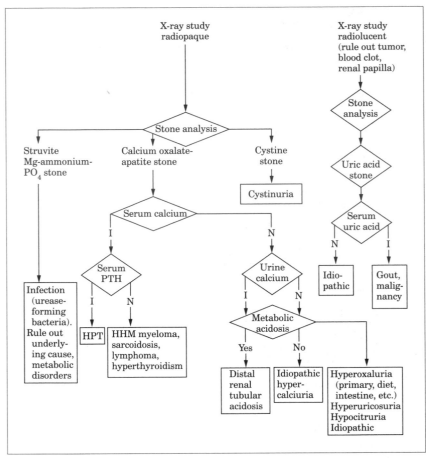

**Fig. 14-2.** Algorithm for diagnosis of renal calculi, as revealed by flank pain, renal colic, hematuria, fever, and urinalysis findings. (HPT = hyperparathyroidism; HHM = humeral hypercalcemia of malignancy.)

Struvite stones (staghorn calculi) occur only when urine pH is high due to infection with urea-splitting bacteria.

Cystine stones form when urine contains >300 mg/day of cystine in congenital familial cystinuria. Cystine-only stones form only in homozygotes. Urine shows cystine crystals. Cyanide-nitroprusside test is positive. Causes 1% of all stones. Heterozygotes form stones with little or no cystine.

Uric acid is present in calculi in 5% of patients.

- Gout—25% of patients with primary gout and 40% of patients with marrow-proliferative disorders have calculi.
- Urine is more acid than normal, often <5.5 (e.g., patients with chronic diarrhea, ileostomy).
- >50% of patients with urinary calculi have normal serum and urine uric acid levels.

Xanthine is present in children with inborn error of metabolism.

Microscopic hematuria
In renal colic, hematuria and proteinuria are present, increased WBC.

Crystalluria is diagnostically useful when there are cystine crystals (occur only in homozygous or heterozygous cystinuria) or struvite crystals. Calcium oxalate, phosphate, and uric acid should arouse suspicion about possible cause of stones but they may occur in normal urines.

## Renal Failure, Acute

### Due to

Prerenal
- Hypotension (e.g., shock)
- Volume contraction (e.g., hemorrhage)
- Severe heart failure

Renal
- Acute tubular necrosis
  Prolonged ischemia
  Toxic agents
    Heavy metals (e.g., lead, mercury, arsenic, cadmium, bismuth)
    Organic solvents (e.g., carbon tetrachloride, ethylene glycol)
    Antibiotics (e.g., aminoglycosides [often nonoliguric], tetracyclines, penicillins, amphotericin)
    X-ray contrast media (especially in diabetic persons or pre-existing renal insufficiency); tends to be oliguric
    Pesticides, fungicides
    Drugs (e.g., phenylbutazone, phenytoin, calcium)
    Acute interstitial nephritis
- Pigment-induced (e.g., hemolysis, rhabdomyolysis)
- Tubular deposition (e.g., multiple myeloma, uric acid)
- Various types of glomerulonephritis
- Large-vessel disease
  Bilateral renal vein occlusion (thrombosis, tumor infiltration)
  Renal artery occlusion

Postrenal
- Bladder obstruction (e.g., benign prostatic hyperplasia [BPH], carcinoma)

*In a patient with two functioning kidneys, obstruction of only one ureter should cause serum creatinine to rise ~50% to 2 mg/dL; acute renal failure that is postrenal with creatinine >2 mg/dL suggests that obstruction is bilateral or patient has only one functioning kidney.*

Total anuria for more than 2 days is uncommon in acute tubular necrosis and should suggest other possibilities (e.g., ruptured bladder, GU tract obstruction, micro- or large-vessel disease, renal cortical necrosis, glomerulonephritis, allergic interstitial nephritis).

### Early Stage

Urine is scant in volume (often <50 mL/day) for ≤ 2 wks; anuria for >24 hrs is unusual.

Usually bloody. Specific gravity may be high because RBCs and protein are present. Urine sodium concentration is usually >50 mEq/L.

WBC is increased even without infection.

BUN rises ≤ 20 mg/dL/day in transfusion reaction. It rises ≤ 50 mg/dL/day in overwhelming infection of severe crushing injuries.

Serum creatinine is increased.

Serum uric acid is often increased; may be >20 mg/dL in some types (e.g., rhabdomyolysis)

Hypocalcemia may occur.

Disproportionately increased serum phosphorus and creatinine indicate tissue necrosis.

Serum amylase and lipase may be increased without evidence of pancreatitis.

Metabolic acidosis is present.

### Second Week

Urine becomes clear several days after onset of acute renal failure, and there is a small daily increase in volume. Daily volume of 400 mL indicates onset of tubular recovery. Daily volume of 1000 mL occurs in ≤ 2 wks. RBCs and large hematin casts are present. Proteinuria is slight or absent.

Azotemia increases. BUN continues to rise for several days after onset of diuresis.

Metabolic acidosis increases.

Serum potassium is increased.

Serum sodium is often decreased, with increased extracellular fluid volume.

Anemia usually appears during second week.

Bleeding tendency is frequent, with decreased platelets, abnormal prothrombin consumption.

### Diuretic Stage

Large urinary potassium excretion may cause decreased serum potassium level.

Urine sodium concentration is 50–75 mEq/L.

Serum sodium and chloride may increase because of dehydration from large diuresis if replacement of water is inadequate.

Hypercalcemia may occur in some patients with muscle damage.

Azotemia disappears 1–3 wks after onset of diuresis.

### Later Findings

Anemia may persist for weeks or months.

Pyelonephritis may first occur during this stage.

Renal blood flow and GFR do not usually become completely normal.

*Suspect urinary tract obstruction, bilateral renal vascular thrombi or emboli, cortical necrosis, or acute glomerulonephritis* if there is complete anuria for >48 hrs.

*Suspect cortical necrosis* if proteinuria is >3–4 gm/L, BUN does not fall, and diuresis does not occur.

*Suspect urinary tract obstruction* if recurrent oliguria and increasing azotemia occur during period of diuresis.

### Urinary Diagnostic Indices in Acute Renal Failure

See Table 14-4 and Fig. 14-3.

**Interpretation**

Urinary sodium levels between 20 mEq/L and 40 mEq/L may be found in all forms of acute renal failure.

$$\text{Fractional excretion of sodium (FENa)} = 100 \times \frac{\text{(urine sodium/plasma sodium)}}{\text{(urine creatinine/plasma creatinine)}}$$

FENa is an index of renal ability to conserve sodium and represents percent of filtered sodium to reach the urine. Is the most reliable test to distinguish prerenal azotemia from acute tubular necrosis with oliguria.

Some causes of FENa <1%
- Prerenal azotemia
- Acute glomerulonephritis
- Early (few hours) acute urinary tract obstruction
- Early sepsis
- Some cases of acute tubular necrosis due to x-ray contrast material or myoglobinuria due to rhabdomyolysis
- 10% of cases of nonoliguric acute tubular necrosis

Some causes of FENa >1% (injured tubules)
- 90% of cases of acute tubular necrosis
- Later urinary tract obstruction (days to months)

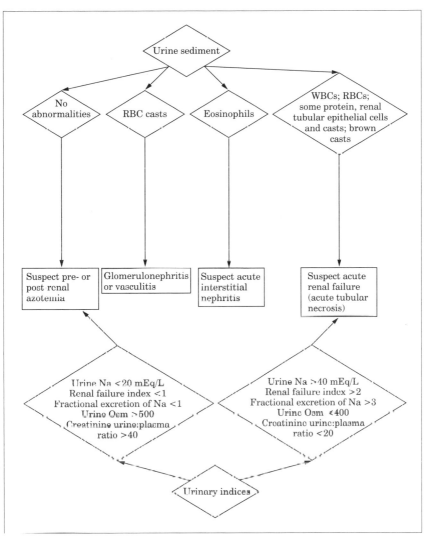

**Fig. 14-3.** Algorithm for differential diagnosis of acute renal failure.

- Diuretic administration
- Pre-existing chronic renal failure
- Diuresis due to mannitol, glycosuria, or bicarbonaturia

Renal failure index (RFI) = urine sodium/(urine creatinine/plasma creatinine) and measures Na conservation and concentrating ability.

**Use**

Indices (especially RFI and FENa) are chiefly of value in *oliguric* patients for the early differentiation of prerenal azotemia from acute tubular necrosis.

Indices are not useful for diagnosis of presence or absence of obstruction in cases of acute renal failure.

**Table 14-4.** Urinary Diagnostic Indices in Acute Renal Failure

| | Prerenal Azotemia | Postrenal (acute obstructive) | Acute Glomerulonephritis and Vasculitis | Acute Interstitial Nephritis | Acute Tubular Necrosis Oliguric | Acute Tubular Necrosis Nonoliguric | Renal Vascular Occlusion Arterial | Renal Vascular Occlusion Venous |
|---|---|---|---|---|---|---|---|---|
| Urine volume (mL/24 hrs) | <500 | Usually <500; fluctuates from day to day | <500 | V | <350 | 1000–2000 | V Anuria if bilateral/complete | V |
| Urine specific gravity | H; >1.015 | | | | L; <1.010 | | | |
| Urine osmolality (mOsm/kg $H_2O$) | >500 | V; usually <500 | <500 | V | <350 | 350 | V | V |
| Urine sodium (mEq/L) | L; <20 | H; >40 | L; usually <20 | V | >40 | V | V | V |
| U/P osmolality | >1.5 | | | | <1.2 | <1.2 | | |
| U/P urea nitrogen | >8 | Usually >8 | >8 | | <3 | <8 | | |

| | | | | | | | | |
|---|---|---|---|---|---|---|---|---|
| U:P creatinine | >40 | <20 | >40 | | <20 | <20 | | |
| Renal failure index | <1 (90% of cases) | >2 (95% of cases) | <1 | | >2 (95% of cases) | >3 | V | |
| FENa | <1 (≤94% of cases) | >3 | <1 | V | >3 | >3 | V | V |
| BUN:creatinine | >20:1 | >20:1 | >20:1 | <20:1 | <20:1 | <20:1 | <20:1 | <20:1 |
| Urine sediment | Hyaline casts | N; RBCs, WBCs, crystals may be present | RBCs, RBC casts | WBCs, WBC casts, eosinophils | Granular casts, renal tubular epithelial cells, cell debris, pigment, crystals | | V | V |
| Comments | Decreased renal perfusion | Evidence of GU tract obstruction | Biopsy findings classify disease | Eosinophilia; thrombocytopenia | Renal hypoperfusion; nephrotoxin | Nephrotoxin | Aortic injury; atheromatous emboli | Renal vein occlusion with nephrotic syndrome |

H = high; L = low; U/P = urine:plasma ratio; FENa = fractional sodium excretion.

### Interpretation

Values ≤ 1 for RFI and FENa strongly suggest prerenal azotemia and values ≥ 3 strongly suggest acute tubular necrosis; values of 1–3 are less definitive but usually indicate tubular necrosis; nonoliguric acute renal failure patients frequently have intermediate values between prerenal azotemia and oliguric renal failure.

Values usually >1 in urinary obstruction or acute interstitial nephritis; values usually <1 in acute glomerulonephritis

Diagnostic indices in patients with reversible acute obstructive uropathy often resemble indices in acute tubular necrosis or prerenal azotemia; indices in obstructive uropathy depend on duration of obstruction and severity of azotemia.

Differences between prerenal azotemia and acute tubular necrosis by these indices are particularly blurred in elderly patients as well as those with hypertensive or diabetic nephrosclerosis or other chronic parenchymal renal diseases.

*These diagnostic indices are often intermediate, and considerable overlapping of values is frequent, especially at time of initial evaluation. Even the total profile may not be useful in the individual case.*

### Interferences

Specimens for urinary indices should be obtained before onset of treatment if possible; therapy (mannitol or furosemide) may make results uninterpretable.

It is not necessary to obtain a timed specimen; a random specimen is sufficient.

### *Urine Sediment in Acute Renal Failure*

Renal tubular cells (or cellular casts) and pigmented granular casts indicate acute tubular necrosis; urine Na >20 mEq/L.

Sediment may be normal in prerenal or postrenal causes with minimal or absent proteinuria.

Eosinophils may be found in acute interstitial nephritis; increased WBC and WBC casts; minimal proteinuria.

RBC casts indicate glomerulonephritis, vasculitis, or microembolic disease; increased RBCs and moderate proteinuria.

RBCs indicate blood from lower GU tract or from glomerulus.

Myoglobin casts indicate myoglobinuria.

WBCs in hyaline casts indicate renal parenchymal infection rather than lower GU tract infection.

## Renal Failure, Chronic

BUN and serum creatinine are increased and renal function tests are impaired.
• Creatinine clearance is decreased.

Loss of renal concentrating ability (nocturia, polyuria, polydipsia) is an early manifestation of progressive renal functional impairment. Specific gravity is usually the same as that of glomerular filtrate.

Abnormal urinalysis is usually the first finding. Variable abnormalities include proteinuria, hematuria, pyuria, granular and cellular casts, and may be found in asymptomatic patients.

*Hypotonic urine unresponsive to vasopressin may occur in*
• Obstructive uropathy
• Chronic pyelonephritis
• Nephrocalcinosis
• Amyloidosis
• Familial nephrogenic diabetes insipidus

Serum sodium is decreased. The decrease is indicated by increased urine sodium (>5–10 mEq sodium/L). It may occur in any renal disease, especially when polyuria is marked, but is more common with obstructive uropathy, chronic pyelonephritis, and interstitial nephritis than with chronic glomerulonephritis.

Serum potassium is increased.

Acidosis is present. Blood organic acids, phenols, indoles, and certain amino acids are increased.

Serum calcium is decreased.

Serum phosphorus increases when creatinine clearance falls to ~25 mL/min.

Serum ALP may be normal or may be increased with renal osteodystrophy.

Serum magnesium increases when glomerular filtration rate falls to <30 mL/min.

Increase in serum uric acid is usually <10 mg/dL. Secondary gout is rare. If serum uric acid level is >10 mg/dL, rule out primary gout nephropathy.

Increased serum amylase occurs frequently.

Serum CK may be increased; a subset of uremic patients have a persistently increased CK-MB fraction without evidence of cardiac disease.

Increased serum triglycerides, cholesterol, and VLDL lipoprotein is common as renal failure progresses.

Normochromic normocytic anemia is usually proportional to the degree of azotemia. Responds to erythropoietin. Burr cells or schistocytes are common.

Bleeding tendency is evident. There may be decreased platelets, increased capillary fragility, abnormal prothrombin consumption (possible platelet defect), normal bleeding and clotting time.

Hemorrhage from ulcers anywhere in GI tract may be severe.

Laboratory findings due to uremic pericarditis, pleuritis, and pancreatitis are noted. Uremic meningitis (BUN is usually >100 mg/dL).

Serum albumin and TP are decreased.

### Chronic Renal Failure with Normal Urine May Occur in

Nephrosclerosis
Renal tubular acidosis
Interstitial nephritis
Hypercalcemia
Potassium deficiency
Uric acid nephropathy
Obstruction

## Renal Pelvis and Ureter, Carcinoma of

Hematuria is present.
Renal calculi are associated.
Urinary tract infection is associated.
Cytologic examination of urinary sediment for malignant cells

## Renal Tubular Acidosis

**(inadequate H$^+$ secretion; glomerular function is either normal or relatively less impaired)**

### Proximal

Low plasma bicarbonate concentration with hyperchloremic acidosis

Alkaline urine that becomes acidic if extracellular bicarbonate level is decreased below the patient's maximum reabsorptive limit

Normal urine pH in the absence of bicarbonate in the urine

**Due to**

Primary (defect in bicarbonate reabsorption)
  • Usually occurs in males.
  • Only clinical manifestation is retarded growth; renal and metabolic complications are absent.
  • Good prognosis with clinical response to alkali therapy, which is usually not permanently required.

Secondary
  • Idiopathic or secondary Fanconi's syndrome (cystinosis, tyrosinemia, glycogen storage disease, Wilson's disease, hereditary fructose intolerance, heavy-metal intoxication, toxic effect of drugs such as outdated tetracycline)
  • Vitamin D–deficient rickets

- Medullary cystic disease
- After renal transplantation
- Nephrotic syndrome, multiple myeloma, renal amyloidosis

### Distal
### (collecting ducts do not secrete sufficient H⁺ to form ammonium)

Hyperchloremic acidosis, low plasma bicarbonate concentration
Alkaline urine (pH 6.5–7.0) that persists at any level of plasma bicarbonate
     Ammonium loading test shows inability to acidify urine below pH 6.5 and
     depressed rates of excretion of titratable acid and ammonium.
No other tubular defects
Laboratory findings due to complications (e.g., nephrocalcinosis, nephrolithia-
     sis, interstitial nephritis)

### Due to
### Hypokalemic or Normokalemic Type
Primary (inability of tubular cell to secrete enough H⁺)
Secondary
- Increased serum globulins (especially gamma) (e.g., SLE, Sjögren's syndrome,
  Hodgkin's disease, sarcoidosis, chronic active hepatitis, cryoglobulinemia)
- Pyelonephritis
- Medullary sponge kidney
- Ureterosigmoidostomy
- Hereditary insensitivity to antidiuretic hormone (vasopressin)
- Various renal diseases (e.g., hypercalcemia, potassium-losing disorders,
  medullary cystic disease, polyarteritis nodosa, amyloidosis, Sjögren's syndrome)
- Various genetically transmitted disorders (e.g., Ehlers-Danlos syndrome,
  Fabry's disease, hereditary elliptocytosis)
- Starvation, malnutrition
- Hyperthyroidism
- Hyperparathyroidism
- Vitamin D intoxication

### Hyperkalemic Type
Hypoaldosteronism
Obstructive nephropathy
SLE
Sickle-cell nephropathy
Cyclosporine toxicity
*An incomplete or mixed tubular acidosis may be seen in obstructive uropathy and
     in hereditary fructose intolerance.*

### Type 4 Renal Tubular Acidosis
Consists of a variety of conditions characterized by
- Mild to moderate renal impairment.
- Hyperchloremic acidosis.
- *Hyper*kalemia.
- Acid urine pH.
- Reduced ammonium secretion.
- Frequently, tendency to lose sodium in urine.
- Decreased mineralocorticoid secretion in some patients due to isolated
  hypoaldosteronism; others have decreased tubular response to aldosterone.

## Tubular Necrosis, Acute

### Due to

Nonoliguric form (one-third to two-thirds of all cases of acute tubular necrosis)
     is usually due to nephrotoxic agents.
Oliguric form is usually due to ischemic events (e.g., renovascular occlusion, bilat-
     eral cortical necrosis), rapidly progressive glomerulonephritis, obstructive
     uropathy.

Usually multiple causes (e.g., hypotension, sepsis, nephrotoxic drugs, x-ray contrast material, volume depletion)

Sudden progressive increase in BUN and serum creatinine with ratio <20:1
In oliguric type without recent diuretic therapy, urine Osm <350 mOsm/kg $H_2O$, spot Na >20 mEq/L
Urine sodium usually >40 mEq/L but may be <20 mEq/L in nonoliguric patients. FENa is usually >1% in both oliguric and nonoliguric patients.

## Tubulointerstitial Nephropathy

Three basic patterns of functional disturbance depending on site of injury: proximal tubular acidosis, distal tubular acidosis, medullary (reduced ability to concentrate urine, causing nephrogenic diabetes insipidus in most severe form)

### Due to

Bacterial infection (e.g., pyelonephritis)
Drugs (e.g., acute interstitial nephritis, analgesic nephropathy)
Immune disorders (e.g., acute interstitial nephritis, transplant rejection, associated with glomerulonephritis, Sjögren's syndrome)
Metabolic disorders (e.g., urate, hypercalcemic, hypokalemic, oxalate nephropathies)
Heavy metals (e.g., lead, cadmium)
Physical factors (e.g., obstructive uropathy, radiation nephritis)
Neoplasia (e.g., myeloma kidney, infiltration in leukemia and lymphoma)
Hereditary renal diseases (e.g., medullary cystic disease, familial interstitial nephritis, Alport's syndrome)
Miscellaneous conditions (e.g., granulomatous diseases [sarcoidosis, TB, leprosy], Balkan nephropathy)

### Laboratory Findings That Favor Chronic Tubulointerstitial Rather Than Glomerulovascular Renal Disease

Minimal or absent proteinuria
Moderate polyuria
Hyperchloremic metabolic acidosis
Severe sodium wasting
Disproportionate hyperkalemia
Mild or absent hypertension

# Nonrenal Genitourinary Diseases

## Benign Prostatic Hypertrophy (BPH)

Laboratory findings due to urinary tract obstruction and secondary infection
Serum PSA may be increased, confusing its use for screening for prostate cancer. Returns to reference range after resection.

## Prostate Carcinoma

See Fig. 14-4.

### Increased serum PSA
*(reference range <4 ng/mL; increases with age; higher in black than white men)*

### Use

Monitor response to total prostatectomy for cancer (failure to decline at least to normal range indicates residual prostatic tissue or metastases; increasing levels indicate recurrent disease).

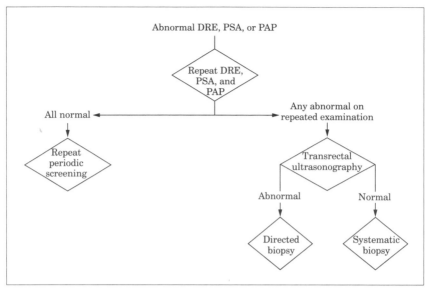

**Fig. 14-4.** Algorithm for prostate cancer screening. (DRE = direct rectal examination.)

Successful radiation or anti-androgen therapy reduce PSA in patients with residual disease. Increasing levels after treatment indicate relapse.

Failure of radiation to decrease PSA to <1 ng/mL indicates likelihood of recurrence.

Is superior to, and increasingly replacing, serum prostatic acid phosphatase (PAP) for routine monitoring.

Now approved for screening by the Food and Drug Administration (FDA) but is controversial because it is also increased in 25–46% of patients with BPH; >10 ng/mL occurs in 2% of cases of BPH and 44% of cases of cancer.

PSA is not sufficiently specific or sensitive to be used *alone* for screening. ~45% of confined cancers and 25% of unconfined cancers have PSA <4.0 ng/mL. Detects only ~2% of cancers in screening healthy asymptomatic men. Physiologic fluctuations ≤ 30%.

PSA >100 ng/mL predicts bone metastases.

Pretreatment doubling time occurs in 4 to >33 months. Correlates with recurrence of disease after radiation therapy.

**Interferences**

Is increased in prostatitis and acute urinary retention and ≤ 2 times by prostatic massage, 4 times by cystoscopy and >50 times by needle biopsy or transurethral resection; should return to normal in 2–6 wks. Digital rectal examination only increases PSA significantly if initial value is >20 ng/mL and is not a confusing factor in falsely elevating PSA. PSA falls 17% in 3 days of lying in hospital; may decrease for >1 wk after ejaculation.

Increased ≤ 2–3 times after vigorous exercise

PSA density (quotient of serum PSA to prostate gland volume by transrectal ultrasound) may help to distinguish BPH and cancer, especially when PSA is 4.0–10.0 ng/mL; low PSA density is unlikely to be cancer but increased density (>0.15) is more likely to be cancer. Additional data are needed.

PSA velocity (rate of change): More rapid rate of increase (>0.75 ng/mL/yr) in early cancer may distinguish carcinoma from BPH. Is not useful for staging. Additional data are needed.

Second generation test measures free PSA divided by total PSA.
- Values of >25% due to cancer in only 5% of patients and 95% are due to BPH.
- Free PSA <7% is found in cancer.
- Free PSA 7–25% is indeterminate and should have biopsy.

### *Increased Serum PAP*

### Use

Identify local extension or distant metastases from prostate carcinoma. It is increased in 60–75% of patients with bone metastases, 20% of patients with extension into periprostatic soft tissue but without bone involvement, 5% of patients with carcinoma confined to gland.

Monitor response to treatment. Increased PAP shows pronounced fall in activity within 3–4 days after castration or within 2 wks after estrogen therapy is begun or return to normal 1 wk after surgery or radiotherapy; failure to fall corresponds to failure of clinical response or presence of metastatic lesions.

Most patients with invasive carcinoma show a significant increase in PAP after massage or palpation; this rarely occurs in patients with normal prostate, BPH, or in situ carcinoma, or in patients with prostate carcinoma who are receiving hormone treatment.

PAP by immunoassay is nearly always increased with a palpable prostatic carcinoma but may be normal in poorly differentiated or androgen-insensitive prostate carcinomas.

More frequently increased with advancing stage and grade of cancer and with lymph node or bone metastases. If PAP assay is elevated in presence of a negative biopsy, the biopsy should be repeated. If PAP is elevated with a normal PSA, the diagnosis lies elsewhere; rule out disseminated malignancy, myeloproliferative or chronic infectious disease.

### Increased in

Prostate carcinoma

Infarction of the prostate (sometimes to high levels).

Operative trauma, instrumentation of the prostate, or prostatic massage may cause transient increase.

Gaucher's disease (only when certain substrates are used in the analysis)

Excessive destruction of platelets, as in idiopathic thrombocytopenic purpura with megakaryocytes in bone marrow

Thromboembolism, hemolytic crises (e.g., sickle-cell disease) due to hemolysis (only when certain substrates are used in the laboratory determination); is said to occur often

Leukemic reticuloendotheliosis ("hairy") cells using a specific assay

### In the Absence of Prostatic Disease, Occurs Occasionally In

- Partial translocation trisomy 21
- Diseases of bone
- Advanced Paget's disease
- Metastatic carcinoma of bone
- Multiple myeloma
- Hyperparathyroidism
- Various liver diseases
    Hepatitis
    Obstructive jaundice
    Laënnec's cirrhosis
- Acute renal impairment (not related to degree of azotemia)
- Other diseases of the reticuloendothelial system with liver or bone involvement (e.g., Niemann-Pick disease)
- In vitro hemolysis

### Decreased in

Not clinically significant

Serum ALP is increased in 90% of patients with bone metastases. Increases with favorable response to estrogen therapy or castration and reaches peak in 3 months, then declines. Recurrence of bone metastases causes new increase.

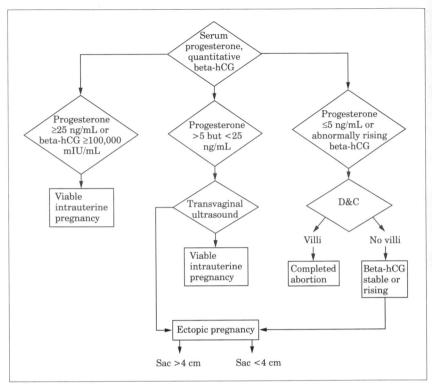

**Fig. 14-5.** Algorithm for diagnosis of unruptured ectopic pregnancy.

Anemia is present.
Carcinoma cells may appear in bone marrow aspirates.
Fibrinolysins are found in some patients with metastatic prostatic cancer with extensive metastases and are usually associated with hemorrhagic manifestations; they show fibrinogen deficiency and prolonged PT.
Needle biopsy of suspicious nodules in prostate is called for.
Cytologic examination of prostatic fluid is not generally useful.

## Pregnancy, Ectopic (Tubal)

See Fig. 14-5.
Serum pregnancy tests are positive in ~50% of patients; however, the beta-subunit hCG assay is positive in ~95% of patients. Can confirm pregnancy in 30 mins. Quantitative hCG >6500 mIU/L without an intrauterine sac on sonography favors ectopic pregnancy because at this titer an intrauterine pregnancy should be visualized. hCG <6000 mIU/L without a sac indicates unknown diagnosis. hCG <6000 mIU with a sac suggests either ectopic or an early normal/abnormal pregnancy. Improved ultrasound instruments may change upper limits of beta-hCG to ~1500 mIU/L for nonvisualization of sac. Newest assays can detect hCG as early as 1 wk before expected menses. In normal pregnancy, serum beta-hCG should rise ≥ 66% of initial titer over 48 hrs; slower increase can identify a pregnancy not developing appropriately (including ectopic pregnancy). hCG titer doubles approximately every 2 days during first 40 days of normal pregnancy; failure indicates abnormal gestation (e.g., ectopic pregnancy, impending abor-

tion). Serum beta-hCG is used to monitor methotrexate treatment of ectopic pregnancy (performed weekly until undetectable).

Urine pregnancy test is variable.

Serum progesterone should be used to screen all patients at risk for ectopic pregnancy at time of first positive pregnancy test. $\geq 25$ ng/mL indicates normal intrauterine pregnancy and $\leq 5$ ng/mL confirms nonviable fetus, permitting diagnostic uterine curettage to distinguish ectopic pregnancy from spontaneous intrauterine abortion. Decrease of beta-hCG of $\geq 15\%$ 12 hrs after curettage is diagnostic of completed abortion but beta-hCG that rises or remains the same indicates ectopic pregnancy.

WBC may be increased; usually returns to normal in 24 hrs. Persistent increase may indicate recurrent bleeding. 75% of the patients have WBC <15,000/cu mm. Persistent WBC >20,000/cu mm may indicate pelvic inflammatory disease.

Anemia depends on degree of blood loss; often precedes the tubal pregnancy. Progressive anemia may indicate continuing bleeding into hematoma.

Culdocentesis fluid with Hct >15% indicates intraperitoneal hemorrhage.

Dilation and curettage shows decidual changes without chorionic villi.

## Cancer, Body of the Uterus

Papanicolaou's (Pap) smear of vagina/cervix is positive in $\leq 70\%$ of patients with endometrial adenocarcinoma. Therefore, a negative Pap smear does not rule out carcinoma.

Pap smear from aspiration of endometrial cavity is positive in 95% of patients.

Endometrial biopsy may be helpful, but a negative result does not rule out carcinoma.

Diagnostic curettage is the only way to rule out carcinoma of the endometrium.

### Trophoblastic Neoplasms

Hydatidiform mole—5% progress to choriocarcinoma.
- Complete mole—normal amount of DNA that is all of paternal origin.
- Partial mole—paternal and maternal DNA present but overabundance of paternal DNA.
- hCG is important to identify 15–20% of hydatidiform moles that persist after curettage.
- Increased incidence of preeclampsia.

Choriocarcinoma—50% are preceded by molar pregnancy, 25% by term pregnancy, 25% by abortion or ectopic pregnancy.

Beta-hCG corresponds to tumor burden. Beta-hCG is used for diagnosis and management of both benign and malignant types. Persistently elevated or slowly declining level indicate persistent trophoblastic disease and the need for systemic therapy for invasive mole or choriocarcinoma.

Amount of hCG produced correlates with amount of trophoblastic tissue.

After evacuation of the uterus, hCG is negative by 40 days. If test is positive at 56 days, 50% have trophoblastic disease. Disease remits in 80% without further treatment. Plateau or rise of titer indicates persistent disease. High-risk patients are indicated by initial serum titer >40,000 mIU/mL.

Measurement of hCG in CSF (ratio of serum:CSF <60:1) is used in diagnosis of brain metastases.

Diagnosis by histologic examination of tissue removed by curettage

RhD-negative patients should receive RhIg at the time of evacuation.

## Cancer, Uterine, Cervix

### Pap Smear

### Use

Routine screening of asymptomatic women to detect carcinoma of cervix or various atypias and to monitor response to therapy for carcinoma

Occasionally detects carcinoma from other gynecologic sites

Often detects presence of various previously undiagnosed infectious agents (e.g., *Trichomonas vaginalis*, HSV, human papillomavirus, *Candida*)

Estimate hormonal status

Occasionally useful in chromosome studies

### Interferences

**(false negative in ~5–10% of cases)**

Sparse cells

Sampling problems (poor fixation or staining), mislabeling, floating cells, obscured cells due to exudate, blood, degeneration, drying, etc.

Certain tumor types are less readily diagnosed (e.g., adenocarcinoma, lymphoma, sarcoma, verrucous carcinoma).

Human error in interpreting difficult cells

### Interpretation

- *Vaginal pool Pap smear has an accuracy rate of ~80% in detecting carcinoma of the cervix. Smears from a combination of vaginal pool, ectocervical, and endocervical scrapings have an accuracy rate of 95%.*
- *After an initial abnormal smear, the follow-up smear taken in the next few weeks or months may not always be abnormal; there is no clear explanation for this finding. Biopsy shows important lesions of the cervix in some of these patients. Therefore, an abnormal initial smear requires further investigation of the cervix regardless of subsequent cytologic reports.*

Laboratory findings due to

- Obstruction of ureters with pyelonephritis, azotemia, etc.
- General effects of cancer

## Carcinoma, Bladder

Hematuria may be gross or only microscopic.

Biopsy of tumor confirms the diagnosis.

Cytologic examination of urine for tumor cells is useful for grades II, III, and IV carcinoma but not for grade I, which has a high false-positive rate. Used in screening chemical dye workers.

Flow cytometry of urine quantitatively measures DNA content or ploidy; cells with normal DNA content are diploid and cells with abnormal DNA content are aneuploid, which is found only in neoplastic cells. Aneuploidy is early indicator of neoplasia and may be present before microscopic evidence of tumor.

Bladder tumor antigen (BTA) in urine is a recent qualitative agglutination test for bladder cancer that detects basement membrane proteins. Positive BTA may occur within 14 days of prostate biopsy or resection, with renal or bladder calculi, symptomatic sexually transmitted disease, other GU tract cancers (e.g., penis, ovary, endometrium, cervix). BTA and cytology may predict relapse of cancer before cystoscopy.

Tumor marker (NMP22) recently approved by FDA to predict recurrence of bladder cancer in first 3–6 months after treatment. Value >10 U/mL has good reported sensitivity and specificity.

Urinary LD level may be useful in screening studies to discover asymptomatic patients with neoplasm of GU tract (e.g., occupational exposure).

## Sexually Transmitted Bacterial Diseases (Including Urethritis, Vulvovaginitis, Pelvic Inflammatory Disease)

### Cervicitis

Cytologic atypia on Pap smear

Cervical Gram's stain >10 PMNs/HPF (1000×) in nonmenstruating women

Tests for appropriate organism (culture, direct antigen test [e.g., chlamydia])

## Human Papillomavirus Infection (HPV)

Suspected in presence of koilocytic changes on Pap smear or cervical biopsy. Low-risk types (e.g., 6, 11) are commonly associated with viral condyloma or mild cervical dysplasia (CIN I) that do not usually progress to invasive disease. High-risk types (e.g., 16, 18, 31, 33, 35) are often associated with moderate dysplasia (CIN II) and severe dysplasia or carcinoma in situ (CIN III) and in most patients with cervical cancer. May be confirmed by antigen detection staining of tissue or DNA hybridization. Can detect HPV types 6, 11, 16, 18, 31, 33, 35 in endocervical or urethral swabs or tissues and detect HPV DNA in genital warts and carcinoma of cervix. Culture is not available. Serologic tests are not useful.

## Bacterial Vaginosis

Polymicrobial infection due to increase in anaerobic organisms and concomitant decrease in lactobacilli
- Vaginal pH >4.5.
- Wet mount of vaginal discharge shows >20% "clue cells" (vaginal epithelial cells coated with bacilli) and curved rods.
- Fishy amine odor on addition of 10% KOH to vaginal fluid.
- Positive culture for *Gardnerella vaginalis* not recommended for diagnosis or test of cure because it may also be found in 40–50% of asymptomatic women with no signs of infection.
- DNA probe test kit simultaneously detects *Trichomonas vaginalis*; allows prompt results.
- Gram's stain and Pap smear may also suggest this diagnosis; gram-negative curved rods and decreased to absent gram-positive rods resembling lactobacilli.
- Homogeneous adherent discharge; mixed with 10% KOH on slide produces a fishy odor.

## Fungi
### (especially *Candida albicans*)
- Wet mount in KOH or Gram's stain of vaginal fluid
- May be seen on Pap smears but culture is needed for definitive identification and is more sensitive

## T. vaginalis
- Recognition of organism in material from vagina. Wet-mount preparation of freshly examined vaginal fluid. Frequently an incidental finding in routine urinalysis. Frequently found in routine Pap smears. The organism is often not identified but may be associated with characteristic concomitant cytologic changes. Not recommended for screening. Culture is the gold standard. DNA probe test kit allows prompt results; excellent method. *Douching within 24 hrs decreases sensitivity of tests.* Do not test during first few days of menstrual cycle.
- Occasionally detected in material from male urethra in cases of nonspecific urethritis. Prostatic fluid usually contains few organisms.
- Serologic tests are not useful.

## HSV

Local cause is most common (e.g., endocrine, poor hygiene, pinworms, scabies, foreign body)

## Atrophic Vaginitis

- pH slightly acidic.
- Mixed nonspecific bacterial flora.
- Vaginal cytology shows atrophic pattern.

## Genital Tuberculosis

Usually tubal. Culture of menstrual fluid is most reliable diagnostic procedure. *Multiple causes may be present and should be sought in each case.*

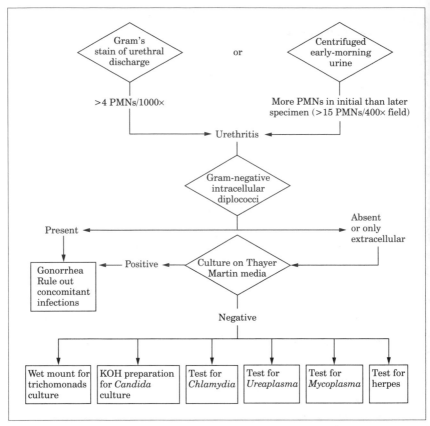

**Fig. 14-6.** Algorithm for diagnosis of urethritis in males.

### Urethritis

See Fig. 14-6.

Is diagnosed if smear of urethral discharge shows >4 PMNs/1000× field

In absence of urethral discharge, an early morning initial 10-mL urine specimen is centrifuged and compared to the rest of the sample. If the first specimen shows >15 PMNs/400× field than the later sample, urethritis is diagnosed. If equal numbers of PMNs are present in both specimens, the inflammation is higher up in the GU tract. If no PMNs are present, urethritis is unlikely. Sediment of the first specimen should also be examined for *T. vaginalis*.

Gram's stains will show gram-negative intracellular diplococci in >95% of cases of gonorrhea.

In males, a positive smear establishes the diagnosis of gonorrhea and a culture is not necessary, but in females, a positive smear should be confirmed by culture on appropriate media (i.e., Gram's stains are highly sensitive and specific in males but not in females).

*Chlamydia* and *Ureaplasma* cannot be identified on smears, and cultures must be performed at specialized laboratories.

When Gram's stains and cultures for gonorrhea are negative, the presumptive diagnosis is nongonococcal urethritis. *Chlamydia trachomatis* causes about 50% of such cases; this is the most frequent venereal disease.

In sexually active young men, acute epididymitis is almost always due to STD; 10% are due to gonorrhea; 50–80% are due to *C. trachomatis* in heterosexuals but *E. coli* is more common in homosexual men and men >35 yrs old.

Women infected with *C. trachomatis* show infection of urethra, rectum, and cervix. Present in <50% of women with cervical gonococcal infection.

- >10 WBC/1000× without microscopic bacteriuria.
- Pap smear may show cytoplasmic inclusion bodies in metaplastic squamous cells of cervix.

Sexually active women with symptoms of lower UTI, pyuria (>15 WBCs/HPF), but sterile urine cultures probably have chlamydial infection. If coliforms or staphylococci are found, bacterial cystitis is likely even if <100,000/mL.

*Ureaplasma urealyticum* probably causes 20–30% of cases of urethritis in males.

*Mycoplasma hominis* may cause pyelonephritis, pelvic inflammatory disease, and postpartum febrile complications. *U. urealyticum* and *M. hominis* are usually diagnosed by culture; DNA probes are less sensitive. Serologic methods are not widely used; diagnosis requires a 4 times rise in IgG titer.

Candida albicans, *T. vaginalis*, herpes simplex, and cytomegalovirus probably cause 10–15% of cases of nongonococcal urethritis.

Laboratory findings of complications (e.g., prostatitis, epididymitis, Reiter's syndrome, salpingitis)

## Toxemia of Pregnancy
### (hypertension, proteinuria, edema after wk 20 of pregnancy)

Proteinuria varies from a trace to very marked (≤ 800 mg/dL, equivalent to 15–20 gm/day).

>15 mg/dL may indicate early toxemia.

In mild preeclampsia there is proteinuria of >300 mg in at least two random clean-catch urine specimens collected 6 hrs apart but <2 gm/24 hrs.

In severe preeclampsia, there is significant proteinuria ≥ 500 mg/24 hrs (2+ on dipstick).

Proteinuria ≥ 5 gm/24 hrs correlates with 3–4+ on dipstick.

Oliguria—urine output <400 mL/24 hrs.

Thrombocytopenia and abnormal liver function tests may be present.

RBCs and RBC casts are not abundant; hyaline and granular casts are present. BUN, renal concentrating ability, and PSP excretion are normal unless the disease is severe or there is a prior renal lesion. *(BUN usually decreases during normal pregnancy because of increase in glomerular filtration rate.)*

Serum uric acid is increased in absence of treatment with thiazides, which can produce hyperuricemia independent of any other disease.

Serum TP and albumin commonly are markedly decreased.

There may be multiple clotting deficiencies in severe cases.

Lupus anticoagulant, antiphospholipid antibodies may be present.

Evidence of microangiopathic hemolysis, abnormal liver function tests, falling platelet count (HELLP syndrome)

Biopsy of kidney can establish diagnosis; rules out primary renal disease or hypertensive vascular disease.

Weekly creatinine clearance to follow renal function

Eclampsia is indicated by occurrence of generalized seizures.

~20% of women develop eclampsia with only mild hypertension and often without proteinuria or edema.

Amniocentesis to determine fetal maturity if induction of labor is required.

Usefulness of monitoring maternal estriols, human placental lactogen and other components is questionable.

MgSO$_4$ treatment requires urine output ≥ 100 mL q4h. Therapeutic mg range = 4–7 mEq/L.

Toxicity begins at 7–10 mEq/L; respiratory depression begins at 10–15 mEq/L; cardiac arrest begins at 30 mEq/L.

*Beware of associated or underlying conditions (e.g., hydatidiform mole, twin pregnancy, prior renal disease, diabetes mellitus, nonimmune hydrops fetalis).*

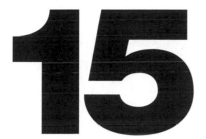

# Infectious Diseases

## Some General Principles for Laboratory Diagnosis of Infectious Diseases

Diagnosis of infectious diseases depends on identifying the causative agent by various methods depending on the suspected cause. The choice of methods and the sequence of work-up is summarized in the included tables and figures. Consultation with the laboratory personnel should be sought in appropriate cases.

1. Site of specimen (e.g., blood, CSF, sputum, wound, abscess, pleural or other body fluid, skin).
2. Smear with appropriate stain—e.g., Gram's stain, acid-fast, methylene blue, Wright, Pap.
   - Organism (bacteria, amebae, fungi). Diagnosis of *parasitic* diseases usually depends on demonstrating the causative organism in specimens concentrated and stained appropriately. Should be considered in patients with eosinophilia.
   - Leukocytes (neutrophils, eosinophils) and RBCs.
   - Cells (inclusion bodies, Tzank smear).
3. Wet preparation of body fluid.
   - Urine for number of bacteria
   - Vaginal fluid for trichomonads
   - CSF (India ink for cryptococcal meningitis)
4. *Bacterial* culture recommendations for optimal use.
   - As soon as possible after onset of chills or fever.
   - Before antimicrobial therapy is started.
     Use resin-assisted blood cultures if patient is already on antimicrobial therapy.
   - Take 2–3 cultures at least 30–60 mins apart if possible; shorter time interval if urgent need to begin therapy. Take 2–3 cultures per septic episode or per 24-hr period.
   - Draw 20–30 mL of blood per culture.
   - Do not draw blood from IV catheter unless no vein sites are available or from umbilical artery catheter in infants.
   - Special methods should be used for suspected fungi or mycobacteria.
   - Use strict aseptic technique. Suspect contamination in the following situations:
     If only one of several cultures is positive
     Type of organism. Common contaminants are *Staphylococcus epidermidis*, *Bacillus* spp., *Propionibacterium acnes*, *Corynebacterium* spp., *Clostridium perfringens*, *Viridans streptococci*, *Candida tropicalis*.
     True infection is almost always present if organism is streptococci (non-*Viridans* group), aerobic and facultative gram-negative rods, anaerobic cocci and gram negative rods, yeasts.
5. *Viral* cultures.
   - Standard viral "tube" culture showing typical cytopathologic changes is the gold standard for proving etiology but may require 10 days to weeks. Shell viral cultures confirmed using fluorescent monoclonal antibodies can

Shell viral cultures confirmed using fluorescent monoclonal antibodies can provide results in 1–2 days.
- Infection by some viruses (e.g., herpesvirus, adenovirus, CMV) may not indicate disease whereas presence of others does indicate disease (e.g., influenza, parainfluenza, RSV).
- Some viruses cannot be cultured and require other techniques.
- Finding enterovirus in stool supports diagnosis but does not prove it is the cause of present illness (e.g., aseptic meningitis, myopericarditis); some viruses can be shed for months in asymptomatic persons (e.g., adenoviruses, HSV, CMV) but unusual for other viruses (e.g., measles, mumps, influenza, parainfluenza, RSV).

6. Serologic tests—evidence of recent *viral* infection may be based on
   - Single serum specimens that show specific IgM antibody within the first few weeks of infection (e.g., EBV, CMV, VZV, rubella, coxsackieviruses) are useful.
   - Seroconversion from negative to positive test is conclusive evidence of recent infection. *Paired sera should always be submitted for diagnosis of viral disease; acute phase serum should be obtained as early as possible; convalescent phase serum is usually obtained 2–4 wks later.* ≥ 4 times rise in antibody titer is usually diagnostic.
   - Various exceptions must be remembered:
     Some may recur with reactivation or reinfection (e.g., herpes, CMV, EBV, VZV).
     Some may persist for 6 or more months (e.g., CMV, rubella).
     Heterotypic response of one virus antibody to another infection (e.g., CMV and EBV)
   - False positives are frequent in sera that contain RF. *Spurious results may also occur in other conditions (e.g., bacterial endocarditis, chronic liver disease, TB and other chronic infections, sarcoidosis, some healthy persons).*
   - False negatives may occur in immunocompromised patients, neonates, infants.
   - For diagnosis of *congenital infection*, serial sera from mother and infant should be submitted.
   - Specific IgM in neonatal blood or cord blood can diagnose congenital infection because mother's IgM does not cross placenta.
   - Single maternal serum negative for IgG may be useful to exclude that particular congenital infection in neonate (e.g., rubella, CMV).
   - Positive IgG titer that does not rise indicates previous exposure and often immunity. Tests to determine immune status may be used for viruses of rubella (in women of childbearing age), CMV (in women of childbearing age working in high-risk environments [e.g., hemodialysis, transplant, pediatric and nursery units]), measles and mumps (IFA indicate prior infection), chickenpox (VZV).

Serologic tests for *bacterial* infection may be based on
- Serologic tests for syphilis.
- Serologic tests for recent streptococcal infections (e.g., ASOT).

Serologic tests for *rickettsial* infection may be based on
- Indirect IFA or ELISA detection of rickettsial-specific IgG and IgM. ELISA is more sensitive and specific for IgM and is now the test of choice; specimens taken at 3- to 4-day intervals will show seroconversion. CF or agglutination tests are positive in most cases but less useful.

7. Direct identification of virus or viral *antigens* in patient tissues by
   - Cytopathology of inclusion bodies. Should confirm virus identification by specific antibody staining.
   - EM identification of viral antigen in tissues (e.g., brain biopsy for HSV particles in encephalitis, Creutzfeldt-Jakob virus) or specimens (e.g., urine for CMV in congenital infection of infants; feces for rotaviruses, Norwalk agents, adenoviruses, coronaviruses, caliciviruses; vesicle fluid for HSV and poxviruses). Is often enhanced by other techniques (e.g., antibody binding).
   - Direct detection of viral antigens.
     DFA and IFA
     EIA—RSV, rotavirus, adenovirus, influenza A, HSV

Agglutination kits for rotavirus
- Histologic appearance of excised lymph node suggests diagnosis and rules out other lesions (e.g., cat-scratch fever in which culture is often sterile and organisms may be demonstrated by special stains and EM); DNA has been detected in tissue biopsies.
8. Testing of suspected source of infection (e.g., rabid animals, food poisoning).
9. Chemical tests (e.g., pleural fluid to distinguish exudate from transudate).
10. Molecular biology—Newer techniques will greatly improve laboratory diagnosis of infectious disease as they become generally available (e.g., PCR for amplifying DNA of microorganisms from AIDS patients) Improvements may include increased sensitivity and specificity, faster turn-around time, identification of organisms for which culture technology is not available or is impractical; fastidious transport is not required. Consult your laboratory director for the current diagnostic availability.
11. Animal inoculation is not often used at present.
12. Xenodiagnosis in chronic Chagas' disease.
13. Nonspecific indicators of infection.
    - Acute phase reactants (e.g., WBC, ESR, CRP).
    - Limulus lysate assay detects trace amounts of endotoxin from all gram-negative bacteria (including *Escherichia coli*, *Neisseria meningitidis*, *Haemophilus influenzae*). Presence in CSF is sensitive indicator of gram-negative bacterial meningitis but serum test is unreliable.
14. Epidemiologic studies may be indicated in certain instances (e.g., various epidemics, occupational exposure).
15. Involvement of specific organs (e.g., hepatitis, meningitis/encephalitis, pneumonitis, endocarditis, arthritis, osteomyelitis) may be important clues to diagnosis.
16. Therapeutic drug monitoring is used
    - Where margin between therapeutic and toxic concentrations is narrow (e.g., aminoglycosides, vancomycin).
    - In patients with renal failure.
17. Serum bactericidal titer is that dilution of serum able to kill >99.9% of the original bacterial inoculum in 18–24 hrs when patient is on antibiotic therapy.
18. Beta-lactamase testing. A positive test
    - Predicts resistance to penicillin, ampicillin, and amoxicillin among *Haemophilus* spp, *Neisseria gonorrhoeae*, and *Moraxella catarrhalis*.
    - Predicts resistance to penicillin and acylamino- and carboxypenicillins among staphylococci and enterococci.

## Organisms Commonly Present in Various Sites

| Site | Normal Flora | Pathogens |
|---|---|---|
| External ear | *Staphylococcus epidermidis* | *Pseudomonas* spp. |
| | Alpha-hemolytic streptococci | *Staphylococcus aureus* |
| | Aerobic corynebacteria | Coliform bacilli |
| | *Enterobacteriaceae* spp. | Alpha-hemolytic streptococci |
| | *Corynebacterium acnes* | *Proteus* spp. |
| | *Candida* spp. | *Streptococcus pneumoniae* |
| | *Bacillus* spp. | *Corynebacterium diphtheriae* |
| | | *Aspergillus* spp. |
| | | *Candida* spp. |
| | | VZV |
| | | HSV |
| | | Papovavirus |
| | | Molluscum contagiosum |
| Middle ear | Sterile | **Acute Otitis Media** |
| | | *H. influenzae* |
| | | *Streptococcus pneumoniae* |

| Site | Normal Flora | Pathogens |
|------|-------------|-----------|
| | | *Moraxella catarrhalis* |
| | | Beta-hemolytic streptococci |
| | | **Chronic Otitis Media** |
| | | *Staphylococcus aureus* |
| | | *Proteus* spp. |
| | | *Pseudomonas* spp. |
| | | Other gram-negative bacilli |
| | | Alpha-hemolytic streptococci |
| | | RSV |
| | | Influenza virus |
| Nasal passages | *Staphylococcus epidermidis* | **Acute Sinusitis** |
| | *Staphylococcus aureus* | *Staphylococcus aureus* |
| | Diphtheroids | *Streptococcus pneumoniae* |
| | *Streptococcus pneumoniae* | *Klebsiella-Enterobacter* spp. |
| | Alpha-hemolytic streptococci | Alpha-hemolytic streptococci |
| | Nonpathogenic *Neisseria* spp. | Beta-hemolytic streptococci |
| | Aerobic corynebacteria | *Moraxella catarrhalis* |
| | | **Chronic Sinusitis** |
| | | *Staphylococcus aureus* |
| | | Alpha-hemolytic streptococci |
| | | *Streptococcus pneumoniae* |
| | | Beta-hemolytic streptococci |
| | | *Mucor, Aspergillus* spp. (especially in diabetics) |
| Pharynx and tonsils | Alpha-hemolytic streptococci | Beta-hemolytic streptococci |
| | *Neisseria* spp. | *Corynebacterium diphtheriae* |
| | *Staphylococcus epidermidis* | *Bordetella pertussis* |
| | *Staphylococcus aureus* (small numbers) | *Neisseria meningitidis* |
| | | *H. influenzae*, type B |
| | *Streptococcus pneumoniae* | *Staphylococcus aureus* |
| | Nonhemolytic (gamma) streptococci | *Candida albicans* |
| | | Respiratory viruses |
| | Diphtheroids | *Mycoplasma pneumoniae* |
| | Coliforms | *Neisseria gonorrhoeae* |
| | Beta-hemolytic streptococci (not Group A) | *Chlamydia pneumoniae* |
| | *Actinomyces israelii* | |
| | *Haemophilus* spp. | |
| | *Marked predominance of one organism may be clinically significant even if it is a normal inhabitant.* | |
| Epiglottis | | *H. influenzae*, type B |
| Larynx | | Respiratory viruses |
| | | *Corynebacterium diphtheriae* |
| | | Infectious mononucleosis |
| | | *Candida albicans* |
| Bronchioli | | RSV |
| Bronchi | | *Mycoplasma pneumoniae* |
| | | Viruses (e.g., influenza, rhinovirus, coronavirus, adenovirus) |
| | | *Corynebacterium diphtheriae* |
| | | *Streptococcus pneumoniae* |
| Lungs | | Bacteria |
| | | *Pseudomonas aeruginosa* |
| | | *E. coli* |
| | | *Klebsiella pneumoniae* |
| | | *Serratia marcescens* |

| Site | Normal Flora | Pathogens |
|------|--------------|-----------|
| | | *Enterobacter* spp. |
| | | *Staphylococcus aureus* |
| | | *Proteus mirabilis* |
| | | *Streptococcus pneumoniae* |
| | | *H. influenzae* |
| | | *Bordetella pertussis* |
| | | *Mycoplasma pneumoniae* |
| | | *Chlamydia pneumoniae* |
| | | *Chlamydia psittaci* |
| | | *Legionella pneumophila* |
| | | *Pneumocystis carinii* |
| | | Tubercle bacilli |
| | | *Francisella tularensis* |
| | | *Yersinia pestis* |
| | | Fungi (e.g., *Histoplasma, Coccidioides* in particular; *Blastomyces, Aspergillus*) |
| | | Viruses (e.g., influenza, para influenza, adenoviruses, RSV, echovirus, coxsackievirus, reovirus, CMV, viruses of exanthems, HSV, hantavirus) |
| | | Rickettsiae (e.g., Q fever, typhus, *Coxiella burnetii*) |
| | | Protozoans (e.g., *Toxoplasma, Pneumocystis carinii*) |
| Pleura | Sterile | *Staphylococcus aureus* |
| | | *Staphylococcus epidermidis* |
| | | *Streptococcus pneumoniae* |
| | | *H. influenzae* |
| | | *Mycobacterium tuberculosis* |
| | | Anaerobic streptococci |
| | | *Streptococcus pyogenes* |
| | | *E. coli* |
| | | *Klebsiella pneumoniae* |
| | | *Actinomyces* spp. |
| | | *Nocardia* spp. |
| Mouth | Alpha-hemolytic streptococci | *Candida albicans* |
| | Enterococci | *Borrelia vincentii* with *Fusobacterium fusiforme* |
| | Lactobacilli | |
| | Staphylococci | |
| | Fusobacteria | |
| | *Bacteroides* spp. | |
| | Diphtheroids | |
| | *Neisseria* spp. (except *Neisseria gonorrhoeae*) | |
| Esophagus | | *Candida albicans* |
| | | CMV |
| | | HSV |
| Stomach | Sterile | *Helicobacter pylori* |
| Small intestine | Sterile in one-third | *Campylobacter jejuni* |
| | Scant bacteria in two-thirds | *Helicobacter pylori* |
| | *E. coli* | |
| | *Klebsiella-Enterobacter* | |
| | Enterococci | |
| | Alpha-hemolytic streptococci | |

| Site | Normal Flora | Pathogens |
|---|---|---|
| | *Staphylococcus epidermidis* | |
| | Diphtheroids | |
| Colon | Abundant bacteria | Enteropathogenic *E. coli* |
| | *Bacteroides* spp. | *Candida albicans* |
| | *E. coli* | *Aeromonas* spp. |
| | *Klebsiella-Enterobacter* | *Salmonella* spp. |
| | Paracolons | *Shigella* spp. |
| | *Proteus* spp. | *Campylobacter jejuni* |
| | Enterococci (group D | *Yersinia enterocolitica* |
| | streptococci) | *Staphylococcus aureus* |
| | Yeasts | *Clostridium difficile* |
| | | *Vibrio cholerae* |
| | | *Vibrio parahaemolyticus* |
| | | Amebae and parasites |
| | | Viruses (e.g., rotavirus, |
| | | CMV, HSV, Norwalk) |
| Rectum | | *Chlamydia* spp. |
| | | *Neisseria gonorrhoeae* |
| | | *Treponema pallidum* |
| | | Lymphogranuloma venereum |
| | | HSV |
| | | *Enterobius vermicularis* (anus) |
| Gallbladder | Sterile | *E. coli* |
| | | *Enterococci* |
| | | *Klebsiella-Enterobacter-* |
| | | *Serratia* |
| | | Occasionally |
| | | Coliforms |
| | | *Proteus* spp. |
| | | *Pseudomonas* spp. |
| | | *Salmonella* spp. |
| Blood | Sterile | *Staphylococci epidermidis* |
| | | *Staphylococci aureus* |
| | | *E. coli* |
| | | Enterococci |
| | | *Pseudomonas* spp. |
| | | Alpha- and beta-hemolytic |
| | | streptococci |
| | | *Streptococcus pneumoniae* |
| | | *H. influenzae* |
| | | *Clostridium perfringens* |
| | | *Proteus* spp. |
| | | *Bacteroides* and related |
| | | anaerobes |
| | | *Neisseria meningitidis* |
| | | *Brucella* spp. |
| | | *Pasteurella tularensis* |
| | | *Listeria monocytogenes* |
| | | *Achromobacter (Herellea)* spp. |
| | | *Streptobacillus moniliformis* |
| | | *Leptospira* spp. |
| | | *Vibrio fetus* |
| | | *Salmonella* spp. |
| | | Opportunistic fungi |
| | | *Candida* spp. |
| | | *Nocardia* spp. |
| | | *Blastomyces dermatitidis* |
| | | *Histoplasma capsulatum* |
| Eye | Usually sterile | *Staphylococcus aureus* |

| Site | Normal Flora | Pathogens |
|---|---|---|
| | Occasionally small numbers of diphtheroids and coagulase-negative staphylococci | *Haemophilus* spp. <br> *Streptococcus pneumoniae* <br> *Neisseria gonorrhoeae* <br> Alpha- and beta-hemolytic streptococci <br> *Achromobacter (Herellea)* spp. <br> Coliform bacilli <br> *Pseudomonas aeruginosa* <br> Other enteric bacilli <br> Morax-Axenfeld bacillus <br> *Bacillus subtilis* (occasionally) <br> *Chlamydia* spp. |
| Spinal fluid | Sterile | *H. influenzae* <br> *Neisseria meningitidis* <br> *Streptococcus pneumoniae* <br> *M. tuberculosis* <br> Staphylococci, streptococci <br> *Cryptococcus neoformans* <br> Coliform bacilli <br> *Pseudomonas* and *Proteus* spp. <br> *Bacteroides* spp. <br> *Listeria monocytogenes* <br> *Leptospira* <br> *Treponema* <br> *Borrelia burgdorferi* <br> Viruses (e.g., coxsackie A and B, echovirus, HSV, mumps, HIV, VZV, lymphocytic, choriomeningitis, CMV, adenovirus) <br> Fungi (e.g., *Histoplasma capsulatum*, *Cryptococcus neoformans*, *Coccidioides immitis*) <br> Free amoebas (e.g., *Naegleria*, *Acanthamoeba*) |
| Urethra, male | *Staphylococcus aureus* <br> *Staphylococcus epidermidis* <br> Enterococci <br> Diphtheroids <br> *Achromobacter wolffi (Mima)* <br> *Bacillus subtilis* | *Neisseria gonorrhoeae* <br> *Chlamydia* spp. <br> *Ureaplasma urealyticum* <br> Enterococci <br> *Gardnerella vaginalis* <br> Beta-hemolytic streptococci (usually group B) <br> Anaerobic and microaerophilic streptococci <br> *Bacteroides* spp. <br> *E. coli* and *Klebsiella-Enterobacter* <br> *Staphylococcus aureus* |
| Urethra, female, and vagina | Lactobacillus (large numbers) <br> Coli-aerogenes <br> Staphylococci <br> Streptococci (aerobic and anaerobic) <br> *Candida albicans* <br> *Bacteroides* sp. <br> *Achromobacter wolffi (Mima)* | Yeasts and *Candida albicans* <br> *Clostridium perfringens* <br> *Listeria monocytogenes* <br> *Gardnerella vaginalis* <br> *Trichomonas vaginalis* <br> *Neisseria gonorrhoeae* <br> *Chlamydia* spp. <br> (See also Urethra, male.) <br> *Ureaplasma urealyticum* <br> *H. ducreyi* |

| Site | Normal Flora | Pathogens |
|------|-------------|-----------|
| Prostate | Sterile | *Streptococcus faecalis* |
| | | *Staphylococcus epidermidis* |
| | | *E. coli* |
| | | *Proteus mirabilis* |
| | | *Pseudomonas* spp. |
| | | *Klebsiella* spp. |
| | | Anaerobic and micro-anaerophilic streptococci (alpha, beta, gamma types) |
| | | *Bacteroides* spp. |
| | | Enterococci |
| | | Beta-hemolytic streptococci (usually group B) |
| | | Staphylococci |
| | | *Proteus* spp. |
| | | *Clostridium perfringens* |
| | | *E. coli* and *Klebsiella-Enterobacter-Serratia* |
| | | *Listeria monocytogenes* |
| Urine | Staphylococci, coagulase negative | *E. coli* |
| | Diphtheroids | *Klebsiella-Enterobacter-Serratia* |
| | Coliform bacilli | *Proteus* spp. |
| | Enterococci | *Pseudomonas* spp. |
| | *Proteus* spp. | Enterococci |
| | Lactobacilli | Staphylococci, coagulase positive and negative |
| | Alpha- and beta-hemolytic streptococci | *Providencia* spp. |
| | | *Morganella morganii* |
| | | *Alcaligenes* spp. |
| | | *Achromobacter (Herellea)* spp. |
| | | *Candida albicans* |
| | | Beta-hemolytic streptococci |
| | | *Neisseria gonorrhoeae* |
| | | *Mycobacterium tuberculosis* |
| | | *Salmonella* and *Shigella* spp. |
| Wound | | *Staphylococcus aureus* |
| | | *Staphylococcus epidermidis* |
| | | Coliform bacilli |
| | | *Pseudomonas* spp. |
| | | Enterococci |
| | | *Streptococcus pyogenes* |
| | | *Clostridium* spp. |
| | | *Bacteroides* spp.; other gram-negative rods |
| | | *Proteus* spp. |
| | | *Achromobacter (Herellea)* spp. |
| | | *Serratia* spp. |
| Pericardium | Sterile | *Staphylococcus aureus* |
| | | *Streptococcus pneumoniae* |
| | | *Enterobacteriaceae* |
| | | *Pseudomonas* spp. |
| | | *H. influenzae* |
| | | *Neisseria meningitidis* |
| | | *Streptococcus* spp. |
| | | Anaerobic bacteria |
| | | *Coccidioides immitis* |
| | | *Actinomyces* spp. |
| | | *Candida* spp. |

| Site | Normal Flora | Pathogens |
|------|-------------|-----------|
| Peritoneum | Sterile | *E. coli* |
| | | Enterococci |
| | | *Streptococcus pneumoniae* |
| | | *Bacteroides* spp.; other gram-negative rods |
| | | Anaerobic streptococci |
| | | *Clostridium* spp. |
| | | *Staphylococcus epidermidis* |
| | | *Staphylococcus aureus* |
| | | *Pseudomonas* spp. |
| | | Alpha-hemolytic streptococci |
| | | *Klebsiella pneumoniae* |
| Bones | Sterile | **Acute Hematogenous** |
| | | *Staphylococcus aureus* |
| | | *H. influenzae*, group B |
| | | Streptococci (groups A and B) |
| | | *Neisseria gonorrhoeae* |
| | | Gram-negative bacilli (e.g., *Pseudomonas aeruginosa, Serratia marcescens, E. coli*) |
| | | *Mycobacterium tuberculosis* |
| | | *Salmonella* spp. in sickle-cell disease |
| | | **Contiguous** |
| | | Anaerobic bacteria (e.g., *bacteroides*, fusobacteria, anaerobic cocci) |
| Joints | Sterile | *Staphylococcus aureus* |
| | | *Staphylococcus epidermidis* |
| | | Beta-hemolytic streptococci |
| | | *Streptococcus pneumoniae* |
| | | *H. influenzae*, group B |
| | | *Klebsiella pneumoniae* |
| | | Gram-negative pathogens in newborns |
| | | *Salmonella* spp. in sickle-cell disease |
| | | *Neisseria gonorrhoeae* |
| | | *Mycobacterium tuberculosis* |
| | | *Mycobacterium kansasii* |
| | | *Mycobacterium intracellulare* |
| | | *Borrelia burgdorferi* |
| | | Viruses (e.g., mumps, rubella, HBV, parvovirus B-19) |
| | | Fungi (e.g., *Candida, Sporothrix schenckii, Coccidioides immitis, Blastomyces dermatitidis*) |
| Skin | *Staphylococcus aureus* *Staphylococcus epidermidis* | *Staphylococcus aureus* (impetigo, folliculitis, furunculosis) |
| | | Group A streptococcus (impetigo, erysipelas) |
| | | *Corynebacterium diphtheriae* |
| | | *Bacillus anthracis* |
| | | *Francisella tularensis* |
| | | *Mycobacterium ulcerans* |

| Site | Normal Flora | Pathogens |
|------|--------------|-----------|
|      |              | *Mycobacterium marinum* |
|      |              | Anaerobic bacteria |
|      |              | Viruses (e.g., papillomavirus, varicella-simplex, HSV, molluscum contagiosum) |
|      |              | Fungi (e.g., *Trichophyton, Microsporum, Epidermophyton, Actinomyces, Nocardia*) |

For amebae and parasites, see Table 15-6.

## Some Organisms Detected by Molecular Biology Methods

### Bacteria

*Mycobacterium tuberculosis*\*
*Mycobacterium avium-intracellulare*†
*Mycobacterium leprae*
*Borrelia burgdorferi* (Lyme disease)
*Treponema pallidum*
*Neisseria gonorrhoeae*†
*Neisseria meningitidis*†
*Bordetella pertussis*
*Legionella pneumophila*
Enteroinvasive *E. coli*
Toxin-genes of toxigenic organisms (e.g., *Clostridium difficile*).
Recognition of transmissible antimicrobial resistance determinants.
Identification of uncultured causative agents not previously known (e.g., ehrlichiosis, Whipple disease, *Rochalimaea henselae*) or only present in tiny amounts. PCR for rapid detection of staphylococcal *mec*A gene, which is associated with penicillin binding protein representing primary mechanism of resistance to methicillin.

### Viruses

CMV†
Enteroviruses†
EBV
Hepatitis B virus DNA†
Hepatitis C virus RNA†
Hepatitis A
Herpes simplex
HIV 1 and 2\*
HTLV-I and HTLV-II
Human papillomavirus
Parainfluenza
Parvovirus B19
Rhinovirus
Rotavirus
Rubella
Varicella-zoster
*Chlamydia/Mycoplasma*
*Chlamydia trachomatis*\*
*Chlamydia pneumoniae*
*Mycoplasma pneumoniae*
*Mycoplasma hominis*

---

\*Approved by FDA.
†Used in other countries.

### Parasites

*Plasmodium falciparum, malariae,* and *vivax*
*Babesia microti* and *divergens*
*Babesia*-like organisms
*Leishmania donovani* and *braziliensis*
*Toxoplasma gondii*
*Trypanosoma cruzi* and *brucei*
*Filaria (Wuchereria bancrofti, Brugia malayi, Loa loa, Onchocerca volvulus)*
*Histoplasma capsulatum*

### Fungi

*Aspergillus* spp.
*Cryptococcus neoformans*
*Blastomyces dermatitidis*
*Coccidioides immitis*
*Candida* spp.
*Pneumocystis carinii*

## Some Organisms Detected by Antibody Tests

### Bacteria

*Bartonella henselae*
*Bordetella pertussis*
*Borrelia* spp. (relapsing fever)
*Borrelia burgdorferi* (Lyme disease)
*Brucella* spp.
*Clostridium botulinum* toxin
*Clostridium tetani* toxin
*Corynebacterium diphtheriae* toxin
*E. coli* O157 toxin
*Francisella tularensis*
*H. influenzae* group b
*Helicobacter pylori*
*Legionella pneumophila*
*Leptospira* spp.
*Salmonella typhi*
*Treponema pallidum*
*Yersinia pestis*

### Viruses

Adenovirus
Colorado tick fever virus
Coronavirus
Coxsackie A and B virus
CMV
Dengue virus
Eastern and Western equine encephalitis virus
Echovirus
EBV
Hantavirus
HAV, HBV, HCV, and HDV
HSV
Human herpesvirus 6
HIV types 1 and 2
HTLV 1 and 2
Influenza A and B virus
Lymphocytic choriomeningitis virus

Mumps virus
Parvovirus B19
Parainfluenza virus
Poliovirus
Reovirus
RSV
Rubella virus
Rubeola virus
St. Louis encephalitis virus
VZV

### Chlamydia/Mycoplasma

*Chlamydia* spp.
*Mycoplasma pneumonia*

### Rickettsia

*Coxiella burnetii* (Q fever)
*Ehrlichia chaffeensis*
Murine typhus
Rocky Mountain spotted fever
Scrub typhus

### Fungi

*Aspergillus* spp.
*Blastomyces dermatitidis*
*Candida* spp.
*Coccidioides immitis*
*Cryptococcus neoformans*
*Histoplasma capsulatum*
*Penicillium marneffei*
*Sporothrix schenckii*
*Zygomycetes*

### Parasites

*Babesia microti*
*Echinococcus* spp.
*Entamoeba histolytica*
*Fasciola hepatica*
*Filaria* spp.
*Giardia lamblia*
*Leishmania* spp.
*Paragonimus westermani*
*Plasmodium* spp.
*Schistosoma* spp.
*Strongyloides stercoralis*
*Taenia solium* (cysticercosis)
*Toxocara canis*
*Toxoplasma gondii*
*Trichinella spiralis*
*Trypanosoma cruzi*

## Some Organisms Detected by Antigen Tests

CIE now largely replaced by latex agglutination. Other sensitive immunologic
tests for rapid identification of specific antigens include coagglutination of
*Staphylococcus aureus*, IF, ELISA.

Provides rapid, specific, reliable detection of certain bacterial antigens in virtually any body fluid obtained from the patient (CSF, serum, urine, joint). In bacterial meningitis, CSF is best specimen; urine is occasionally useful in establishing diagnosis; serum is usually not helpful. In contrast to cultures, results can be obtained within several hours. Is most useful for identification of *H. influenzae* type B, *Staphylococcus pneumoniae*, *Neisseria meningitidis* (groups A and C), group B streptococcus. Sensitivity may be improved by testing serum and urine and CSF. Is especially valuable when patient has received antibiotics before cultures and Gram's stains are taken and whenever smear and culture are negative.

A negative test does not unequivocally exclude infection due to that organism. Larger amounts of antigen correlate with more complications and poorer prognosis. *Cross reaction and nonspecific precipitation may occur with some antisera.*

For all of these tests, false positives may occur due to a number of different organisms. False negatives can occur early in disease; repeat specimens are often useful. Do not use grossly lipemic or hemolyzed specimens, which may give inaccurate results.

## *Other Organisms Detected Include*

### Bacteria
*Bacillus anthracis*
*Bartonella henselae*
*Bordetella pertussis*
*Borrelia* spp. (relapsing fever)
*Borrelia burgdorferi* (Lyme disease)
*Brucella* spp.
*Chlamydia trachomatis*
*Clostridium difficile* toxins A and B
*Francisella tularensis*
*Klebsiella pneumoniae*
*Legionella* spp.
*Listeria monocytogenes* in CSF
*Mycobacterium tuberculosis*
*Neisseria gonorrhoeae*
*Pseudomonas aeruginosa*
*Staphylococcus aureus* in pleural fluid
*Tropheryma whippleii* (Whipple's disease)
*Yersinia pestis*

### Viruses
Adenovirus
Colorado tick fever virus
Coronavirus
Creutzfeldt-Jakob virus
EBV
HAV
HBV
HCV
HDV
HSV
Human papillomavirus
HIV type 1
HTLV 1 and 2
Influenza A virus
Parainfluenza virus
Parvovirus B19
RSV
Rotavirus
VZV

## Fungi

*Candida* precipitin titer = 1:8 or 4 times increase in titer indicates invasive candidiasis rather than *Candida* colonization.

*Cryptococcus neoformans*

*Pneumocystis carinii* pneumonitis

## Parasites

*Cryptococcus neoformans* meningitis in CSF, urine, or serum

*Cryptosporidium parvum*

*Entamoeba histolytica*, especially in liver abscess material

*Giardia lamblia*

*Taenia solium* (cysticercosis)

*Toxoplasma gondii*

*Trichinella spiralis*

See Tables 15-1 through 15-7 and Figs. 15-1 through 15-6.

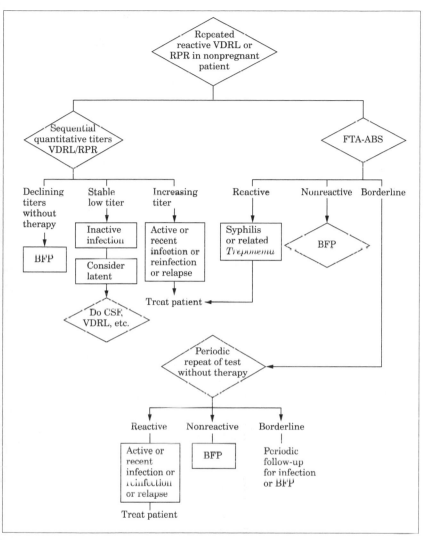

**Fig. 15-1.** Algorithm for positive serologic test for syphilis. Rule out underlying causes of biological false positive (BFP). (RPR = rapid plasma reagin test.)

**Table 15-1.** Stages of Syphilis

| Stage | Symptom | Time After Exposure | Laboratory Changes | Response to Treatment | | |
| --- | --- | --- | --- | --- | --- | --- |
| | | | | **VDRL** | **FTA-ABS/MHA-TP** | |
| Primary | Chancre | Average 3 wks (11–90 days) | Dark-field positive<br>Serologic tests often negative<br>Rising titers VDRL and FTA-ABS | Remains negative | Remains negative | |
| | Lymph nodes | Average 4 wks | Dark-field positive<br>Rising antibody titers | Usually becomes negative within 6 mos | After seroconversion, usually remains positive indefinitely without regard for stage of disease or adequacy of treatment | |
| Secondary | | 6–20 wks | Dark-field positive<br>Peak antibody titers<br>CSF abnormal in 25–50% of patients without CNS findings<br>Increased serum ALP (due to pericholangitis) in 20%<br>Proteinuria | Usually becomes negative within 12–24 mos | | |

| | | | |
|---|---|---|---|
| Latent | Early: 3–12 mos<br>Late: >12 mos | CSF VDRL negative<br>Serum treponemal test positive<br>Falling VDRL titers | |
| Late (tertiary) | Neurosyphilis (asymptomatic) | Usually >4 yrs | CSF VDRL positive or increased cells and protein<br>Serum treponemal test positive; nontreponemal test positive or negative<br>Without treatment, CNS disease occurs within 10 yrs in 20% of patients | |
| Late (tertiary) | Symptomatic | >4 yrs | Same as asymptomatic<br>Treatment does not reverse nontreponemal test in 25–75% of patients | Usually remains positive indefinitely with gradually declining titer |

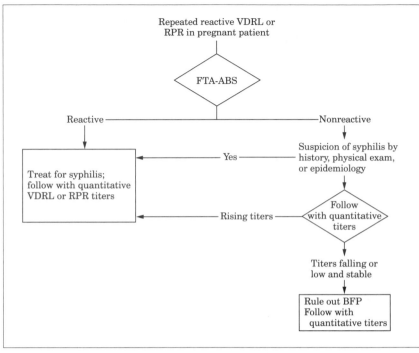

**Fig. 15-2.** Algorithm for reactive serologic test for syphilis in the pregnant patient. (RPR = rapid plasma reagin test; BFP = biological false positive.)

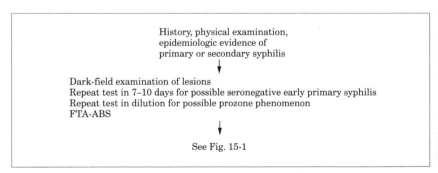

**Fig. 15-3.** Algorithm for nonreactive serologic test for syphilis in the nonpregnant patient.

**Table 15-2.** Correlation of CD4 Count and Disease in HIV Infection

| CD4 Count (per cu mm) | Disease |
| --- | --- |
| 500–800 | Aggressive bacterial, respiratory, skin, enteric infections |
| >500 | Kaposi's sarcoma |
| 200–500 | Weight loss, fever, sweats<br>Hairy leukoplakia<br>*Candida* (oral, esophageal)<br>TB reactivation |
| <200 | Pneumocystosis<br>*Mycobacterium avium-intracellulare*<br>Cryptococcosis<br>Dementia |
| <50 | Toxoplasmosis<br>CMV<br>Death |

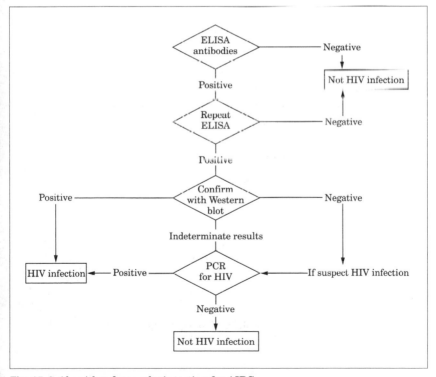

**Fig. 15-4.** Algorithm for serologic testing for AIDS.

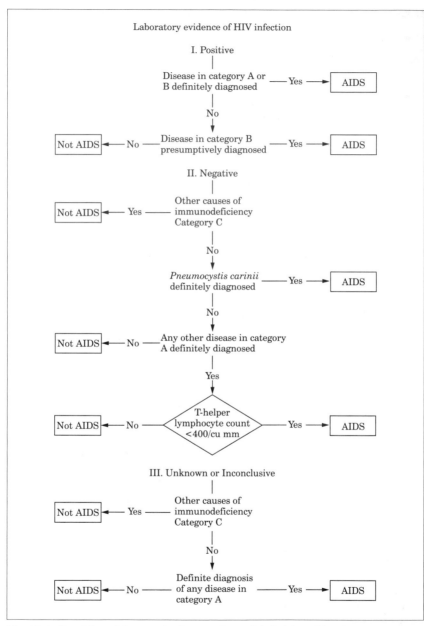

**Fig. 15-5.** Algorithm of Centers for Disease Control definition of AIDS. I, II, and III refer to criteria on pp. 769, 771 of Wallach, J. *Interpretation of Diagnostic Tests* (6th ed). Lippincott–Raven, Philadelphia, 1996.

**Table 15-3.** 1993 Revised Classification System for HIV Infection and Expanded AIDS Surveillance Case Definition for Adolescents and Adults (≥ 13 Yrs)

| CD4+ T-Cell Categories | | Clinical Categories | | |
|---|---|---|---|---|
| **Number** | **%** | **A** | **B** | **C** |
| (1) ≥ 500/cu mm | ≥ 29 | A1 | B1 | C1 |
| (2) 200–499/cu mm | 14–28 | A2 | B2 | C2 |
| (3) <200/cu mm | <14 | A3 | B3 | C3 |

Notes: Groups A3, B3, C3 with CD4+ T-cell counts <200/cu mm are reported as AIDS.
Groups C1, C2, C3 with AIDS-indicator conditions are reported as AIDS. T-cell count <200/cu mm is an AIDS indicator.
The lowest accurate CD4+ T-cell count is used for classification; need not be the most recent count.

**Table 15-4.** Methods for Diagnosis of Chlamydial Infections

| Method | Application | Sensitivity/Specificity |
|---|---|---|
| Culture | All chlamydial infections<br>Is only acceptable method for medicolegal cases (e.g., suspected sexual assault or abuse) | Gold standard; most valuable to screen low-risk patients; ≤ 80% sensitivity |
| Cytology | Inclusion conjunctivitis, trachoma | ~95% sensitivity |
| Serology | Invasive infection (pneumonia, psittacosis, lymphogranuloma venereum). Not for genital or superficial eye infections. | |
| Complement fixation | *Chlamydia psittaci* infection; not for infantile pneumonia | |
| Microimmuno-fluorescence | Pneumonia 4× increase in acute and convalescent titers (IgM ≥ 1:16 of single IgG ≥ 1:512) | 50–90% sensitivity, specificity unknown |
| Antigen detection | | |
| Direct fluorescent antibody | Specimens from GU tract, conjunctiva, rectum, nasopharynx | ~75% sensitivity, 95% specificity |
| Enzyme immuno-assay | Specimens from GU tract, conjunctiva | 81% sensitivity, 99% specificity from endocervix; rapid turnaround |
| Nucleic acid DNA probes | Method of choice for genital specimen<br>Not good for urine specimens<br>Same specimen can be used to test for *Neisseria gonorrhoeae* | Very high sensitivity and specificity |
| Amplification (PCR ligase chain reaction) | Specimens from GU tract<br>Method of choice for urine specimens | ≤ 100% sensitivity and specificity |

Note: Positive nonculture results should be verified by culture or another nonculture technology.

**Table 15-5.** Summary of Laboratory Findings in Fungus Infections

| Disease | Causative Organism | Blood | CSF | Stool | Urine | Nasopharynx, throat | Sputum, lung | Gastric washings | Vagina, cervix | Exudates, lesions, sinus tracts, etc. | Skin, nails, hair | Bone marrow | Lymph node | Fresh unstained material | Stained material | Culture | Animal inoculation | Serologic tests | Histologic examination |
|---|---|---|---|---|---|---|---|---|---|---|---|---|---|---|---|---|---|---|---|
| | | Source of Material | | | | | | | | | | | | Diagnostic Methods | | | | | |
| | | | | | | | | | | | | | | Microscopic examination | | | | | |
| Cryptococcosis | *Cryptococcus neoformans* | + | + | + | + | | + | | | | + | + | | | + | + | + | + | + |
| Coccidioidomycosis | *Coccidioides immitis* | + | + | + | | | + | + | | | + | + | + | + | | + | + | + | + |
| Histoplasmosis | *Histoplasma capsulatum* | + | | | | | + | + | | | + | + | + | | + | + | + | + | + |

| Disease | Organism |
|---|---|
| Actinomycosis | *Actinomyces israelii* |
| Nocardiosis | *Nocardia asteroides* |
| North American blastomycosis | *Blastomyces dermatitidis* |
| South American blastomycosis | *Paracoccidioides brasiliensis* |
| Moniliasis | *Candida albicans* |
| Aspergillosis | *Aspergillus fumigatus*, others |
| Geotrichosis | *Geotrichum candidum* |
| Chromoblastomycosis | *Fonsecaea pedrosoi*, *Phialophora verrucosa*, *compactum*, etc. |
| Sporotrichosis | *Sporotrichum schenckii* |
| Rhinosporidiosis | *Rhinosporidium seeberi* |

**Table 15-6.** Summary of Laboratory Findings in Protozoan Diseases

| Disease | Causative Organism | Blood | CSF | Stool | Urine | Vagina | Urethra | Exudates, ulcers, skin lesions | Bone marrow | Spleen | Lymph node aspirate |
|---|---|---|---|---|---|---|---|---|---|---|---|
| Malaria | *Plasmodium species* | + | | | | | | | + | | |
| Babesiosis | | + | | | | | | | | | |
| Trypanosomiasis Acute sleeping sickness | *T. rhodesiense* | + | + | | | | | | + | | + |
| Chronic sleeping sickness | *T. gambiense* | + | + | | | | | | + | | + |
| Chagas' disease | *T. cruzi* | + | | | | | | | | | + |
| Leishmaniasis Kala-azar | *L. donovani* | + | | | | | | | + | + | + |
| American mucocutaneous | *L. brasiliensis* | | | | | | | + | | | |
| Oriental sore | *L. tropica* | | | | | | | + | | | |
| Toxoplasmosis | *T. gondii* | | + | | | | | | | | + |
| Interstitial plasma cell pneumonia | *Pneumocystis carinii* | | | | | | | | | | |
| Amebiasis | *Entamoeba histolytica* | | | + | | | | | | | |
| Giardiasis | *G. lamblia* | | | + | f | | | | | | |
| Balantidiasis | *B. coli* | | | + | | | | | | | |
| Coccidiosis | *Isospora hominis* or *belli* | | | + | | | | | | | |
| Trichomoniasis | *T. vaginalis* | | | | + | + | + | | | | |

[a]Liver, lymph node.
[b]Hemagglutination, Sabin-Feldman dye test.
[c]Lymph node, muscle.
[d]Special stains.

| | Diagnostic Methods | | | | | | Other Significant Laboratory Abnormalities | | | | | | | | | |
| --- | --- | --- | --- | --- | --- | --- | --- | --- | --- | --- | --- | --- | --- | --- | --- | --- |
| | Microscopic examination | | | | | | | | | | | | | | | |
| | Fresh unstained material | Stained material | Culture | Animal inoculation | Xenodiagnosis | Histologic examination | Anemia | WBC decreased | Monocytosis | Serum globulin increased | CSF abnormalities | Renal function abnormalities | Liver function abnormalities | Skeletal muscle abnormalities | Cardiac abnormalities | Other |
| | | − | | | | | + | + | + | + | + | + | + | | | |
| | + | | + | | | + | + | | | | | + | + | | | |
| | + | + | rare | + | | + | + | | + | + | + | | + | | | |
| | | + | rare | + | | + | + | | + | + | + | | + | | | |
| | | + | + | + | + | a | | | | | + | | | + | + | |
| | | + | + | | | | + | + | | + | | + | | | | |
| | | + | + | + | | − | − | | | | | | | | | |
| | | + | + | | | + | | | | | | | | | | |
| | | + | | + | | c | | | | + | | | | | | b |
| | | + | | | | + | | | | | | | | | | d |
| | | + | | | | e | | | | | | | + | | | |
| | | + | | | | | | | | | | | | | | |
| | | + | | | | | | | | | | | | | | |
| | | + | | | | | | | | | | | | | | |
| | + | + | | | | | | | | | | | | | | |

[e]Rectum.
[f]Also duodenal washings.
Notes: Serologic tests can be performed at the Centers for Disease Control (Atlanta, GA) on specimens submitted through state health department laboratories that do not perform such tests. See Table 15-7.

**Table 15-7.** Serologic Tests in Diagnosis of Parasitic Diseases

| Disease | Tests |
| --- | --- |
| Amebiasis | EIA, IHA |
| Babesiasis | IF |
| Chagas' disease | EIA, IF, CF, IHA |
| Cryptosporidiosis | Ag |
| Cysticercosis | IB, EIA |
| Echinococcosis | EIA, IHA, IB |
| Fascioliasis | EIA |
| Filariasis | EIA |
| Giardiasis | EIA, IF (Ag in stool) |
| Leishmaniasis | IF, CF |
| Malaria | IF |
| Paragonimiasis | EIA, IB |
| Pneumocystosis | Ag |
| Schistosomiasis | EIA, IB |
| Strongyloidiasis | EIA |
| Toxocariasis | EIA |
| Toxoplasmosis | EIA, IF, EIA-IgM |
| Trichinosis | BF, EIA |
| Trichomoniasis | Ag |
| *Trypanosoma cruzi* | EIA, IF, CF |

IB = immunoblot; BF = bentonite flocculation.

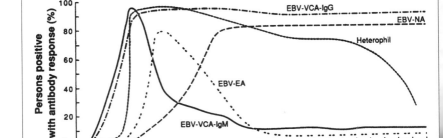

**Fig. 15-6.** Percentage of persons with positive antibody response at specified time intervals. (EA = early antigen; NA = nuclear antigen.)

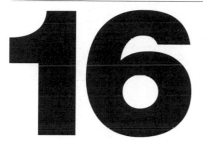

# Miscellaneous Diseases

# Laboratory Tests for Collagen/Vascular Diseases

## Antineutrophil Cytoplasmic Antibodies (ANCA)

### Use

Aid in diagnosis and classification of various vasculitis-associated and autoimmune disorders

### Interpretation

c-ANCA (anti-proteinase 3; coarse diffuse cytoplasmic pattern) is highly specific for active Wegener's granulomatosis. High titer may persist during remission for years. Occasionally found in other vasculitides.

p-ANCA (against various proteins [e.g., myeloperoxidase, elastase, lysozyme]; perinuclear pattern). Positive result should be confirmed by ELISA. Pulmonary small vessel vasculitis is strongly linked with myeloperoxidase antibodies.

Both p-ANCA and c-ANCA may be found in non–immune-mediated polyarteritis and other vasculitides.

Atypical pattern (neither c-ANCA nor p-ANCA; unknown target antigens) has poor specificity and unknown sensitivity in various conditions (e.g., HIV infection, endocarditis, cystic fibrosis, Felty syndrome, ulcerative colitis, Crohn's disease).

## Antinuclear Antibodies

### Use

Mainly to exclude SLE. See Table 16-1.

### Interpretation

*ANA is the most sensitive laboratory test for detecting SLE* but low specificity. Negative ANA in patient with active multisystem disease is strong evidence against SLE; positive ANA without other manifestations is not diagnostic. High titers are most often associated with SLE. ANA may become negative during remission. Titers correlate poorly with remission/relapse. Persistently negative ANA tests occur in ~5% of SLE.

Pattern of ANA immunofluorescence is of limited value. Anti-ENA detects only 2 ENAs: ribonucleoprotein (RNP) and Sm.

### ANA Profile in SLE

*Multiple (3 or more) antibodies are characteristic of SLE.*
*High titers of dsDNA are characteristic of and very specific for SLE.*
*High titers of anti-Sm is the most specific diagnostic test for SLE but not sensitive.*

**Table 16-1.** ANA Disease Profiles*

| ANAs | SLE | Drug-Induced Lupus Erythematosus | Mixed Connective Tissue Disease | Scleroderma Syndrome | CREST | Sjögren's Syndrome | Dermatomyositis and Polymyositis | RA |
|---|---|---|---|---|---|---|---|---|
| ANA screen | >95 | >95 | >95 | 70–90 | 70–90 | 75–90 | 40–60 | R |
| Native DNA | **60** | R | R | R | R | R | R | 40 |
| Histones | 30 | **>95** | R | R | R | R | R | 20 |
| Sm | **30** | R | R | R | R | R | R | R |
| Nuclear RNP | 40–50 | R | **>95** | 15 | 10 | R | 15 | 10 |
| Scl-70 | R | R | R | **30–70** | R | R | R | R |
| SS-A (Ro) | 40–60 | R | R | R | R | **≤90** | 10 | R |
| SS-B (La) | 15 | R | R | R | R | **≤60** | R | R |
| Centromere | R | R | R | 30 | **70–85** | R | R | R |
| Nucleolar | 25 | R | R | **40–70** | R | R | R | R |
| PM-Scl (PM-1) and Jo-1 | R | R | R | ~20 | R | R | **10–50** | R |

CREST = calcinosis, *R*aynaud's syndrome, *e*sophageal dysmotility, *s*clerodactyly, *t*elangiectasia; R = rare; Sm = Smith; SS = Sjögren's syndrome; RNP = ribonucleoprotein; PM-Scl = polymyositis-scleroderma.
*Reported frequency of ANAs in various diseases is given as a percentage. Boldface indicates significant correlation.

*High titers are characteristic of SLE and rarely found in other conditions.*
Anti–single-stranded DNA is not specific for SLE, but it is a sensitive indicator.

### ANA Profile in Drug-Induced Lupus

*Antihistone antibodies are present in >95% of cases*; if negative, drug-induced
lupus is unlikely.

### ANA Profile in Sjögren's Syndrome

SS-A and SS-B without other antibodies indicates probable Sjögren's syndrome;
with other ANA probably indicates SLE.

### ANA Profile in Mixed Connective Tissue Disease (MCTD)
*(combines clinical features of RA, polymyositis, SLE, and especially scleroderma; ~10% of SLE patients fulfill criteria for MCTD)*

*High titer of anti-RNP without anti-Sm and other antibodies is characteristic*; is
found in 100% of MCTD.

### ANA Profile in Scleroderma and CREST Syndrome

Centromere is only antibody in CREST (acronym for calcinosis, Raynaud's syndrome, esophageal dysmotility, sclerodactyly, telangiectasia) syndrome patients.
PM-1/Scl-70 is highly specific for scleroderma.
High titer nucleolar antibodies in 40–50% of patients

### ANA Profile in Rheumatoid Arthritis

RA nuclear antigen in 85–95% of patients. RF present.
ANAs absent; low titer anti-native DNA may be present.

## Hematoxylin Bodies
**(homogeneous round extracellular material)**

May be found in SLE, RA, multiple myeloma, cirrhosis

## Lupus Band Test (LBT)

Direct IF on biopsy of normal skin

### Use

In patients without sufficient clinical manifestations of SLE (e.g., only renal or
CNS findings)
In patients whose symptoms and other laboratory tests show remission due to
steroid therapy
In differentiation of early SLE from RA

### Interpretation

Is positive in 50% of all SLE patients and ≤ 80% with active multisystem (especially renal) disease; in discoid lupus is found only in skin lesions
May be positive in dermatomyositis, undifferentiated collagen-vascular disease,
and other nonrheumatic diseases, but usually only one immunoglobulin is found

# Collagen/Vascular/Rheumatic Diseases; Miscellaneous Disorders

## Amyloidosis

Diagnosis is established by demonstration of amyloid in tissue.

- Biopsy of gingiva, rectum, kidney, bone, liver, skin, tissue from carpal tunnel decompression, etc.
- Other areas of involvement include GI tract, spleen, respiratory tract.
- EM is the most specific diagnostic method.
- Congo red stain under polarized and transmitted light is positive in one-third of patients with primary and approximately two-thirds of patients with secondary amyloidosis.
- Immunohistochemical staining shows reaction of fibrils with kappa or lambda antisera.
- Evans blue dye is retained in serum.

### *Classification*

### (AL) Light-Chain Amyloid (Primary)
**(paraprotein disorder characterized by monoclonal light-chain deposits in tissues; BJ proteinuria occurs; derived from malignant clone of plasma cells in neoplastic type or small nonproliferative population of plasma cells in non-tumor type)**
One-third of cases show overt myeloma; occurs in ~15% of cases of multiple myeloma. Primary when there is no evidence of associated disease.
One organ usually shows predominant involvement.
- Cardiovascular system.
- Proteinuria and azotemia occur in most cases; nephrotic range proteinuria (>3 gm/day) occurs. Should always be ruled out in patients >age 30 yrs with unexplained nephrotic syndrome.
- Tongue is enlarged in 20% of cases.
- Respiratory system.
- Peripheral neuropathy; CNS is not involved.
- Carpal tunnel syndrome.
- GI tract (e.g., malabsorption).
- Bone marrow.
Serum protein electrophoresis shows hypogammaglobulinemia in 25% and an abnormal immunoglobulin (monoclonal spike) in another 45% of cases.
Immunoelectrophoresis/immunofixation detects a monoclonal protein in two-thirds of cases.
Urine contains free light chains. Low levels of urine monoclonal light chains (<200 mg/24 hrs) may indicate an immunocytic malignancy (multiple myeloma, chronic lymphocytic leukemia or non-Hodgkin's lymphoma) even when serum is negative for M proteins. *Monoclonal proteins are not found in secondary, senile, familial, or localized amyloidosis.*
Some renal insufficiency in ~50% of cases. Mild anemia in 50% of cases.
WBC is frequently increased.
ESR is increased.
Bone marrow shows >5% plasma cells in 50% of cases.

### (AA) Reactive (Secondary) Systemic (Amyloid A Protein)
**(no BJ proteinuria)**
Due to
- RA
- Juvenile RA
- Ankylosing spondylitis
- Chronic infections
- Osteomyelitis, burns, decubital ulcers
- Leprosy
- TB
- Heroin use with chronic infection of skin injection sites
- Chronic inflammation (e.g., bowel disease)
- Neoplasms
    Hodgkin's disease
    Nonlymphoid solid tumors (e.g., renal and bladder adenocarcinoma)
- Heredofamilial systemic amyloidosis
    Familial Mediterranean fever (AA type)

Neuropathic types (I, II, III, IV)—serum protein electrophoresis and immunoelectrophoresis are normal.

**Local Amyloidosis Types**
**(BJ proteinuria is absent)**
(SSA) Senile cardiac amyloid
(AF) Familial amyloid
(CAA) Cerebral amyloid

# Giant Cell Arteritis

Biopsy of involved segment of temporal artery is diagnostic.

Classic triad of increased ESR, anemia, and increased serum ALP is strongly suggestive of giant cell arteritis.

Normocytic normochromic anemia is rough indicator of degree of inflammation.

ESR is markedly increased in virtually all patients. A normal ESR excludes the diagnosis when there is little clinical evidence for temporal arteritis.

WBC is usually normal or slightly increased with shift to the left.

# Polyarteritis Nodosa

Tissue biopsy is basis for diagnosis
- Findings in random skin and muscle biopsy is confirmatory in 25% of patients.
- Testicular biopsy is useful when local symptoms are present.
- Renal biopsy is not specific; often shows glomerular disease.

Increased WBC ($\leq$ 40,000/cu mm) and PMNs. Eosinophils are increased usually with pulmonary manifestations.

ESR and CRP are increased.

Mild anemia is frequent; may be hemolytic anemia with positive Coombs' test.

Urine is frequently abnormal.

Uremia occurs in 15% of patients.

Serum globulins are increased.

Abnormal serum proteins occasionally occur. Circulating anticoagulants, cryoglobulins, macroglobulins, biological false-positive (BFP) test for syphilis occurs.

HBsAg is present in 20–40% of adult patients. p-ANCA is positive in 70% of patients.

# Sarcoidosis

Diagnosis is established by tissue biopsy that shows noncaseous granulomas at several sites for which a specific cause (e.g., fungal, acid-fast bacillus infection, or berylliosis) has been excluded. Kveim test may be used in place of another tissue biopsy.
- Needle biopsy of liver shows granulomas.
- Lymph node biopsy is likely to be positive if lymph node is enlarged.
- Muscle biopsy is likely to be positive if arthralgia or muscle pain is present.
- Skin lesions may occur.
- Other sites of biopsy are synovium, eye, lung, minor salivary glands of lower lip.

Kveim reaction (skin biopsy 4–6 wks after injection of human sarcoid tissue shows a noncaseating granulomatous reaction at that site).
- Positive Kveim tests may occur in other diseases with enlarged lymph nodes (e.g., TB, leukemia). Kveim test material is not available commercially; a few medical centers have limited quantities with variable specificities.

## *Serum Angiotensin-Converting Enzyme (ACE)*
*(Note—values vary between labs even with same method.)*

### Use
Monitor activity of sarcoidosis and response to therapy
Little diagnostic value because of poor specificity

## May Be Increased in

- Active pulmonary sarcoidosis
- Gaucher's disease
- Diabetes mellitus
- Hyperthyroidism
- Leprosy
- Chronic renal disease
- Cirrhosis
- Silicosis
- Berylliosis
- Amyloidosis
- TB

## Normal in

- Lymphoma
- Lung cancer

Serum globulins are increased producing reduced A:G ratio and increased TP.

Serum protein electrophoresis shows decreased albumin and increased globulin (especially gamma) with characteristic "sarcoid-step" pattern.

WBC is decreased.

Eosinophilia may occur.

Mild normocytic, normochromic anemia occurs.

ESR is increased.

Serum calcium may be mild to markedly increased in ~10% of patients; often transiently.

Increased urine calcium occurs twice as often as hypercalcemia. Increased frequency of renal calculi and nephrocalcinosis.

Increased serum 1,25-hydroxyvitamin D in hypercalcemic patients

Increased serum uric acid may occur.

Mumps CF that is positive in presence of negative mumps skin test supports the diagnosis but is not specific.

# Systemic Lupus Erythematosus (SLE)

## Criteria for Classification of SLE
### (American Rheumatism Association, 1982)

Presence of ≥ 4 criteria at same or different times allows the diagnosis of SLE and excludes other disorders.

| Manifestation | Sensitivity (%) | Specificity (%) |
|---|---|---|
| Malar rash | 57 | 96 |
| Discoid lupus | 18 | 99 |
| Oral/nasopharyngeal ulcers | 27 | 96 |
| Photosensitivity | 43 | 96 |
| Arthritis | 86 | 37 |
| Proteinuria (>0.5 gm/day or 3+ qualitative) or cellular casts | 51 | 94 |
| Seizures or psychosis not due to other causes | 20 | 98 |
| Pleuritis or pericarditis | 56 | 86 |
| Cytopenia (any of the following four findings) | 59 | 89 |
|   Autoimmune hemolytic anemia | 15 | |
|   Neutropenia (<4,000/cu mm on two or more occasions) | | |
|   Lymphopenia (<1,500/cu mm on two or more occasions) | | |
|   Thrombocytopenia (<100,000/cu mm in absence of causative drugs) | | |

| | | |
|---|---|---|
| Immunologic findings (any of the following four findings)<br>Anti-nDNA antibodies<br>Anti-Sm antibodies<br>LE cells<br>False-positive serologic test for syphilis >6 months' duration confirmed by FTA-ABS or *Treponema pallidum* immobilization test | 85 | 93 |
| Positive ANA in the absence of known causative drugs | 99 | 49 |
| **Overall** | **96** | **96** |

*ANA is the most sensitive laboratory test for SLE.* Most patients with SLE will have multiple (≥ 3 antibodies) present but drug-induced lupus and other connective tissue diseases are likely to have fewer ANA present. *Combination of positive ANA test, positive dsDNA antibodies, and hypocomplementemia has diagnostic specificity of virtually 100%.*

Traditional parameters of disease activity (Hb, WBC, ESR, CRP, urinalysis, serum creatinine) do not distinguish activity from superimposed infection or drug toxicity.

Current indicators of disease activity *do not predict which manifestations are likely to become active or the time interval, and some patients never manifest active disease. The strongest correlation is with active nephritis, but these tests do not substitute for renal biopsy.*

* Decrease in early complement components (C3, C4; C4 is most sensitive) and total hemolytic complement (THC), occurring in ~70% of patients with active SLE, are not specific for diagnosis but are helpful in managing patients who are at risk for renal and CNS involvement; may be helpful in following response to therapy. THC should be part of initial evaluation of SLE patients. Reduced C3, C4, CH50 are rarely seen without immune complex diseases; therefore, strongly supports diagnosis of SLE in patient with suggestive history and physical examination.
* Presence of circulating immune complexes.
* Presence of cryoglobulins correlates well with disease activity.
* C1q binding.

SLE may present as "idiopathic" thrombocytopenic purpura.

Anemia is most commonly anemia of chronic disease or may be due to iron deficiency. Autoimmune hemolytic anemia occurs in ~15% of patients and correlates with disease activity.

* Abnormal serum proteins frequently occur.
* BFP test for syphilis is very common. *This may be the first manifestation of SLE and may precede other features.*
* Serum gamma globulin is increased in 50% of patients; a continuing rise may indicate poor prognosis. Alpha$_2$ globulin is increased; albumin is decreased. Immunoglobulins may be increased.

Tissue biopsy of skin, muscles, kidney, and lymph node may be useful.

SLE should be ruled out in asymptomatic patients with false-positive VDRL, various unexplained conditions (e.g., thrombocytopenia, leukopenia, proteinuria, abnormal urine sediment, positive Coombs' test, or prolonged aPTT).

# Malignant Diseases

## Tumor Markers

### Use

Not generally useful to establish a definite diagnosis or for screening
May be useful to monitor effect of therapy, detect recurrence, to follow the clinical course, to pinpoint the tissue of origin

Sometimes useful to assess the extent of tumor and to estimate prognosis

## Interpretation

Enzymes increased

- Serum ALP and GGT in liver metastases. Also in bone metastases, osteogenic sarcoma, myeloid leukemia. Placental isoenzyme of ALP increased in ovarian cancer, some cancers of endometrium, lung, breast, and seminoma; may also be increased in smokers. Intestinal isoenzyme is associated with hepatomas and malignant tumors of GI tract.
- Serum GGT in metastatic carcinoma of liver.
- Serum LD in metastatic carcinoma of liver, acute leukemia, lymphomas.
- Serum LD total and LD-1 in testicular cancer.
- Serum CK total and CK-BB in various cancers (e.g., prostate, breast, ovary, colon, small cell carcinoma of lung).
- Serum acid phosphatase in metastatic prostate cancer.
- Neuron-specific enolase in APUD (amine precursor uptake [and] decarboxylation) tumors, including small cell carcinoma of lung, neuroblastoma, medullary carcinoma of thyroid.
- Serum amylase in carcinoma of pancreas.
- Terminal deoxynucleotidyl transferase—large amounts in blast cells of acute lymphoblastic leukemia but little or none in nonlymphoid leukemia or nonleukemic cells; useful to differentiate acute lymphoid and acute myeloid leukemia.

Oncofetal antigens

- Serum AFP in hepatoma, teratoblastoma, yolk sac tumor
- Serum CEA in carcinoma of GI tract, breast, small cell carcinoma of lung

Specific products of hormone-producing tumor of primary organ or ectopic

- Renin-producing tumor of kidney.
- VMA, catecholamines in pheochromoblastoma, neuroblastoma, neural crest tumors, pheochromocytoma.
- Urinary 17-KS in adrenal cortical carcinoma, androgenic arrhenoblastoma.
- HIAA in carcinoid.
- Erythropoietin in paraneoplastic erythrocytosis.
- Thyroglobulin detectable in patients with total thyroidectomy indicates recurrent thyroid cancer.
- Prolactin.
- ACTH in Cushing's syndrome.
- Beta-hCG subunit (in blood or urine).
- C-peptide in insulinoma.
- Estrogen and progesterone receptors.
- Parathormone-related protein produced by lung, ovarian, thymoma, carcinoid, islet cell tumor of pancreas, medullary carcinoma of thyroid.
- Anti-diuretic hormone produced by small cell cancer of lung, carcinoid, Hodgkin's disease, bladder.
- Calcitonin produced by medullary carcinoma of thyroid, breast, liver, kidney, lung carcinoid.
- Gastrin in gastrinoma, gastric carcinoma; part of MEN-1 syndrome, carcinoma of pancreas, parathyroid, pituitary.
- Isoenzymes of ALP (Regan, Nagao).

Other proteins

- PSA.
- CA-125.
- CA 19-9.
- CA 15-3.
- Immunoglobulins in multiple myeloma, lymphomas, Waldenström's macroglobulinemia.
- Interleukin 2 receptor may be increased in serum in adult T-cell leukemia.
- Antigen from squamous cell carcinoma.
- Plasma chromogranin A in pheochromocytoma.

Philadelphia chromosome in chronic myeloid leukemia

Paraneoplastic syndromes
- One-third of these patients show ectopic hormone production (e.g., bronchogenic carcinoma).
- One-third show evidence of connective tissue (e.g., polymyositis, dermatomyositis) and dermatologic (e.g., acanthosis nigricans) disorders.
- One-sixth show psychiatric and neurologic syndromes.
- Remainder show immunologic, GI (e.g., malabsorption), renal (e.g., nephrotic syndrome), hematologic (e.g., anemia of chronic disease, DIC), paraproteinemias (e.g., multiple myeloma), amyloidosis.

## Alpha-Fetoprotein (AFP)

### Use

Tumor marker for hepatoma
- Screening high prevalence populations (e.g., Chinese, Eskimos)
- Patients with chronic active hepatitis or cirrhosis positive for HBsAg

Tumor marker for germ cell tumors of ovary and testis
- Embryonal carcinoma.
- Malignant teratoma.
- *Should be used in conjunction with hCG and LD and LD-1; more often increased with advanced disease. These are useful to monitor therapy; may predict relapse before clinical or x-ray evidence.*

To distinguish neonatal hepatitis (>40 ng/mL in most patients) from neonatal biliary atresia (<40 ng/mL in most patients)

Screening for fetal defects and placental disease during pregnancy

### Interpretation
*(>50 ng/mL is essentially diagnostic of AFP-producing tumor)*

Primary cancer of liver in 50% of whites and 75–90% of nonwhites; may be very increased (>1000 ng/mL in ~50% of cases usually indicates tumor >3 cms in size). Increased in almost 100% of cases in children and young adults. In benign liver diseases, AFP >400 ng/mL is extremely rare.

Failure to return to normal after surgery indicates incomplete resection or presence of metastases.

Increases associated with nonmalignant conditions are usually temporary and concentrations subsequently fall, but in malignant disease, concentrations continue to rise.

### Increased In

Ataxia-telangiectasia
Hereditary tyrosinemia
Hereditary persistence of AFP
Some patients with liver metastases from carcinoma of stomach or pancreas

### Absent In

Normal persons after first weeks of life
Various types of cirrhosis and hepatitis in adults
Seminoma of testis
Choriocarcinoma, adenocarcinoma, and dermoid cyst of ovary

## Carcinoembryonic Antigen (CEA)

### Use

Primarily for monitoring for persistent, metastatic, or recurrent cancer of colon after surgery; less frequently for breast or other cancers
Not usually useful for diagnosis of local recurrence
Not recommended for screening

Not used alone to establish the diagnosis
Determine prognosis in patients with colon cancer

### Interpretation

After complete removal of colon cancer, CEA becomes normal in 6–12 wks. Fail-ure to become normal suggests incomplete resection.

Predicts recurrence (by progressive increase) earlier than other methods; increas-ing concentrations may precede recurrence by 2–6 months. 20% change in serum concentration is concordant with change in the tumor.

Serum concentrations at time of diagnosis are related to stage of disease and likelihood of recurrence. CEA concentrations <5 ng/mL before therapy suggest localized disease and a favorable prognosis, but >10 ng/mL sug-gest extensive disease and a poor prognosis. Serum CEA >20 ng/mL cor-relates with tumor volume in breast and colon cancer and is usually associated with metastatic disease or with a few types of cancer (e.g., can-cer of the colon or pancreas); however, metastases may occur with concen-trations <20 ng/mL. Values <2.5 ng/mL do not rule out primary, metastatic, or recurrent cancer.

### Increased in

Cancer. There is a wide overlap in values between benign and malignant disease.
- 75% of patients with carcinoma of entodermal origin (colon, stomach, pan-creas, lung) have CEA titers >2.5 ng/mL, and two-thirds of these titers are >5 ng/mL. Increased in approximately one-third of patients with small cell carcinoma of lung and approximately two-thirds of patients with non–small cell carcinoma of lung.
- 50% of patients with carcinoma of nonentodermal origin (especially breast, head and neck, ovary) have CEA titers >2.5 ng/mL, and 50% are >5 ng/mL. Increased in >50% of cases of breast cancer with metastases, 25% of cases without metastases, but not associated with benign lesions.
- 40% of patients with noncarcinomatous malignant disease have increased CEA concentrations, usually 2.5–5.0 ng/mL.
- Effusion fluid due to these cancers.

Active nonmalignant inflammatory diseases (especially of the GI tract [e.g., ulcer-ative colitis, regional enteritis, diverticulitis, peptic ulcer, chronic pancreati-tis]) frequently have elevated concentrations that decline when the disease is in remission.

Liver disease (alcoholic, cirrhosis, chronic active hepatitis, obstructive jaundice)
Others
- Renal failure
- Fibrocystic disease of breast

Smoking
- 97% of healthy nonsmokers have plasma CEA concentrations <2.5 ng/mL.
- 19% of heavy smokers and 7% of former smokers have CEA concentrations >2.5 ng/mL.

### Interferences

*Heparinized patients or plasma collected in heparinized tubes*

## Serum CA-125
**(increased in benign or malignant conditions that stimulate peritoneal synthesis)**

### Use

To monitor for persistent or recurrent serous carcinoma of ovary in postopera-tive period or during chemotherapy
Not for screening for serous carcinoma of ovary

Not useful to distinguish benign from malignant pelvic masses even at high concentrations

### Interpretation

Remains increased in stable or progressive serous carcinoma of ovary. Rising concentrations may precede recurrence by many months and may be indication for second-look operation; but lack of increased values does not indicate absence of persistent or recurrent tumor. Greater concentration is roughly related to poorer survival; >35 U/mL is highly predictive of tumor recurrence. Normal concentration does not exclude tumor.

### Increased in
### (upper limit of normal <35 U/mL)

Malignant disease
- Nonmucinous epithelial ovarian carcinoma
- Fallopian tube tumors
- Cervical adenocarcinoma
- Endometrial adenocarcinoma
- Trophoblastic tumors
- Squamous cell carcinomas of vulva or cervix

Conditions that affect the endometrium
- Pregnancy
- Menstruation
- Endometriosis

Pleural effusion or inflammation (e.g., cancer, congestive heart failure)
Peritoneal effusion or inflammation (e.g., pelvic inflammatory disease, ovarian hyperstimulation syndrome, cirrhosis, other diseases of liver, pancreas, GI tract). *Especially increased in bacterial peritonitis in which ascitic concentration > serum concentration.*

Some nonmalignant conditions
- Cirrhosis, severe liver necrosis
- Other disease of liver, pancreas, GI tract
- Renal failure

*Not increased in mucinous adenocarcinoma*

## Serum CA 19-9

### Use

Utility is still being evaluated.
May be a useful adjunct to CEA for diagnosis and to detect early recurrence of cancer.
May indicate development of cholangiocarcinoma in patients with primary sclerosing cholangitis.

### Increased in
### (>37 U/mL)

Carcinoma of pancreas. Very high concentrations predict unresectable cancer—only 5% of patients with concentrations >1000 U/mL can be resected. Postsurgical recurrence correlates with increased concentrations.
Pancreatitis—concentrations are usually <120 U/mL; are much higher in pancreatic cancer.
Hepatobiliary cancer
Gastric cancer
Colon cancer

## Serum CA 15-3
**(glycoprotein expressed on various adenocarcinomas, especially breast)**

### Use

To detect tumor recurrence before symptoms and to monitor response to treatment

### Interpretation

Increased in ~20% of stage I or II disease and 70–80% of patients with metastatic or recurrent breast cancer

Increases in 75% of patients with progressive disease and decreases in 38% of those responding to therapy

### Increased in

Benign breast and liver diseases causing low specificity

## Serum Human Chorionic Gonadotropin (beta-hCG)

### Use

Routine pregnancy test; may also be used to gauge success of artificial insemination or in vitro fertilization.

Diagnosis and monitor course of gestational trophoblastic tumors

Differentiation of ectopic pregnancy from other causes of acute abdominal pain

In ectopic pregnancy and in abortion, serial hCG levels will usually decrease over 48 hrs.

Prenatal screening for Down syndrome

### Increased in

Normal pregnancy (secreted first by trophoblastic cells of conceptus and later by placenta). hCG levels double approximately every 48 hrs during early normal pregnancy.

Gestational trophoblastic tumors, benign or malignant. Is valuable marker for management.
* Hydatidiform mole (sometimes markedly increased; after 12 wks of pregnancy, >500,000 IU/24 hrs usually are associated with moles; >1,000,000 are almost always associated with moles).
* Choriocarcinoma in virtually 100% of cases, sometimes markedly. Increased levels are most useful for monitoring remission after treatment; failure to fall to an undetectable level or a rise after an initial fall signals residual tumor or progression of disease and need for another form of therapy.

Germ cell tumors of testicle and in 10% of patients with pure seminoma

Some nontrophoblastic neoplasms (e.g., cancers of ovary, cervix, GI tract, lung, breast)

## Neuron-Specific Enolase (NSE)

### Increased in

Neuroendocrine tumors
* Especially small cell carcinoma of lung
* Monitor patients with neuroblastoma, carcinoid, pancreatic islet cell tumor, pheochromocytoma, medullary carcinoma of thyroid

Wilms' tumor, malignant lymphoma, seminoma; 20% of cancers of breast, GI tract, prostate

Occasional patients with benign liver diseases

## Prostate-Specific Antigen (PSA) and Prostatic Acid Phosphatase (PAP)

(See Prostate Carcinoma, Chapter 14.)

# Neoplastic Diseases

## Breast Cancer

Serum CEA increase becomes more frequent with increasing stage and tumor burden.
* An increasing concentration usually reflects disease progression and a decreasing concentration usually reflects remission.
* An increased or rising concentration may precede recurrence by months.
* May be increased in CSF in metastases to CNS, meninges, or spine, but not in primary brain tumors.
* Not useful for screening or diagnosis of early breast cancer.
Serum CA 15-3

### *Steroid Receptor Assays*

#### Use

Prognosis and treatment of breast carcinoma. Determination of both receptors yields best information on response to hormone therapy.

Estrogen receptor (ER) is positive (>10 fmol/mg cytoplasmic protein) in 60% of breast tumor specimens; higher in post- than in premenopausal patients but this is not so for progesterone receptors (PGRs).

When ER is negative, there is <10% chance of obtaining a favorable response to any endocrine therapy; thus chemotherapy would be the primary approach. There is a greater likelihood of visceral metastases (>50%) with ER-negative than with ER-positive patients (<6%).

When ER is positive, there is 55–60% chance of favorable response (i.e., tumor shrinkage and/or clinical improvement).

When ER and PGR assays are both positive, response to endocrine therapy is 75–80%. No response in 10–15% of patients with ER/PGR-positive tumors.

Prognostic value
* Recurrence rate is significantly greater for ER-negative tumors, both Stage I and II.

Predictive value of assay is increased if ER and PGR levels are both high.
* ER titer >100 fmol/mg protein.
* PGR is also positive, especially >100 fmol/mg.

Receptor assay should also be performed on recurrent carcinoma, even when the original tumor has been previously assayed. Initial ER positives are later negative in 19%, and initial ER negatives are later positive in 13%. Initial PGR negatives are later positive in 8% and initial PGR positives are later reported negative in 28–44% of cases. These discordance rates may be ≤ 75% in patients receiving antiestrogen tamoxifen within 2 months.

Receptor assay may be useful in differential diagnosis of metastatic undifferentiated carcinoma in women.

*Unfixed tissue specimen should be frozen immediately after removal.*

DNA aneuploidy predicts shorter mean survival, independent of stage. ER- and PR-assay negative tumors are more likely to be DNA aneuploid.

DNA ploidy strongly correlates with histopathologic grade: poorly differentiated tumors are more likely to be DNA aneuploid.

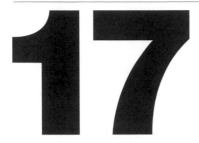

# Disorders Due to Physical and Chemical Agents

## Acetaminophen Poisoning

Blood levels
- 200 μg/mL within 4 hrs after ingestion or >50 μg/mL at 12 hrs predicts severe liver damage.
- <150 μg/mL at 4 hrs or <30–35 μg/mL at 12 hrs indicates no liver damage will occur.
- *Liver toxicity cannot be predicted from blood levels earlier than 4 hrs.*
- *Patients taking other drugs or with concomitant cirrhosis may develop liver toxicity at different blood levels.*
- *Toxicity is less common in children <5 yrs old, and changes in liver function tests may be mild when serum drug levels are in toxic range.*

With hepatotoxicity
- During first 12–24 hrs, increased AST and ALT are found in only ~50% of patients and serum drug levels are the chief guide to therapy; this is the only stage when treatment can prevent liver damage.
- During next 24–48 hrs, AST, ALT, serum bilirubin, and PT are increased. AST and ALT are very high (typically >4000 U/L); AST/ALT ratio <2 in ~90% of cases.
- On days 3–4, liver function abnormalities peak; hypoglycemia, secondary renal failure may occur.

## Alcoholism

Laboratory findings due to alcohol ingestion
- Blood alcohol level >300 mg/dL at any time or >100 mg/dL in routine examination. *(Blood alcohol level >150 mg/dL without gross evidence of intoxication suggests alcoholic patient's increased tolerance.)* In high-dose coma, blood alcohol should be >300 mg/dL; otherwise rule out other etiologies, especially diabetic acidosis and hypoglycemia.
- Breath test has certain constraints and limitations.
- Alcohol content in saliva—Enzyme strip is compared with a color scale to determine level of intoxication.
- Serum osmolality—22.4 increment >200 mOsm/L reflects 50 mg/dL alcohol. Increased osmolar gap (difference between measured and calculated osmolality is increased >10). Absence of increased gap is evidence against elevated blood level of ethanol, methanol, or ethylene glycol.

*Alcoholic ketoacidosis is preponderantly due to beta-hydroxybutyrate; therefore, increased ketone levels in blood and urine are often negative or only weakly positive because nitroprusside test detects acetoacetic but not beta-hydroxybutyric acid.*

Increase in these blood values with no other known cause that should arouse suspicion of alcoholism
- MCV >97 with round macrocytosis
- GGT

- Uric acid
- ALT, AST
- ALP
- Bilirubin
- Triglycerides

After 4 wks of abstention, alcohol challenge in "moderate drinkers" causes increased AST and GGT in 24 hrs with slow decline thereafter. ALT, LD, and ALP show little or no change.

Decrease of GGT after 1 wk of abstinence or decrease of MCV after 1–12 months are markers of alcoholism in cirrhosis; persistent decrease of GGT to <2.5 times upper limit of normal is marker of abstinence in alcoholic liver disease.

Declining serum potassium level to hypokalemia during alcohol withdrawal is said to be a reliable predictor of delirium tremens.

## Barbiturate Overdosage

Correlation between serum concentrations of barbiturates and state of intoxication in patients who have taken only a short-acting barbiturate, who are not habitual drug users, and who have no medical complications:

| | |
|---|---|
| <6 μg/mL | Alert |
| 6–10 μg/mL | Drowsy |
| 11–17 μg/mL | Stuporous |
| 16–20 μg/mL | Coma 1 |
| 20–24 μg/mL | Coma 2 |
| 24–28 μg/mL | Coma 3 |
| 28–40 μg/mL | Coma 4 |

*If the serum drug level is less than expected for the state of intoxication, look for medical complications (e.g., aspiration pneumonia, head trauma) or presence of other drugs.*

## Lead Poisoning (Plumbism)

See Tables 17-1 and 17-2.

Rapid micromethods for measurement of zinc protoporphyrin (ZPP) and free erythrocyte protoporphyrin (FEP) in blood are more sensitive indicators of lead poisoning than delta-ALA acid in urine. Especially useful for screening children. ZPP is good indicator of total body burden of lead. After therapy or removal

**Table 17-1.** Centers for Disease Control Classification of Whole-Blood Lead in Children 6–72 Months Old for Prevention and Control

| Level (μg/dL) | Classification |
|---|---|
| ≤ 9 | Not considered lead poisoning |
| >10* | Rescreen. Intervention. Search for source. |
| 10–14 | Need for more frequent screening of child and search for source |
| 15–19 | Rescreen; educational and nutritional intervention |
| 20–44 | Evidence of increased lead exposure; remedy environment; consider chelation |
| 45–69 | Chelation therapy; environmental intervention |
| >70 | Emergency treatment should begin immediately. |

*Centers for Disease Control, Atlanta, GA, has lowered the intervention level from 25 to 10 μg/dL.

**Table 17-2.** Screening for Lead Poisoning in High-Risk Children

| Lead (µg/dL) | FEP (µg/dL)[a] | | | |
|---|---|---|---|---|
| | ≤ 34 | 35–109 | 110–249 | ≥ 250 |
| ≤ 24 | Retest in 1 year. | Rule out other causes of I FEP[b] Retest in 3 mos. | Rule out iron deficiency. Retest in 3 mos. | Rule out erythropoietic protoporphyria. Retest in 3 mos. |
| 25–49 | Retest next visit. | Retest in 1–3 mos, then every 3–6 mos.[c] | Rule out iron deficiency. Retest in 2–4 wks.[c] | |
| 50–69 | Usual pattern. Retest to confirm. | Retest in 2 wks, then every 1–3 mos.[d] | Retest stat. Rule out iron deficiency.[d] | Retest stat. Mobilization test or treat. |
| ≥ 70 | Unusual pattern. Retest to rule out contaminated specimen. | Retest stat and treat. | Retest stat and treat. | Hospitalize stat. |

FEP = free erythrocyte protoporphyrin.

[a]Other causes of increased FEP are iron deficiency, anemia of chronic disease, sickle-cell disease, and erythropoietic protoporphyria.

[b]Iron deficiency and thalassemia should be ruled out even if lead level is increased because iron deficiency and lead poisoning can occur together. Use blood lead and zinc protoporphyrin (ZPP) together for possible lead poisoning; blood ZPP with serum iron and ferritin for iron deficiency.

[c]Consider mobilization test if lead ≥ 35 µg/dL.

[d]Consider mobilization test if lead = 35–55 µg/dL. Treat if lead = 56–69 µg/dL.

of exposure, blood lead becomes normal weeks to months before RBCs. Centers for Disease Control (Atlanta, GA) now recommends determination of whole-blood lead in children because ZPP is not reliable below ~25 $\mu$g/dL.

Other causes of increased FEP are iron deficiency, anemia of chronic disease, sickle-cell disease, erythropoietic protoporphyria. FEP $\geq$ 190 $\mu$g/dL is almost always due to lead intoxication. Iron deficiency and thalassemia should be ruled out even if lead level is increased. Use blood lead and ZPP together for possible lead poisoning; blood ZPP with serum iron and ferritin for iron deficiency.

Delta-ALA is increased in urine. Because it is increased in 75% of asymptomatic lead workers who have normal coproporphyrin in urine, it can be used to detect early excess lead absorption. Is not increased until blood lead >40 $\mu$g/dL.

Confirm diagnosis with determination of blood lead—a single determination cannot distinguish chronic from acute exposure. *All blood and urine specimens must be collected in special containers.*

Blood lead concentration in adults
* <10 $\mu$g/dL: Without occupational exposure.
* <20 $\mu$g/dL: Considered normal.
* 25 $\mu$g/dL: Report to state occupational health agency.
* >60 $\mu$g/dL: Remove from occupational exposure; chelation therapy.

Urine lead
* <150 $\mu$g/L is normal for adults.
* <80 $\mu$g/L is normal for children.
* >500 $\mu$g/24 hrs in children indicates excess mobile total body lead burden and suggests chelation therapy.

Increased coproporphyrin in urine is a reliable sign of intoxication and is often demonstrable before basophilic stippling.

Anemia is common. Mild (rarely <9 gm/dL), normochromic, normocytic, but may be hypochromic and microcytic, especially in children. MCHC is reduced only moderately. Is often the first manifestation of chronic lead poisoning. In acute lead poisoning, hemolytic crisis may occur. Anemia may be seen at blood lead levels of 50–80 $\mu$g/dL in adults and 40–70 $\mu$g/dL in children.

Anisocytosis and poikilocytosis and a few nucleated RBCs may be seen. Some polychromasia is usual.

Stippled RBCs occur later. Basophilic stippling is not pathognomonic of lead poisoning.

Bone marrow shows erythroid hyperplasia, and erythroid cells show stippling.

Hematologic changes of lead poisoning are more marked in patients with iron deficiency.

Urine urobilinogen and uroporphyrin are increased.

Porphobilinogen is normal or only slightly increased in urine (in contrast to acute intermittent porphyria).

Renal tubular damage occurs with Fanconi's syndrome, usually in very severe or very chronic cases. Increased serum uric acid is most frequent renal finding; causes saturnine gout.

CSF protein is increased, and frequently up to 100 mononuclear cells/cu mm are present in encephalopathy.

In children, acute encephalopathy may be seen with blood lead $\geq$ 80 $\mu$g/dL; abdominal and GI symptoms may occur with levels of 50 $\mu$g/dL, but usually indicate levels $\geq$ 70 $\mu$g/dL.

# Narcotics Addiction (Usually Heroin) and Chronic Usage; Drugs of Abuse

Persistent absolute and relative lymphocytosis occurs, with lymphocytes, often bizarre and atypical, that may resemble Downey cells.

Eosinophilia in 25% of patients.

Liver function tests commonly show increased serum AST and ALT. HBsAg is found in 10% of patients; liver biopsy is abnormal in 25% of patients.

Laboratory findings due to sexually transmitted diseases

Positive screening tests should always be confirmed by gas chromatography/mass spectroscopy (GC/MS) in the same laboratory.

RIA of hair for cocaine or heroin has high specificity and sensitivity. Assay of hair permits estimate of cocaine use for previous several months and can indicate isolated or steady pattern.

Blood levels only detect recent ingestion, but do not predict toxicity. Has no clinical value but can be used to calculate when drug was used. Higher ratio of cocaine to benzoylecgonine (cocaine metabolite) indicates more recent use.

Toxicologic urine screen will detect cocaine exposure within past 6–9 days in neonate and within past 24 hrs in adult.

False-negative immunoassays may result from adding drain opener, bleach, or table salt to urine.

### Laboratory Findings Due to Complications of Cocaine Abuse

Catecholamine blood levels may reach several thousand ng/mL.
Sudden death due to AMI
Acute myocarditis, acute cardiomyopathy
Bacterial endocarditis
Aortic rupture
Pneumopericardium
Acute rhabdomyolysis that may cause acute renal failure and DIC, etc.
Cerebral vasculitis with cerebral and subarachnoid hemorrhage
Hyperthyroidism
Pulmonary hemorrhage and hemoptysis, pulmonary edema, "crack lung"

### Cannabinoids (Marijuana, Hashish)

Testing (for tetrahydrocannabinol) is done to detect drug abuse rather than for therapeutic monitoring. Lower limit of detectability <15 ng/mL by definitive GC/MS. ≤ 25 mg/mL can be due to passive inhalation.

May be detected in plasma up to 6 days after smoking one marijuana cigarette.

In chronic marijuana users, cannabinoid metabolites have been detected in the urine up to 46 days after last use.

Urines adulterated with bleach, detergent, blood, salt, or vinegar may produce negative tests with EMIT methods.

Screening tests positive with one method (e.g., EMIT, RIA) should be confirmed with another method (e.g., GC/MS). Qualitative EMIT screen has occasional false positives.

### Laboratory Findings Due to Phencyclidine (PCP)

Massive ingestion may cause
- Rhabdomyolysis
- Acute tubular necrosis
- Hypoglycemia

## Salicylate Intoxication

Increased serum salicylate

Peak serum level is reached 2 hrs after therapeutic and >6 hrs after toxic dose. Serum levels drawn <6 hrs after ingestion cannot be used with Done's nomogram. Done's nomogram cannot be used for enteric-coated aspirin.

When awaiting laboratory measurement, can estimate peak salicylate levels:

mg/dL of salicylate = mg of salicylate ingested × 100/70% of body weight (gm)*

*Total body water.

*In older children and adults, serum salicylate level corresponds well with severity; in younger children, correlation is more variable.*

Early, serum electrolytes and $CO_2$ are normal.

Early respiratory alkalosis followed by metabolic acidosis; 20% of patients have either one alone.

Later, progressive decrease in serum sodium and $pCO_2$ occurs. 80% of patients have combined primary respiratory alkalosis and primary metabolic acidosis; change in blood pH reflects the net result. *(Infants may show immediate metabolic acidosis with the usual initial respiratory alkalosis. In older children and adults, the typical picture is respiratory alkalosis.)*

Hypokalemia accompanies respiratory alkalosis.

Dehydration occurs.

Urine shows paradoxic acid pH despite the increased serum bicarbonate.

- Ferric chloride test is positive on boiled as well as unboiled urine (thus differentiating salicylate from ketone bodies); it may have a false-positive result because of phenacetin.
- Tests for glucose, reducing substances, or ketone bodies are positive. All positive urine screening tests should be confirmed by serum sample.
- RBCs may be present.

Hypoglycemia occurs, especially in infants on restricted diet and in diabetics.

Serum AST and ALT may be increased.

Hypoprothrombinemia after some days of intensive salicylate therapy is temporary and occasional.

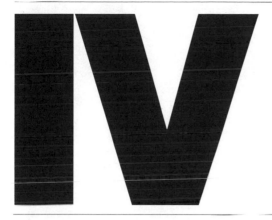

# IV

**Drugs and Laboratory Test Values**

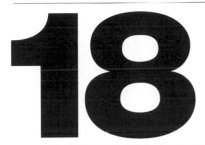

# Effects of Drugs on Laboratory Test Values

## Effect of Artifacts on Laboratory Test Values

Spurious values are false results due to interferences in laboratory analysis but not due to clerical error, improper performance of tests, instrument failure, or poor reagents. They are sufficiently frequent to require awareness of them *especially in the face of discrepant laboratory results.*

Common causes of spurious laboratory values are

- Hemolysis releases RBC analytes and enzymes into serum characteristically increasing serum LD, potassium, acid phosphatase and PAP, cholesterol if hemolysis is marked; AST, ALT, CK, iron, and magnesium may be affected to a lesser extent. It is not possible to correct for these changes based on an estimate of the degree of hemolysis.
- Lipemia may cause hyponatremia, hypokalemia, hyperchloremia, negative ion gap by three mechanisms:

  Turbidity (due to light scattering by lipid particles interfering with photometry)

  Partitioning errors that cause the analyte to enter the lipid, nonpolar phase making it inaccessible for the chemical reaction

  Fat-replacing serum water altering the distribution and concentration of electrolytes in the total volume of the specimen. This does not become a problem until triglycerides >1500 mg/dL, at which time serum is milky rather than just cloudy. Serum sodium decreases ~1.5 mEq/L for every 1000 mg/dL increase in triglycerides. Decreased serum iron may occur.

- Osmotic effect of hyperglycemia decreases sodium 1.6 mEq/L for each 100 mg/dL increase in serum glucose.
- Cationic effect of paraproteins, which displace sodium and decrease sodium 0.7 mEq/L for each 1 gm/dL of monoclonal protein.
- Glucose decreases at rate of 7 mg/dL/hr at room temperature if blood cells are not separated from serum even with a normal blood count.
- 0.8 mg of calcium is bound to 1.0 gm of albumin in serum allowing for correction of serum calcium values. Binding to globulin only affects total calcium if globulin >6 gm/dL. Serum albumin and TP should always be measured simultaneously with calcium determinations.

Other causes of artifactual results may be due to

- Underfilling or overfilling of blood collection tubes.
- Specimen drawn adjacent to or through infusion lines.
- Presence of abnormal blood components (e.g., RF, cryoglobulins, temperature, or ethylenediaminetetraacetic acid–dependent agglutinins).

The reader must also remember physiologic changes (e.g., diurnal variation), and other pre-analytical variations.

Only those spurious results with the most clinical significance and frequency are included here.

For more details on the manifestations, causes, and diagnostic clues or modes of confirmation, the reader is referred elsewhere.*

*Wallach, J. *Interpretation of Diagnostic Tests* (6th ed). Lippincott–Raven, Philadelphia, 1996.

## Effects of Drugs on Laboratory Test Values

With the coincident ingestion of a large number of drugs and the performance of
many more laboratory tests, abnormal results may be due to drugs as often as
to disease. Correct interpretation of laboratory tests requires awareness of all
drugs that the patient is taking. Patients often do not tell their physician about
medications they are taking (prescribed by other doctors or by the patients
themselves).

The classes of drugs most often involved include the anticoagulants, anticonvulsants, antihypertensives, anti-infectives, oral hypoglycemics, hormones,
and psychoactive agents.

The frequency of such modified laboratory test values is variable. A number of
causative mechanisms may operate, sometimes simultaneously. Some changes
are due to interference with the chemical reaction used in the testing procedure. Other changes reflect damage to a specific organ. In some cases, specific
metabolic alterations are induced, such as accelerated or retarded formation
or excretion of a specific chemical, competition for binding sites, stimulation
or suppression of degradative enzymes. Often the mechanism of these altered
laboratory test values is not known.

The list of the more frequently performed laboratory test values that may be
altered by commonly used drugs is so lengthy as to preclude inclusion in this
pocket guide. The reader is referred elsewhere.* For the most specific information, the reader should consult detailed sources about individual drugs,
such as the manufacturer's insert sheets and data, computer file–based data,
and the most current literature published since this and other compilations.

*Wallach, J. *Interpretation of Diagnostic Tests* (6th ed). Lippincott–Raven, Philadelphia,
1996.

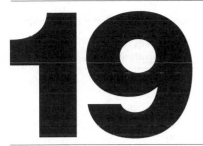

# Therapeutic Drug Monitoring and Toxicology

The determination of toxic and effective therapeutic concentration of drugs has become one of the most important and widely used functions of the laboratory. In the past, drugs were measured by their effects (e.g., coumadins prolonged PT, antimicrobials inhibited growth of microorganisms). Newer methodologies now permit direct determination of drug concentrations in the blood.

The clinician must be aware of the various influences on pharmacokinetics, factors such as half-life, time to peak and to steady state, protein binding, and excretion, that are not within the province of this book but are needed to prescribe these drugs appropriately.

The route of administration and sampling time after last dose of drug must be known for proper interpretation. For some drugs, different assay methods produce different values (e.g., quinidine), and the clinician must know the normal range for the test method used.

In general, peak concentrations alone are useful when testing for toxicity, and trough concentrations alone are useful for demonstrating a satisfactory therapeutic concentration. Trough concentrations are commonly used with such drugs as lithium, theophylline, phenytoin, carbamazepine, quinidine, tricyclic antidepressants, valproic acid, and digoxin. Trough concentrations can usually be drawn at the time the next dose is administered *(this does not apply to digoxin)*. Both peak and trough concentrations are used to avoid toxicity but ensure bactericidal efficacy (e.g., gentamicin, tobramycin, vancomycin). IV and IM administration should usually be sampled 30 mins to 1 hr after administration is ended to determine peak concentration.

Concentrations are meant only as a general guide; the laboratory performing the tests should supply its own values.

Blood should be drawn at a time specified by that laboratory (e.g., 1 hr before the next dose is due to be administered). This trough concentration should ideally be greater than the minimum effective serum concentration.

If a drug is administered by IV infusion, blood should be drawn from the opposite arm.

The drug should have been administered at a constant rate for at least 4–5 half-lives before blood samples are tested. (See Table 19-1.)

The reader is referred to the full Chapter 19 of *Interpretation of Diagnostic Tests* (6th ed) and to other texts for further information (e.g., drug interactions, preparatory screening before prescribing the drug, monitoring organ systems for toxic effects, etc.).

## Indications for Therapeutic Drug Monitoring (TDM)

Symptoms or signs of toxicity occur.
Therapeutic effect not obtained.
Noncompliance is suspected.
Drug has a narrow therapeutic range.
To provide or confirm an optimal dosing schedule
To confirm cause of organ toxicity (e.g., abnormal liver or kidney function tests)
Other diseases or conditions exist that affect drug utilization.

**Table 19-1.** Reported Reference Ranges of Some Common Therapeutic Drugs

| Drug | Therapeutic Concentration | Toxic Concentration |
|---|---|---|
| Acetaminophen (e.g., Anacin, Dristan, Excedrin, Nyquil, Sinutab, Tylenol) | $<50\ \mu g/mL$ | $>120\ \mu g/mL$ |
| Amitriptyline + nortriptyline | 75–225 ng/mL | >500 ng/mL |
| Nortriptyline (only) | 50–150 ng/mL | >500 ng/mL |
| Bromide | $1000–2000\ \mu g/mL$ | $\geq 3000\ \mu g/mL$ |
| Butabarbital | $1–5\ \mu g/mL$ | $\geq 10\ \mu g/mL$ |
| Butalbital | $10–20\ \mu g/mL$ | $\geq 40\ \mu g/mL$ |
| Caffeine | $5–15\ \mu g/mL$ | $\geq 30\ \mu g/mL$ |
| Carbamazepine (P) (Tegretol for seizures) | $2–10\ \mu g/mL$ | $\geq 12\ \mu g/mL$ |
| Carbamazepine-10-11-epoxide (P) | $0.4–4.0\ \mu g/mL$ | $\geq 8.0\ \mu g/mL$ |
| Carotene (S) | $48–200\ \mu g/dL$ | |
| Chlordiazepoxide (S) (Librium) | $5–10\ \mu g/mL$ | $\geq 15\ \mu g/mL$ |
| Chlorpromazine (S) (Thorazine) | >50 ng/mL | $\geq 1500$ ng/mL |
| Clonazepam (for seizures) | 10–50 ng/mL | $\geq 100$ ng/mL |
| Cyclosporine (B) | 100–300 mg/mL | $\geq 400$ ng/mL |
| Diazepam | $0.2–0.8\ \mu g/mL$ | |
| Nordiazepam | $0.2–1.0\ \mu g/mL$ | |
| Total for both | $0.4–1.8\ \mu g/mL$ | $\geq 5.0\ \mu g/mL$ |
| Dicumarol (P) (Warfarin) | $2–5\ \mu g/mL$ | $\geq 10\ \mu g/mL$ |
| Digoxin | 0.5–2.0 ng/mL | $\geq 3.0$ ng/mL |
| Digitoxin | 15–30 mg/mL | >30 ng/mL |
| Disopyramide (P) | $2.0–4.5\ \mu g/mL$ | $\geq 8.0\ \mu g/mL$ |
| Doxepin (combined with determination of metabolite desmethyldoxepin) | 100–275 ng/mL | $\geq 500$ ng/mL |
| Ethchlorvynol (S) | $5–10\ \mu g/mL$ | $\geq 20\ \mu g/mL$ |
| Ethosuximide (P) | $40–75\ \mu g/mL$ | $\geq 100\ \mu g/mL$ |
| Folate, RBC (B) | | |
| $\geq 12$ yrs old | 150–800 ng/mL | |
| 1–11 yrs old | 96–362 ng/mL | |
| <1 yr old | 74–995 ng/mL | |
| Folate (S) | $\geq 3.5\ \mu g/L$ | |
| Fluoride (P) | | $\geq 15\ \mu mol/L$ |
| Glutethimide (S) | 0.2–7.0 mg/mL | >10 mg/mL |
| Gold | | |
| (S) | $1.0–2.0\ \mu g/mL$ | $>5.0\ \mu g/mL$ |
| (24-hr urine) | $<1.0\ \mu g/specimen$ | $>5000\ \mu g/specimen$ |
| Imipramine + | | |
| Desipramine (P) | 125–225 ng/mL | $\geq 500$ ng/mL |
| Desipramine only | 75–225 ng/mL | |
| Lidocaine (P) (Xylocaine) | $2.0–5.0\ \mu g/mL$ | $\geq 6.0\ \mu g/mL$ |
| Lithium (S) | 0.8–1.2 mEq/L | $\geq 1.5$ mEq/L |
| Mephobarbital (P) | $1–7\ \mu g/mL$ | $\geq 15\ \mu g/mL$ |
| (Phenobarbital determination should be determined on same sample) | See Phenobarbital | |
| Meprobamate (S) | $<10\ \mu g/mL$ | $\geq 100\ \mu g/mL$ |

| Drug | Therapeutic Concentration | Toxic Concentration |
|---|---|---|
| Methaqualone (S) | 1–5 $\mu$g/mL | $\geq$ 10 $\mu$g/mL |
| Methotrexate (S) | <0.1 $\mu$mol/L after 48 hrs | $1.0 \times 10^{-5}$ at 24 hrs<br>$1.0 \times 10^{-6}$ at 48 hrs<br>$1.0 \times 10^{-7}$ at 72 hrs |
| Methsuximide (S) | <1.0 $\mu$g/mL | >55 $\mu$g/mL |
| Normethsuximide (should be performed with methsuximide determination) | 20–40 $\mu$g/mL | >55$\mu$g/mL |
| Methyprylon (S) | <10 $\mu$g/mL | $\geq$ 30 $\mu$g/mL |
| Mexiletine (S or P) | 0.75–2.0 $\mu$g/mL (trough) | $\geq$ 2.0 $\mu$g/mL (trough) |
| Pentobarbital (S) | 1–5 $\mu$g/mL | $\geq$ 10 $\mu$g/mL |
| For reducing intracranial pressure | 30–40 $\mu$g/mL | |
| Phenobarbital (P) | | |
|   Adults | 20–40 $\mu$g/mL | $\geq$ 55 $\mu$g/mL |
|   Infants and children | 15–30 $\mu$g/mL | |
| Phenytoin | | |
|   Total (P) | 10–20 $\mu$g/mL | $\geq$ 25 $\mu$g/mL |
|   Free (P) | 1–2 $\mu$g/mL | $\geq$ 2.5 $\mu$g/mL |
| Primidone (P) (should be performed with phenobarbital determination) | 9–12.5 $\mu$g/mL (adults); 7–10 $\mu$g/mL (children <5 years old) | $\geq$ 15 $\mu$g/mL |
| Procainamide (P) (should be performed with NAPA determination) | 4–8 $\mu$g/mL; <46 $\mu$g/mL (both) | $\geq$ 16 $\mu$g/mL; >46 $\mu$g/mL (both) |
| N-Acetylprocainamide (P) (NAPA) | $\leq$ 30 $\mu$g/mL | >30 $\mu$g/mL |
| Propoxyphene (S) | 0.2–0.5 $\mu$g/mL | $\geq$ 2 $\mu$g/mL |
| Propranolol (P) | 50–100 ng/mL | $\geq$ 1000 ng/mL |
| Quinidine (P) | 2.0–5.0 $\mu$g/mL | $\geq$ 7.0 $\mu$g/mL |
| Salicylates (S) | 2–20 mg/dL (adults) | $\geq$ 50 mg/dL |
| Secobarbital (S) | 1.0–5.0 $\mu$g/mL | $\geq$ 7.0 $\mu$g/mL |
| Theophylline (P) | 10–20 $\mu$g/mL (adults); 5–20 $\mu$g/mL (children) | $\geq$ 20 $\mu$g/mL |
| Thiocyanate (S) | 4–20 $\mu$g/mL | > 60 $\mu$g/mL |
| Thioridazine (S) | >50 ng/mL | $\geq$ 1500 ng/mL |
| Tocainide (S) | 5–12 $\mu$g/mL | $\geq$ 15 $\mu$g/mL |
| Trazodone (S) | 500–1100 ng/mL | $\geq$ 1500 ng/mL |
| Trifluoperazine (S) | <10 ng/mL | > 50 ng/mL |
| | N.B. Lower limit for detection is 20 ng/mL. Only useful to detect toxic concentration. | |
| Valproic acid (P) | 40 $\mu$g/mL (trough); 100 $\mu$g/mL (peak) | $\geq$ 120 $\mu$g/mL |

| Antimicrobial Drug | Therapeutic Concentration ($\mu$g/mL) | High or Toxic Concentration ($\mu$g/mL) | Low Concentration ($\mu$g/mL) |
|---|---|---|---|
| Amikacin | | | |
|   Peak | 20–25 | 30 | 14 |
|   Trough | 5–10 | 10 | |

**Table 19-1.** (continued)

| Antimicrobial Drug | Therapeutic Concentration ($\mu$g/mL) | High or Toxic Concentration ($\mu$g/mL) | Low Concentration ($\mu$g/mL) |
|---|---|---|---|
| Chloramphenicol | | | |
| Peak | 15–25 | 30 | 15 |
| Trough | 8–10 | 15 | 8 |
| 5-Flucytosine | | | |
| Peak | 100 | 125 | 50 |
| Trough | 50 | 125 | 30 |
| Gentamicin | | | |
| Peak | 4–8 | 8 | 3 |
| Trough | 1–2 | 2 | |
| Netilmicin | | | |
| Peak | 4–8 | 8 | 3 |
| Trough | 1–2 | 2 | |
| Streptomycin | | | |
| Peak | 5–20 | 40 | |
| Trough | <5 | 40 | |
| Sulfadiazine (S) | 100–120 | ≥ 300 | |
| Sulfamethoxazole (S) | 90–100 | ≥ 300 | |
| Sulfapyridine (S) | 75–90 | ≥ 300 | |
| Sulfisoxazole (S) | 90–100 | ≥ 300 | |
| Trimethoprim/sulfamethoxazole (TMP/SMX) | | | |
| Peak (trimethoprim) | ≥ 5 | | 5 |
| Peak (sulfamethoxazole) | ≥ 100 | | 100 |
| Tobramycin | | | |
| Peak | 4–8 | 8 | 3 |
| Trough | 1–2 | >2 | |
| Vancomycin | | | |
| Peak | 20–40 | 40 | 15 |
| Trough | 5–10 | 15 | 5 |

P = plasma; S = serum; B = blood.

Drug interactions altering a desired or previously achieved therapeutic concentration are suspected.

Drug shows large variations in utilization or metabolism between individuals.

Need medicolegal verification of treatment, cause of death or injury (e.g., suicide, homicide, accident investigation), detect use of forbidden drugs (e.g., steroids in athletes, narcotics).

Differential diagnosis of coma

### Drugs for Which TDM May Be Useful

Anticonvulsive drugs (phenobarbital, phenytoin)

Theophylline

Antimicrobials (aminoglycoside, chloramphenicol, vancomycin, flucytosine [5-fluorocytosine])

Antipsychotic drugs

Antianxiety drugs
Cyclic antidepressants
Lithium
Cardiac glycosides (digoxin)
Cardiac antiarrhythmics and antianginal drugs
Antihypertensive drugs
Antineoplastic drugs
Cannabinoids
Other drugs of abuse (cocaine, etc.)
Androgenic anabolic steroids
Immunosuppressant drugs (cyclosporine)
Anti-inflammatory drugs
  • Nonsteroidal (salicylates, propionic acids, oxicams, indoleacetic acids)
  • Steroids
Total parenteral nutrition
Four drugs (digoxin, phenytoin, phenobarbital, and theophylline) now account
  for ~50% of drug monitoring.

## Antiarrhythmic Agents

### Amiodarone (Cordarone)/Desethylamiodarone

Therapeutic range = 1.5–2.5 μg/mL.
Toxic concentration ≥ 3.5 μg/mL

### Diltiazem

Therapeutic range: Plasma concentration 40–200 ng/mL

### Flecainide (Tambocor)

Therapeutic range: Trough plasma concentration of 0.2–1.0 μg/mL
Toxic concentration >1.0 μg/mL

### Lidocaine (Xylocaine)

Draw blood 12 hrs after beginning therapy.
Indications for monitoring
  • Repeat every 12 hrs when drug clearance is altered by liver disease, heart
    failure, AMI.
  • Toxicity is suspected.
  • Ventricular arrhythmias occur despite therapy.
Therapeutic range = 2–5 μg/mL
Toxic concentration ≥ 6 μg/mL

### Mexiletine (Mexitil)

Therapeutic range: Plasma trough concentration of 0.75–2.00 μg/mL
Toxic concentration >2.0 μg/mL

### Nifedipine

Therapeutic range: Serum concentration 25–100 ng/mL

### Procainamide

Is measured along with its active metabolite N-acetylprocainamide (NAPA)
Therapeutic range: Procainamide = 4–8 μg/mL; NAPA ≤ 30 μg/mL; both ≤ 30 μg/mL
Toxic concentration: Procainamide ≥ 16 μg/mL; NAPA >30 μg/mL

### Quinidine

Therapeutic range = 2.0–5.0 μg/mL
Toxic concentration ≥ 7.0 μg/mL

### Tocainide (Tonocard)

Therapeutic range: Plasma concentration of 5–12 $\mu$g/mL
Toxic concentration $\geq$ 15 $\mu$g/mL (peak)

### Verapamil (Calan) or Norverapamil

Therapeutic range: Serum concentration 50–200 ng/mL (peak)
Toxic concentration $\geq$ 400 ng/mL (peak)

## Antihypertensive Drugs

There is little correlation between plasma concentration and clinical effect.

## Antineoplastic Drug Monitoring

Despite the large number of classes and drugs available, is clinically useful only in the following instances and the clinical result is improved only with methotrexate.

### Doxorubicin

To determine kinetics in patients with liver dysfunction

### 5-Fluorouracil

To monitor systemic concentration with intrahepatic or intraperitoneal use

### Melphalan

To monitor absorbance of oral drug

### Methotrexate

Therapeutic concentration $\leq$ 1.0 $\times$ 10$^{-7}$ mol/L
Toxic concentration = 1.0 $\times$ 10$^{-5}$, 1.0 $\times$ 10$^{-6}$, 1.0 $\times$ 10$^{-7}$ mol/L at 24, 48, and 72 hrs, respectively

## Cyclic Antidepressants

TDM is usually requested because of lack of clinical response.
Utility is decreased by the lack of objective monitoring criteria, poor correlation of plasma concentration with clinical response, and the presence of active metabolites.

## Cyclosporine (Sandimmune)

Initial oral dose 4–12 hrs before transplantation surgery. Oral dose needs to be decreased (e.g., 5%) during the following weeks or months to maintain constant blood concentration. Half-life = 4–6 hrs. Peak concentration 2–6 hrs after oral dose. Trough concentration 12–18 hrs after maintenance oral dose but longer after initial oral dose. Trough concentration about 12 hrs after one IV dose.

Therapeutic range = 100–300 ng/mL (trough) in whole blood for kidney transplants. No immunosuppression with trough whole blood <100 ng/mL. For first weeks after transplantation, rejection occurs with trough values <170 ng/mL; quiescence is usually maintained at $\geq$ 200 ng/mL; requirements diminish to 50–75 ng/mL by about 3 months and are maintained for rest of patient's life.

Monitoring: Draw blood just before next dose (trough concentration). Periodic monitoring (e.g., daily for liver transplant, three times/wk for kidney transplant) should be performed but this is not recommended as a stat procedure.

## Digitoxin

Draw blood just before next dose or >6 hrs after last dose.
Therapeutic range = 15–30 ng/mL.
Toxicity is common with concentration >30 ng/mL.

## Digoxin

Draw blood 6–8 hrs (or 8–24 hrs) after last oral dose after steady state has been achieved in 1–2 wks.
Therapeutic range: 0.5–2.0 ng/mL.
Toxic range ≥ 3.0 ng/mL but 10% of patients may show toxicity at <2 ng/mL.
* Pediatric toxic concentration may be higher. Therapeutic index is very low (i.e., small difference between therapeutic and toxic blood concentration). However, ~10% of patients have serum concentration 2–4 ng/mL without evidence of toxicity. On dose of 0.25 mg/day, mean serum concentration = 1.2±0.4 ng/mL; on dose of 0.5 mg/day, mean serum concentration = 1.5±0.4 ng/mL; on dose of 0.1 mg/day, mean serum concentration = 17±6 ng/mL. Digitalis leaf dose of 0.1 gm/day produces same serum concentration as 0.1 mg/day of crystalline digitoxin. Electrocardiographic evidence of toxicity in one-third to two-thirds of patients with no symptoms or signs.
Toxicity may occur at a lower blood concentration in presence of hypokalemia, hypercalcemia, hypomagnesemia, hypoxia, chronic heart disease.
Because most methods measure both endogenous digoxin-like substances and inactive metabolites of digoxin, therapeutic monitoring should mostly be used to assess patient compliance and to confirm drug toxicity.

## Ethanol

Lower limit for detection = 100 $\mu$g/mL
For treatment of methanol or ethylene glycol poisoning, desirable blood concentration = 100 mg/dL
For diagnosis of alcoholism
* A major criterion:
    Blood concentration >150 mg/dL without gross evidence of intoxication
* Minor criteria are
    Blood concentration >300 mg/dL at any time
    Blood concentration >100 mg/dL in routine examination
Toxic concentration ≥ 200 mg/dL

## Flucytosine (5-Fluorocytosine)
**(used as antimycotic agent [e.g., *Cryptococcus neoformans*, *Candida*])**

Therapeutic range: Serum concentration of 50–100 mg/L. Most susceptible organisms are killed at 0.5–12.5 mg/L concentrations. Serum and CSF fungistatic concentration of 10–40 mg/L. Bone marrow toxicity becomes prominent at serum concentration >125 mg/L or in presence of renal dysfunction.

## Haloperidol
**(used for treatment of psychoses, Tourette's syndrome, unresponsive hyperexcitable children)**

TDM is used to distinguish unresponsiveness from noncompliance or to detect high concentration in patients with abnormal liver function.
Therapeutic range = 5–16 ng/mL
Routine monitoring not indicated with good response to low-dose therapy
Allow >1 wk for steady state. Collect serum 12 hrs after last dose.

## Lithium

Therapeutic concentration = 0.8–1.2 mEq/L based on serum trough concentration drawn 12 ± ½ hrs after evening dose. Blood should be drawn after steady state (3–10 days) has been achieved.
Toxic concentration >1.5 mEq/L. >3.0 mEq/L can be lethal.
Peak concentration occurs 1–2 hrs after lithium carbonate or citrate, 4 hrs after slow-release preparations.

## Nonsteroidal Anti-Inflammatory Drugs

Salicylates (aspirin, diflunisal)
    Therapeutic range = 2–20 mg/dL
    Toxic concentration ≥ 50 mg/dL
Propionic acids (ibuprofen, diclofenac, naproxen, oxicams, piroxicam)
Indoleacetic acids (indomethacin, sulindac)
Except for salicylates, routine drug monitoring is not clinically useful.

## Pentobarbital

Therapeutic range = 1–5 $\mu$g/mL
Target for reducing intracranial pressure = 30–40 $\mu$g/mL
Toxic concentration ≥ 10 $\mu$g/mL

## Phenobarbital (Luminal)

Draw blood just before next oral dose, after steady state has occurred (11–25 days in adults; 8–15 days in children).
Therapeutic range = 20–40 $\mu$g/mL in adults; 15–30 $\mu$g/mL in children
Toxic concentration >55 $\mu$g/mL
Monitoring is indicated when patients are poorly controlled, have toxic symptoms, or 2–3 wks after change in dose or drug (e.g., primidone and mephobarbital, which are metabolized to phenobarbital).

## Phenytoin (Dilantin)

Patient should be on stable dose for at least 1 wk; draw blood just before next dose. Draw trough sample 1 wk after beginning treatment and again in 3–5 wks. After IV administration, draw blood 2–4 hrs after loading dose.
TDM is indicated when
  • Medication or dosage has changed (allow 1 wk to reach steady state).
  • Seizures are poorly controlled.
  • Toxic symptoms occur.
  • Children (10–13 yrs old) every 3–4 months until stable concentration occurs.
Therapeutic range: Total = 10–20 $\mu$g/mL. Free = 1–2 $\mu$g/mL
Toxic concentration: Total ≥ 25 $\mu$g/mL. Free ≥ 2.5 $\mu$g/mL

## Theophylline

Therapeutic range = 10–20 $\mu$g/mL (adults), 5–20 $\mu$g/mL (children); <5 $\mu$g/mL is usually ineffective.
Toxic concentration >20 $\mu$g/mL is toxic in 75% of persons.
Concentrations are usually measured at peak rather than trough.
Peak occurs 2 hrs after oral standard form and ~5 hrs after sustained release form.

# Appendices

# Abbreviations
# and Acronyms

| | |
|---|---|
| AA | atomic absorption |
| Ab | antibody |
| ABG | arterial blood gas |
| ACh | acetylcholine |
| ACTH | adrenocorticotropic hormone |
| ADH | antidiuretic hormone |
| AF | amniotic fluid |
| AFB | acid-fast bacillus |
| AFP | alpha-fetoprotein |
| Ag | antigen |
| AG | anion gap |
| A/G | albumin-globulin ratio |
| AHF | antihemophilic factor |
| AIDS | acquired immunodeficiency syndrome |
| ALA | aminolevulinic acid |
| ALL | acute lymphoblastic leukemia |
| ALP | alkaline phosphatase |
| ALT | alanine aminotransferase (SGPT) |
| AMI | acute myocardial infarction |
| AML | acute myeloblastic leukemia |
| | acute myelocytic leukemia |
| | acute myelogenous leukemia |
| ANA | antinuclear antibody |
| aPTT | activated partial thromboplastin time |
| ARC | AIDS-related complex |
| ARDS | acute respiratory distress syndrome |
| ASOT | antistreptolysin-O titer |
| AST | aspartate aminotransferase (SGOT) |
| BAL | bronchoalveolar lavage |
| BCG | bacillus Calmette-Guérin |
| BJ protein | Bence Jones protein |
| BT | bleeding time |
| BUN | blood urea nitrogen |
| CA-125 | C125 tumor antigen |
| CAH | chronic active hepatitis |
| | congenital adrenal hyperplasia |
| CEA | carcinoembryonic antigen |
| CF | complement fixation |
| ChE | cholinesterase |
| CIE | counterimmunoelectrophoresis |
| CK | creatine kinase |
| CLL | chronic lymphocytic leukemia |
| CMV | cytomegalovirus |
| CNS | central nervous system |

| | |
|---|---|
| COPD | chronic obstructive pulmonary disease |
| CRP | C-reactive protein |
| CSF | cerebrospinal fluid |
| | |
| D | decreased |
| DFA | direct fluorescent antibody |
| DHEA-S | dehydroepiandrosterone sulfate |
| DIC | disseminated intravascular coagulation |
| DKA | diabetic ketoacidosis |
| DNA | deoxyribonucleic acid |
| DOC | deoxycorticosterone |
| | |
| EBV | Epstein-Barr virus |
| ECG | electrocardiogram |
| EIA | enzyme immunoassay |
| ELISA | enzyme-linked immunosorbent assay |
| EM | electron microscopy |
| EMIT | enzyme multiplied immunoassay technique |
| ENA | extractable nuclear antigen |
| ERCP | endoscopic retrograde cholangiopancreatography |
| ESR | erythrocyte sedimentation rate |
| | |
| Fab | antigen-binding fragment of immunoglobulin |
| FAB | French-American-British classification for acute leukemias |
| FBS | fasting blood sugar |
| Fc | crystallizable fragment of immunoglobulin |
| fL | femtoliter |
| FNA | fine-needle aspiration |
| FSH | follicle-stimulating hormone |
| FTA | fluorescent treponemal antibody |
| FTA-ABS | fluorescent treponemal antibody absorption test |
| FTI | free thyroxine index |
| $FT_4$ | free thyroxine |
| | |
| GFR | glomerular filtration rate |
| GGT | gamma-glutamyl transferase |
| GI | gastrointestinal |
| gm | gram |
| G6PD | glucose-6-phosphate dehydrogenase |
| GTT | glucose tolerance test |
| GU | genitourinary |
| | |
| hr(s) | hour(s) |
| HA | hemagglutination |
| HAA | hepatitis-associated antigen |
| HAI | hemagglutination inhibition |
| HAV | hepatitis A virus |
| Hb | hemoglobin |
| HbA1c | glycosylated hemoglobin, hemoglobin $A_{1c}$ |
| HBcAb | hepatitis B core antibody |
| HBcAg | hepatitis B core antigen |
| HBeAb | hepatitis B e antibody |
| HBeAg | hepatitis B e antigen |
| HBIG | hepatitis B immune globulin |
| HBsAb | hepatitis B surface antibody |
| HBsAg | hepatitis B surface antigen |
| HBV | hepatitis B virus |
| hCG | human chorionic gonadotropin |
| Hct | hematocrit |
| HCV | hepatitis C virus |

| | |
|---|---|
| HDN | hemolytic disease of the newborn |
| HDV | hepatitis delta virus |
| hGH | human growth hormone |
| HI | hemagglutination inhibition |
| HIAA | hydroxyindoleacetic acid |
| HIV | human immunodeficiency virus |
| HLA | human leukocyte antigen histocompatibility antigen |
| HPF | high-power field |
| HPLC | high-performance liquid chromatography |
| HSV | herpes simplex virus |
| HTLV | human T-cell leukemia virus |
| | human T-cell lymphotropic virus |
| HVA | homovanillic acid |
| | |
| I | increased |
| ICDH | isocitric dehydrogenase |
| IEP | immunoelectrophoresis |
| IF | immunofluorescence |
| IFA | indirect immunofluorescent assay |
| Ig | immunoglobulin |
| IgA | immunoglobulin A |
| IgD | immunoglobulin D |
| IgE | immunoglobulin E |
| IgG | immunoglobulin G |
| IgM | immunoglobulin M |
| IHA | indirect hemagglutination |
| IM | infectious mononucleosis |
| | intramuscular |
| INH | isoniazid |
| IRMA | immunoradiometric assay |
| ITP | idiopathic thrombocytopenic purpura |
| IV | intravenous |
| | |
| 17 KGS | 17-ketogenic steroids |
| 17-KS | 17-ketosteroids |
| | |
| L | liter |
| LA | latex agglutination |
| LAP | leucine aminopeptidase |
| | leukocyte alkaline phosphatase |
| LD | lactate dehydrogenase |
| LDL | low-density lipoprotein |
| LE | lupus erythematosus |
| LH | luteinizing hormone |
| | |
| MAO | monoamine oxidase |
| MCH | mean corpuscular hemoglobin |
| MCHC | mean corpuscular hemoglobin concentration |
| MCV | mean corpuscular volume |
| MEN | multiple endocrine neoplasia (syndrome) |
| mEq | milliequivalent |
| mg | milligram |
| MHA-TP | microhemagglutination test (for *Treponema pallidum*) |
| min(s) | minute(s) |
| mm Hg | millimeters of mercury |
| mmol | millimole |
| mol | mole |
| MoM | multiple of the median (replaces mean of SD from mean when results are skewed rather than gaussian distribution [e.g., see alpha-fetoprotein]) |

| | |
|---|---|
| N | normal |
| NANB | non-A, non-B hepatitis (hepatitis C) |
| NBT | nitroblue tetrazolium |
| NIDDM | non-insulin-dependent diabetes mellitus |
| 5'-NT | 5'-nucleotidase |
| | |
| OGTT | oral glucose tolerance test |
| 17-OHKS | 17-hydroxyketosteroids |
| O & P | ova and parasites |
| | |
| PA | pernicious anemia |
| Pap | Papanicolaou's smear (stain) |
| PAP | prostatic acid phosphatase |
| PAS | $p$-aminosalicylic acid |
| $pCO_2$ | partial pressure of carbon dioxide |
| PCR | polymerase chain reaction |
| PCV | packed cell volume |
| PDW | platelet distribution width |
| pH | hydrogen ion concentration |
| PKU | phenylketonuria |
| PMN | polymorphonuclear neutrophil |
| PNH | paroxysmal nocturnal hemoglobinuria |
| $pO_2$ | partial pressure of oxygen |
| PRA | plasma renin activity |
| PSA | prostate-specific antigen |
| PSP | phenolsulfonphthalein |
| PTH | parathyroid hormone |
| PT | prothrombin time |
| | |
| RA | rheumatoid arthritis |
| RAIU | thyroid uptake of radioactive iodine |
| RAST | radioallergosorbent test |
| RBC | red blood cells |
| RDW | red cell distribution width |
| RE | reticuloendothelial |
| RF | rheumatoid factor |
| Rh | rhesus factor |
| RIA | radioimmunoassay |
| RNA | ribonucleic acid |
| ROC | receiver-operating characteristic |
| RSV | respiratory syncytial virus |
| $rT_3$ | reverse $T_3$ |
| | |
| sec(s) | second(s) |
| SBE | subacute bacterial endocarditis |
| SGOT | serum glutamic oxaloacetic transaminase (aspartate aminotransferase [AST]) |
| SGPT | serum glutamic-pyruvic transaminase (alanine amino-transferase [ALT]) |
| SI | Système International d'Unités |
| SIADH | syndrome of inappropriate ADH secretion |
| SLE | systemic lupus erythematosus |
| STD | sexually transmitted disease |
| | |
| $T_3$ | triiodothyronine |
| $T_4$ | thyroxine |
| TB | tuberculosis |
| TBG | thyroxine-binding globulin |
| TDM | therapeutic drug monitoring |
| TGT | thromboplastic generation time |

| | |
|---|---|
| THC | marijuana (delta-9-tetrahydrocannabinol) |
| TIBC | total iron-binding capacity |
| TLC | thin-layer chromatography |
| TORCH | toxoplasma, others, rubella, cytomegalovirus, herpes simplex |
| TP | total protein |
| TPN | total parenteral nutrition |
| TRH | thyrotropin-releasing hormone |
| TSH | thyroid-stimulating hormone |
| TSI | thyroid-stimulating immunoglobulin |
| TTP | thrombotic thrombocytopenic purpura |
| | |
| U | units |
| ULN | upper limit of normal |
| URI | upper respiratory infection |
| UTI | urinary tract infection |
| UV | ultraviolet |
| | |
| V | variable |
| VCA | viral capsid antigen |
| VDRL | Venereal Disease Research Laboratory (test for syphilis) |
| VIP | vasoactive intestinal polypeptide |
| VLDL | very-low-density lipoprotein |
| VMA | vanillylmandelic acid |
| vWF | von Willebrand's factor |
| VZV | varicella-zoster virus |
| | |
| WBC | white blood cell, white blood cell count |
| wk(s) | week(s) |
| | |
| yr(s) | year(s) |
| | |
| Z-E | Zollinger-Ellison (syndrome) |

## Symbols

| | |
|---|---|
| > | greater than |
| $\geq$ | equal to or greater than |
| < | less than |
| $\leq$ | equal to or less than |
| $\pm$ | plus or minus |
| ~ | approximately |

# Conversion Factors Between Conventional and Système International d'Unités

This list is included to assist the reader in converting values between conventional units and the newer SI units (Système International d'Unités), which have been mandated by some journals. Only common analytes are included.

**Table A-1.** Hematology

| Analyte | Conventional Units | SI Units | Conversion Factors Conventional to SI Units | SI to Conventional Units |
|---|---|---|---|---|
| WBC count (leukocytes) | | | | |
| (B) | /$\mu$L or /cu mm or /mm$^3$ | cells $\times$ 10$^9$/L | 0.001 | 1000 |
| (CSF) | /cu mm or | 10$^6$/L | 1 | 1 |
| | /cu $\mu$L | 10$^6$/L | 10$^6$ | 10$^{-6}$ |
| (SF) | /$\mu$L | /L | 10$^6$ | 10$^{-6}$ |
| Platelet count | 10$^3$/cu mm | 10$^9$/L | 1 | 1 |
| Reticulocytes | /cu mm | 10$^9$/L | 0.001 | 1000 |
| RBC count (erythrocytes) | | | | |
| (B) | 10$^6$/$\mu$L or /cu mm or /mm$^3$ | 10$^{12}$/L | 1 | 1 |
| (CSF) | /cu mm | 10$^6$/L | 1 | 1 |
| Hct (packed cell volume [PCV]) | % | Volume fraction | 0.01 | 100 |
| MCV (volume index) | $\mu^3$ (cubic microns) | fL | 1 | 1 |
| MCH (color index) | pg (or $\mu\mu$g) | pg | 1 | 1 |
| | pg | fmol | 0.06206 | 16.11 |
| MCHC (saturation index) | gm/dL | gm/L | 10 | 0.1 |
| | gm/dL | mmol/L | 0.6206 | 1.611 |
| Hb | gm/dL | gm/L | 10 | 0.1 |
| (Whole blood) | gm/dL | mmol/L | 0.155 | 6.45 |
| (Plasma) | mg/dL | $\mu$mol/L | 0.155 | 6.45 |
| Fetal hemoglobin | % | mol/mol (may omit symbol) | 0.01 | 100 |
| Haptoglobin | mg/dL | mg/L | 10 | 0.1 |
| Fibrinogen | mg/dL | gm/L | 0.01 | 100 |

For abbreviations, see Table A-2 footnotes.

**Table A-2.** Chemistry

| Analyte | Conventional Units | SI Units | Conversion Factors Conventional to SI Units | Conversion Factors SI to Conventional Units |
|---|---|---|---|---|
| ACTH | pg/mL | ng/L | 1 | 1 |
| | pg/mL | pmol/L | 0.2202 | 4.541 |
| Aldosterone | | | | |
| (S) | ng/dL | nmol/L | 0.277 | 36.1 |
| (U) | mEq/24 hrs | mmol/day | 1 | 1 |
| (U) | $\mu$g/24 hrs | nmol/day | 2.77 | 0.36 |
| Androstenedione | ng/dL | pmol/L | 34.92 | |
| Angiotensin II | ng/dL | ng/L | 10 | 0.1 |
| Angiotensin-converting enzyme (ACE) | nmol/min/mL | U/L | 1 | 1 |
| Antidiuretic hormone (ADH; vasopressin) | pg/mL | ng/L | 1 | 1 |
| Albumin | | | | |
| (S) | gm/dL | gm/L | 10 | 0.1 |
| (CSF, AF) | mg/dL | mg/L | 10 | 0.1 |
| Alpha$_1$-antitrypsin | mg/dL | gm/L | 0.01 | 100 |
| AFP | | | | |
| (S) | ng/mL | $\mu$g/L | 1 | 1 |
| | ng/dL | ng/L | 10 | 0.1 |
| | mg/dL | gm/L | 0.01 | 100 |
| | mg/dL | mg/L | 10 | 0.1 |
| | $\mu$g/dL | $\mu$g/L | 10 | 0.1 |
| Ammonia | $\mu$g/dL | $\mu$mol/L | 0.714 | 1.4 |
| (P) | $\mu$g/dL | $\mu$mol/L | 0.5872 | 1.703 |
| Anion gap | mEq/L | mmol/L | 1 | 1 |
| Base excess | mEq/L | mmol/L | 1 | 1 |
| Bicarbonate | mEq/L | mmol/L | 1 | 1 |
| Bilirubin | mg/dL | $\mu$mol/L | 17.1 | 0.0584 |
| Calcitonin | pg/mL | ng/L | 1 | 1 |
| Catecholamines (U) | | | | |
| Norepinephrine | $\mu$g/24 hrs | nmol/day | 5.91 | 0.169 |
| | $\mu$g/mg creatinine | $\mu$mol/mol creatinine | 669 | 0.00149 |
| | pg/mL | pmol/L | 5.91 | 0.169 |
| | ng/mL | nmol/L | 5.91 | 0.169 |
| Epinephrine | $\mu$g/24 hrs | nmol/day | 5.46 | 0.183 |
| | $\mu$g/mg creatinine | $\mu$mol/mol creatinine | 617 | 0.00162 |
| | pg/mL | pmol/L | 5.46 | 0.183 |
| | ng/mL | nmol/L | 5.46 | 0.183 |
| Normetanephrine | ng/mL | nmol/L | 5.46 | 0.183 |
| | mg/gm creatinine | $\mu$mol/mmol creatinine | | |
| Dopamine | $\mu$g/24 hrs | nmol/day | 6.53 | 0.153 |
| | $\mu$g/mg creatinine | $\mu$mol/mol creatinine | 738 | 0.00136 |

**Table A-2.** (continued)

| Analyte | Conventional Units | SI Units | Conversion Factors Conventional to SI Units | Conversion Factors SI to Conventional Units |
|---|---|---|---|---|
| | pg/mL | pmol/L | 6.53 | 0.153 |
| | ng/mL | nmol/L | 6.53 | 0.153 |
| Metanephrines | mg/24 hrs | $\mu$mol/day | 5.07 | |
| | mg/gm creatinine | $\mu$mol/mol creatinine | 0.5736 | |
| Catecholamines (P) | | | | |
| Epinephrine | pg/mL | pmol/L | 5.458 | |
| Norepinephrine | pg/mL | nmol/L | 0.0059 | |
| hCG, beta-subunit | mU/mL | IU/L | 1 | 1 |
| | U/24 hrs | IU/day | 1 | 1 |
| Calcium | | | | |
| (S) | mg/dL | mmol/L | 0.25 | 4.0 |
| | mEq/L | mmol/L | 0.5 | 2.0 |
| (U) | mg/24 hrs | mmol/day | 0.025 | 40 |
| Carbon dioxide total (content $CO_2$ + bicarbonate) | mEq/L | mmol/L | 1 | 1 |
| $CO_2$ partial pressure, tension ($pCO_2$) | mm Hg | kPa | 0.133 | 7.52 |
| Standard bicarbonate (hydrogen carbonate) | mEq/L | mmol/L | 1 | 1 |
| Carotene | $\mu$g/dL | $\mu$mol/L | 0.0186 | |
| Chloride | mEq/L or mg/dL | mmol/L | 1 | 1 |
| CEA | ng/mL | $\mu$g/L | 1 | 1 |
| | $\mu$g/mL | mg/L | 1 | 1 |
| Ceruloplasmin | mg/dL | mg/L | 10 | 0.1 |
| Cholesterol | mg/dL | mmol/L | 0.0259 | 38.61 |
| HDL-cholesterol | mg/dL | mmol/L | 0.0259 | 38.61 |
| LDL-cholesterol | mg/dL | mmol/L | 0.0259 | 38.61 |
| Apolipoprotein A-1 or B | mg/dL | mg/L | 10 | |
| Copper | | | | |
| (S) | $\mu$g/dL | $\mu$mol/L | 0.157 | 6.37 |
| (U) | $\mu$g/24 hrs | $\mu$mol/day | 0.0157 | 63.69 |
| Coproporphyrins (I and III) | $\mu$g/dL | nmol/L | 15 | 0.067 |
| (U) | $\mu$g/24 hrs | nmol/day | 1.5 | 0.67 |
| (F) | $\mu$g/gm | nmol/gm | 1.5 | 0.67 |
| Cortisol (S) | $\mu$g/dL | $\mu$mol/L | 0.028 | 35.7 |
| | ng/mL | nmol/L | 2.76 | 0.362 |
| 17-OHKS (cortisol) (U) | mg/24 hrs | $\mu$mol/day | 2.759 | 0.3625 |
| | $\mu$/24 hrs | nmol/day | 2.759 | 0.3625 |
| Creatine (S) | mg/dL | $\mu$mol/L | 76.3 | 0.0131 |

| Analyte | Conventional Units | SI Units | Conversion Factors | |
|---|---|---|---|---|
| | | | Conventional to SI Units | SI to Conventional Units |
| Creatinine | | | | |
| (S, AF) | mg/dL | $\mu$mol/L | 88.4 | 0.0133 |
| (U) | gm/24 hrs | mmol/day | 8.84 | 0.1131 |
| (U) | mg/24 hrs | mmol/day | 0.00884 | 113.1 |
| (U) | mg/kg/24 hrs | $\mu$mol/kg/day | 8.84 | 0.113 |
| (C) | mL/min/1.73 m$^2$ | mL/s/m$^2$ | 0.00963 | 104 |
| Cyclic adenosine monophosphate (cAMP) | | | | |
| (S) | $\mu$g/L | nmol/L | 3.04 | 0.329 |
| (B) | ng/mL | nmol/L | 3.04 | 0.329 |
| (U) | mg/24 hrs | $\mu$mol/day | 3.04 | 0.329 |
| (U) | mg/gm creatinine | $\mu$mol/mol creatine | 344 | 0.00291 |
| DHEA-S | | | | |
| (S) | $\mu$g/mL | $\mu$mol/L | 2.6 | 0.38 |
| (AF) | ng/mL | nmol/L | 2.6 | 0.38 |
| 17-KS (as dehydro-epiandrosterone) (U) | mg/24 hrs | $\mu$mol/day | 3.467 | 0.2904 |
| 17-KGS (as dehydroepian-drosterone) (U) | mg/24 hrs | $\mu$mol/day | 3.467 | 0.2904 |
| 17-Hydroxycortico-steroids (17-OHCS) (U) | mg/day creatinine | mg/mol creatinine | 113.1 | 0.00884 |
| 11-Deoxycortico-sterone (DOC) (S) | pg/mL | pmol/L | 3.03 | 0.33 |
| Ferritin | ng/mL | $\mu$g/L | 1 | 1 |
| Gastrin | pg/mL | ng/L | 1 | 1 |
| Glucose | mg/dL | mmol/L | 0.0555 | 18.02 |
| Growth hormone | ng/mL | $\mu$g/L | 1 | 1 |
| HVA (U) | mg/24 hrs | $\mu$mol/day | 5.49 | 0.182 |
| | $\mu$g/24 hrs | $\mu$mol/day | 0.00549 | 182 |
| | $\mu$g/mg creatinine | mmol/mol creatinine | 0.621 | 1.61 |
| 5-HIAA (U) | mg/24 hrs | $\mu$mol/day | 5.2 | 0.19 |
| Hormone receptors (T) | | | | |
| Estrogen receptor assay | fmol/mg protein | nmol/kg protein | 1 | 1 |
| Progesterone receptor assay | fmol/mg protein | nmol/kg protein | 1 | 1 |
| Iron | $\mu$g/dL | $\mu$mol/L | 0.179 | 5.587 |
| Iron-binding capacity | $\mu$g/dL | $\mu$mol/L | 0.179 | 5.587 |
| Iron saturation | % | Fraction saturation | 0.01 | 100 |
| Lactate | mg/dL | mmol/L | 0.111 | 9.01 |
| Lead | | | | |
| (S) | $\mu$g/dL | $\mu$mol/L | 0.0483 | 20.72 |

**Table A-2.** (continued)

| Analyte | Conventional Units | SI Units | Conversion Factors Conventional to SI Units | SI to Conventional Units |
|---|---|---|---|---|
| (S) | mg/dL | μmol/L | 48.26 | |
| (U) | μg/24 hrs | μmol/day | 0.00483 | |
| Lipids (total) | mg/dL | gm/L | 0.01 | 100 |
| Magnesium (S) | mEq/L | mmol/L | 0.5 | 2 |
| (S) | mg/dL | mmol/L | 0.411 | 2.433 |
| (U) | mg/24 hrs | mmol/day | 0.411 | 2.433 |
| Osmolality | mOsm/kg | mmol/kg | | |
| Osteocalcin | ng/mL | μg/L | 1 | |
| $O_2$ partial pressure ($p[a]O_2$) | mm Hg | kPa | 0.133 | 7.5 |
| PTH (S) | pg/mL | ng/L | 1 | 1 |
| (P) | μLEq/mL | mLEq/L | 1 | 1 |
| pH | nEq/L | nmol/L | 1 | 1 |
| Phosphate (inorganic phosphorus) | | | | |
| (S) | mg/dL | mmol/L | 0.323 | 3.10 |
| (U) | gm/24 hrs | mmol/day | 32.3 | 0.031 |
| Porphobilinogen (U) | mg/24 hrs | μmol/day | 4.42 | 0.226 |
| Potassium | | | | |
| (S) | mEq/L | mmol/L | 1 | 1 |
| (U) | mEq/24 hrs | mmol/L | 1 | 1 |
| (U) | mg/24 hrs | mmol/day | 0.02558 | 39.1 |
| Protein, total | | | | |
| (S) | gm/dL | gm/L | 10 | 0.1 |
| (U) | mg/24 hrs | gm/day | 0.001 | 1000 |
| (CSF) | mg/dL | mg/L | 10 | 0.1 |
| Renin (PRA) | ng/mL/hr | μg/L/hr | 1 | 1 |
| Serotonin (S) | ng/mL | μmol/L | 0.00568 | 176 |
| Sodium | | | | |
| (S) | mEq/L | mmol/L | 1 | 1 |
| (U) | mEq/24 hrs | mmol/L | 1 | 1 |
| (U) | mg/24 hrs | mmol/day | 0.0435 | 22.99 |
| Testosterone (total) (S) | ng/dL | nmol/L | 0.0347 | 28.8 |
| TBG | mg/dL | mg/L | 10 | 0.1 |
| | μg/dL | μg/dL | 10 | 0.1 |
| TSH | μU/mL | mIU/L | 1 | 1 |
| Thyroglobulin | ng/mL | μg/L | 1 | 1 |
| TRH | pg/mL | ng/L | 1 | 1 |
| | pg/mL | pmol/L | 2.759 | |
| $T_3$ total | ng/dL | nmol/L | 0.0154 | 65.1 |
| Free | pg/dL | nmol/L | 15.4 | |
| Reverse $T_3$ ($rT_3$) | ng/dL | nmol/L | 0.0154 | 65.1 |
| $T_4$ total | μg/dL | nmol/L | 12.9 | 0.0775 |
| Free | ng/dL | pmol/L | 12.9 | |

| Analyte | Conventional Units | SI Units | Conventional to SI Units | SI to Conventional Units |
|---|---|---|---|---|
| | | | **Conversion Factors** | |
| Transferrin | mg/dL | gm/L | 0.01 | 100 |
| Triglycerides | mg/dL | mmol/L | 0.0113 | 88.5 |
| Urea nitrogen | | | | |
| (S) | mg/dL | mmol/L | 0.357 | 2.8 |
| (U) | gm/24 hrs | mol/day | 0.0357 | 28 |
| Uric acid | | | | |
| (S) | mg/dL | mmol/L | 0.05948 | 16.9 |
| (U) | mg/24 hrs | mmol/day | 0.0059 | 169 |
| Uroporphyrin (U) | $\mu$g/24 hrs | nmol/day | 1.204 | |
| | $\mu$g/gm creatinine | nmol/mol creatinine | 1.1362 | |
| VMA (U) | mg/24 hrs | $\mu$mol/day | 5.05 | 0.198 |
| | $\mu$g/gm creatinine | mmol/mol creatinine | 0.571 | 1.75 |
| Viscosity (S) | Centipoise | Same | | |
| Vitamin $B_6$ | ng/mL | nmol/L | 5.982 | |
| Folate | ng/mL | nmol/L | 2.266 | |
| Vitamin $B_{12}$ (cyanocobalamin) | pg/mL | pmol/L | 0.738 | 1.355 |
| Unsaturated $B_{12}$ binding capacity (S) | pg/mL | pmol/L | 0.738 | 1.355 |
| Vitamin C (ascorbic acid) | mg/dL | $\mu$mol/L | 56.78 | 0.176 |
| Vitamin A | $\mu$g/dL | $\mu$mol/L | 0.0349 | 28.65 |
| Vitamin D (calcitrol; 1,25-dihydroxy) | pg/mL | pmol/L | 2.4 | 0.417 |
| (25-hydroxy) | ng/mL | nmol/L | 2.496 | |
| Vitamin E (alpha-tocopherol) | ng/mL | nmol/L | 23.22 | |
| Xylose (U) | mg/dL | mmol/L | 0.0666 | 15.01 |
| | gm/5 hrs | mmol/5 hrs | 6.66 | 0.15 |

S = serum; U = urine; P = plasma; C = clearance; F = feces; SF = synovial fluid; B = blood; T = tissue. All reference is to serum unless otherwise stated.

# Index

in nephrotic syndrome, 265
proteinuria in, 68
renal failure in, 395
Renin
in adrenal hyperplasia, 345
hyporeninemia, hyponatremia in, 368
plasma activity, 17, 355–356
in aldosteronism, 339
in Bartter's syndrome, 343
conventional and SI units, 482
in Cushing's syndrome, 350
in pheochromocytoma, 354
ratio to aldosterone, 341
in renovascular hypertension, 354, 388
production by tumor of kidney, 446
Renin-angiotensin system
blocking sites, 343
hyperactivity in aldosteronism, 342
Renovascular hypertension, 354
Reovirus
antibody tests, 423
in lungs, 417
Reserpine
and plasma renin activity, 355
and prolactin, 374
Resorcinol, urine color from, 57
Respiratory disorders, 83–96
Respiratory distress, acute, protein C in, 239
Respiratory viruses
in larynx, 416
in pharynx and tonsils, 416
Reticulin, antibodies to, 53
Reticulocyte count, 8, 178–179
in anemia
aplastic, 185
from blood loss, 185
myelophthisic, 201
pernicious, 198
pure red cell, 201
conventional and SI units, 478
in hemoglobinopathies, 173
in hemolysis, 207
in iron deficiency, 196
in myelofibrosis, 208
in polycythemia vera, 206
in spherocytosis, 209
in thrombotic thrombocytopenic purpura, 250
Reticulocyte index, 179
Reticuloendotheliosis, leukemic, prostate-
specific antigen in, 405
Reye's syndrome
creatine kinase isoenzymes in, 34
hypoglycemia in, 328
Rhabdomyolysis
aspartate transaminase in, 25
BUN:creatinine ratio in, 29
calcium in, 29, 30, 31
in cocaine abuse, 456
creatine kinase in, 32, 34
in phencyclidine abuse, 456
renal failure in, 395
Rheumatic fever, 81–82
erythrocyte sedimentation rate in, 51
Rheumatoid arthritis. See Arthritis, rheumatoid
Rheumatoid factor
antibodies to, 18, 53
and artifacts in laboratory tests, 461
in joint diseases, 165–166

latex agglutination, 18
in pericarditis, 81
in polymyositis, 161
rate nephelometry, 18
in rheumatoid arthritis, 168
in Sjögren's syndrome, 168
Rhinitis, allergic, eosinophilia in, 184
Rhinosporidiosis, laboratory findings in, 419
Rhinovirus
in bronchi, 416
detection with molecular biology, 422
*Rhodococcus equi* in pneumonia, 95
Riboflavin, urine color from, 57
Ribonucleoprotein, antibodies to, 18, 440
in mixed connective tissue disease, 441
Rickets, 104
alkaline phosphatase in, 23
calcium in
in serum, 30
in urine, 55
25-hydroxyvitamin D in, 310
laboratory findings in, 312
renal, 312
phosphorus in, 38
vitamin D–deficient, renal tubular acidosis
in, 403
vitamin D in, 50
Rickettsiae
antibody tests, 424
in lungs, 417
Rickettsial diseases
monocytosis in, 183
pericarditis in, 81
pleural effusions in, 84
serologic tests in, 414
Rifampin
and free thyroxine, 291
and sputum color, 93
and urine color, 56
Ristocetin cofactor, 9
in hemophilia, 248
in von Willebrand's disease, 252
Ristocetin-induced platelet aggregation in von
Willebrand's disease, 251
Ristocetin-Willebrand factor, 9
RNA of hepatitis C virus, 130
*Rochalimaea henselae* detection with molecular biology, 422
Rocky Mountain spotted fever, monocytosis
in, 183
Rotavirus
antigen tests, 425
in colon, 418
in diarrhea, 104
in gastroenteritis, 109
and intestinal inflammation, 106
molecular biology, 422
Rotor's syndrome, 138, 264
bilirubin in, 26
Rouleaux formation
in macroglobulinemia, 222
in multiple myeloma, 221
Rous sarcoma virus
antibody tests, 423
antigen tests, 425
in bronchioli, 416
cultures of, 414
in lungs, 417